Periodontitis: Clinical Advances

Periodontitis: Clinical Advances

Editor: Norman Waltz

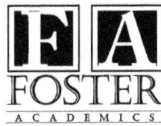

FA
FOSTER
ACADEMICS

www.fosteracademics.com

www.fosteracademics.com

EA
FOSTER
ACADEMICS

Cataloging-in-Publication Data

Periodontitis : clinical advances / edited by Norman Waltz.
      p. cm.
Includes bibliographical references and index.
ISBN 978-1-63242-611-6
1. Periodontitis. 2. Inflammation. 3. Dentistry. I. Waltz, Norman.
RK450.P4 P47 2019
617.632--dc23

Foster Academics,
118-35 Queens Blvd., Suite 400,
Forest Hills, NY 11375, USA

ISBN 978-1-63242-611-6 (Hardback)

Contents

Preface

A set of medical conditions in which the tissues surrounding the teeth exhibit inflammation is known as periodontal disease. Bacteria present in the mouth can infect the tissues around the teeth and cause periodontal disease. Some common symptoms include bleeding of gums, halitosis, swelling of gums, deep pockets between teeth and gums, etc. Periodontal probe is a device used by dentists in order to evaluate periodontitis. A standard treatment to prevent the progression of periodontitis is the use of special instruments to clean the teeth, especially below the gum line. Periodontal disease may be prevented by regular brushing, daily flossing, regular dental check-ups, professional teeth cleaning, etc. The topics included in this book on periodontitis are of utmost significance and bound to provide incredible insights. It will serve as a valuable source of reference for graduate and post graduate students, and dentists.

This book is a comprehensive compilation of works of different researchers from varied parts of the world. It includes valuable experiences of the researchers with the sole objective of providing the readers (learners) with a proper knowledge of the concerned field. This book will be beneficial in evoking inspiration and enhancing the knowledge of the interested readers.

In the end, I would like to extend my heartiest thanks to the authors who worked with great determination on their chapters. I also appreciate the publisher's support in the course of the book. I would also like to deeply acknowledge my family who stood by me as a source of inspiration during the project.

Editor

Discriminating Life Forms in Oral Biofilms

Vishakha Grover and Anoop Kapoor

Abstract

The bacteria colonizing the hard and soft tissues of the oral cavity are known to significantly influence oral health and disease. Recent studies of subgingival dental plaque, based on different identification methods, provide direct evidence of substantial diversity of plaque microbiota. Till date only about 280 bacterial species have been isolated by cultivable methods, characterized and formally named out of this enormous microbial diversity of oral biofilms. As a consequence, there is a complete lack of information about the properties of a substantial proportion of the plaque microbiota, apart from their position in the taxonomic hierarchy of bacteria. This limited knowledge about the behavior and properties, combined with recognition of the considerable diversity that exists within individual species, raises serious questions to the foundations on which previous conclusions, concerning the etiology of periodontal diseases, rest. The emerging realization is it is impossible to fully understand oral health and disease without identifying and understanding the pathogenic potential of all of the bacteria that colonize the oral cavity. The current chapter shall provide an update on current status of oral microbiota, ecological significance of their biofilm life style and various methods to study microbes residing in oral biofilms.

Keywords: biofilm, dental plaque, microbes, methods, identification

1. Introduction

Upon formation of earth about 3.5 billion years ago life began under anaerobic conditions, which resulted in current form as a result of evolution that is continued with the time. Initially, earth was colonized by unicellular prokaryotic bacteria that could survive under anaerobic conditions and eventually facilitated aerobic conditions that turned into evolution. However, till date we can find these microbes in various anaerobic environments. The estimated microbial diversity on earth constitutes 1.2×10^{29} in oceans, 2.6×10^{29} in terrestrial environment [1].

Remarkably, much more diversity was observed in subsurface environment with an estimate of 2.5×10^{30}, suggesting the adaptation of these microbes to such conditions at the formation of earth. Thus, microbial diversity constitutes a significant mass on earth among living organisms. However, most of the microbial diversity remained undisclosed due to limited knowledge on their adaption strategies and functions under diverse environments. In fact, their association has been observed with higher forms of living organisms including plants, animals and humans. There were various projects dealt with understanding the role of these microbes in host. Among those human microbiome project is considered to be important that helped in understanding the ecology of microbes in human including their disease causing abilities. Various habitats on human body are composed of vast microbial flora which include both autochthonous and allochthonous populations. Among those the oral microbiome is known to contain more than 700 different prokaryotic species with distinct subsets prevailing at different habitats of oral niche including periodontic and endodontic environments. Attempts were made for extensive characterization of this microbiome using both cultivation and culture-independent molecular methods. Unfortunately, most of the culture-independent methods revealed vast majority of oral taxa as uncultured clone and referenced by their 16S rRNA GenBank accession numbers [2, 3]. Application of recent advances in technology provided new insights in understanding the oral microbiome complexity and their role in both health and disease. In this chapter we have made an attempt to compile all updated information and current status of oral microbiota their biofilms, ecological significance and various methods to study microbes residing in oral biofilms. In 1978, Costerton invented the word "biofilm", referring to the matrix-enclosed bacterial community [4]. However, the first biofilm described by Antonie van Leeuwenhoek.

2. Oral microflora – general aspects

The "oral microbiome" represents a group of microorganisms that includes mutualistic, symbiotic, commensal and pathogenic microorganisms which determine oral health and disease1. Though babies are protected inside the amniotic sac during pregnancy and born with germ free oral cavity, various microbes of the vaginal environment of the mother comes into contact at the time of birth and subsequently establish their niche in oral cavity. Thus, the initial microbial flora of oral cavity resembles the mother's vaginal flora. Despite the possibility of contamination from the environment and surrounding personnel, the mouth of a newborn baby is usually sterile and microbes start invading with residential flora during feeding process. The natural history of oral bacteria acquisition and potential determinants of oral microbial composition are beyond the scope of this chapter. With direct exposure to the environment, oral cavity possesses a complex microbial ecosystem where wide variety of microbes including bacteria and fungi are continually involved in their establishment upon attachment to the surfaces like teeth, tongue, restorations and soft tissues. These varying colonizers primarily cause polymicrobial infection in the form of biofilm i.e., dental plaque with ecologic succession and inter-bacterial interactions between commensals, opportunistic pathogens and pathogenic microbes leading toward homeostasis in oral microflora [5]. Microbial studies of human dental plaque carried out by Socransky clearly showed that the oral health depends on the type of microorganisms present [6], however, interspecies interactions among these microbes determines healthy or diseased condition [7]. In fact, dysbiosis of microbial communities leads to dental caries or periodontitis [8, 9]. Commensal bacteria persist in oral habitat for long duration upon colonization and thus, they co-evolve with host and prevent access to pathogenic microorganisms by stimulating the immune response [10]. Dental caries are actually result of disequilibrium between acid and alkali producing microorganisms or acid producers and utilizers [11].Thus, paradigm of microbial dysbiosis revealed significance of autochthonous or resident microflora in maintaining healthy oral environment [11, 12].

3. Dental plaque

Dental plaque is a sticky film comprising multiple bacteria assembled as biofilm on surface or periphery of teeth. It consists of highly structured complex that allows sequential bacterial/ microbial succession. Dental plaque development studies under in vitro and in vivo investigations revealed occurrence of early and late colonizers. While early colonizers with ability to produce biochemical components that adhere to target tissue initiates biofilm formation on tooth surface including periodontal tissue. Subsequently, they allow the adhesion of late colonizers that are capable to adhere with early colonizers to impart metabolic and competitive advantages to biofilm. Usually, early colonizers include species of *Streptococcus, Lactobacillus, Lactococcus, Eikenella, Veillonella, Provetella, Propionobacterium* and *Hemophilus*. Late colonizers represented by members of the genera like *Actinomycetes, Eubacterium, Treponema* and *Porphyromonas*. A mature dental plaque biofilm contain bacterial species that are well bound to bacterial strains located adjacent to form a unique structure that improves their adherence ability and provides protection from adverse conditions. Previous comprehensive reviews by Kolenbrander et al. should be consulted for assessment of these important properties [13–15].

3.1. Microbial composition of dental plaque

Dental plaque represents a microbial community with high genetic diversity. Moreover, it maintains a stable structural complexity, despite the continuous exposure to external environment and various stress factors. The microbial composition largely remains constant as a result of balanced antagonistic and synergistic associations [16, 17]. This indicates specific contribution of physiological functions by individual participating microorganisms in biofilms. In addition, their physiological functions contribute to facilitate growth of other organisms such as anaerobic microbes. The biofilms formed on tooth are divided into supra- and subgingival biofilms. While supragingival biofilm is formed above the gum, subgingival biofilm formed under the gum. Most of the bacterial strains described from oral environment were isolated from these biofilms. With more than 700 Gram-positive and Gram-negative bacterial species oral ecosystem represents a complex ecosystem after gut environment [18, 19]. It is often observed that supragingival plaque contained Gram-positive bacteria, including members belonging to genera *Streptococcus Lactococcus, Lactobacillus, Veillonella* and the subgingival plaque revealed primarily gram negative anaerobic bacteria such as *Actinobacteria, Tannerella, Campylobacter, Treponema, Fusobacterium, Porphyromonas, Prevotella,*. Majority of these microbes belongs to the phyla like *Firmicutes, Bacteroidetes, Proteobacteria, Actinobacteria, Spirochaetes, Fusobacteria* as well as uncharacterized phyla like SR1and TM7 [18, 20]. Despite such huge diversity, only very limited number of bacterial species have been isolated and characterized by cultivable methods till date and this may be due to lack of understanding of microenvironment associated with these microbes [3, 19].

3.2. Dental plaque – a highly specialized host associated biofilm

As mentioned earlier, dental plaque is a biofilm attached not only to tooth surface but also under gums. Diverse community of microbes exists in the form of biofilm where all microbial strains bound tightly between them as well as to the tooth surface. Dental plaque is a form of biofilms, which engulf diverse bacterial populations adherent to each other and primarily results in formation of dental caries. Their structure is influenced with high and low bacterial biomass interlaced with aqueous channels formed to provide nutrients to the bacterial strains [21, 22]. Biofilms permit association of diverse species with increased metabolic efficiency, enhanced virulence and higher resistance to stress and antimicrobials as a result of entirely different expression of genes in comparison to planktonic form. Ability to adhere on surface, strong binding between cells gene regulation and genetic transfer are some of the important properties that define biofilm formation. In fact, extensive metabolites exchanges, signaling trafficking and different levels of interactions among different species were usually observed in biofilms [16, 23, 24]. However, introduction of biofilm theory into oral microbiology provided insights to understand the roles of different bacterial species at different time intervals. Most important is these biofilms proven to provide protection by increasing the antibiotic and acid tolerance, a property indicating it as a marker for caries production. Though biofilms consist of millions of cells of multiple species in thousands of layers, they behave like a single organism. These microbial cells are also encompassed in polysaccharide complex to stay together and acquire resistant properties to survive under stress environment.

4. Clinical relevance of biofilms in disease etiology

Planktonic microbes existing in dental ecosystem often involved in acute infections that can be diagnosed and treated appropriately before the establishment of disease. In contrast, bacteria existing in biofilms demonstrate an infectious course in disease establishment as observed in dental caries, where large quantities of acid formed as a result of increased acid tolerance. Dental plaque biofilm also increase the expression of virulence factors as differential expression of participants lead to formation of noxious products that initiates inflammation and development of periodontal disease. Biofilm exhibit all genetic network required for these activities as evident in global analysis of gene expression during biofilm formation. This state also imparts global adaptation to stress condition i.e. crowded environment. Thus, this lifestyle appears most important adaptation to any form of environmental stress and gain increased tolerance. This cooperative behavior among the participating species in a biofilm covered by extracellular matrix with coordinated management between cells using quorum sensing signal molecules for communication mimics an integrated multicellular organism. Additionally, the virulence was increased in multispecies participating biofilms in comparison to their mono-species counterparts [24]. Most of the bacterial cells exhibit attachment sites on their surface for an effective attachment to abiotic and/or neighbor microbial cells and thereby multiplies inside the extracellular matrix. This amplification in biofilms results in formation of aggregates that play important role in virulence in establishment of diseases like endocarditis, dental caries, middle ear infections, osteomyelitis, chronic lung infections in cystic fibrosis patients [25–27]. Remarkably about 80% of all microbial infections are found to develop biofilms on host tissues associated with different organs. Cells residing in biofilms termed as persister cells that are mostly exist in dormant stage with minimal active metabolism to cause chronic infections. These infections include production of exo- and endotoxins, metabolites like acids and other products involved in inflammation of dental tissue. However, the intensity of infection is directly related to their antibiotic resistance and ability to modulate host immune system [28, 29].

5. Biofilm characterization methods

5.1. Methods to discriminate oral microbial flora

Several attempts made to discriminate oral microbial flora by cultivable and non-cultivable methods have provided limited information. Though several taxa have been reported to present, only few microbes could grow in pure culture. Cultivation of individual strains in pure culture through the perspective of Koch's postulates. Further, identification of these microbial isolates helps in understanding infection process and disease establishment. To achieve this numerical taxonomy was practiced earlier, however, it has been replaced with molecular taxonomy and polyphasic taxonomy (**Table 1**).

However, in the recent past microbiologists have refocused on microbial communities' identification instead of planktonic form as they developed disease in the form of biofilm. In fact, oral diseases like caries and periodontitis are reported to be outcome of a consortia of organisms in a biofilm. Therefore, detailed analysis of a microbial community is essential to understand their pathogenicity. It is pertinent to mention that our understanding of the microbial world is very limited due to the intrinsic limitation of the culture-dependent methods. Thus, only less than 1% organisms could be revived in pure culture form under in vitro conditions. Considering the fact that several microbial species involved in biofilm formation, comprehensive understanding on complexity and genetic diversity of these communities are severely hampered due to non-availability of cultivation techniques [30]. Furthermore, uncultured status of these microbes also intervening in completion of understanding human microbiome and thereby effects on human health and disease [31]. Various culture-independent techniques such as cloning and amplification of total DNA obtained from samples can be used to understand the total microbial taxa. For which various housekeeping genes like 16S rRNA gene have been employed in molecular cloning and sequence methods to reveal their exact

Phenotypic methods	Genotypic methods
Expressed, Characteristics	Amplification of housekeeping genes like 16S rRNA and rpoB genes
Colony morphology Size Shape Color	
Cell morphology Gram Staining Shape	Phylogenetic analysis of gene sequences
Motility	Analysis of fragments obtained from random amplification of polymorphic DNA (RAPD)
Biochemical, enzymology acid-gas Production, Oxidation – Fermentation	DNA separation by pulsed-field gel electrophoresis (PFGE)
Whole cell protein analysis	Multilocus sequence typing (MLST)
Utilization of Carbon compounds	Restriction fragment length polymorphism (RFLP) of DNA
Antibiotic sensitivity	
Susceptibility to phages	Nucleic acid base composition Mole % G + C
Susceptibility to bacteriocins	DNA–DNA hybridization
Chemotaxonomic (Lipids, Fatty acid methyl esters (FAMEs), Isoprenoid quinones, Mycolic acids, Pigments, Peptidoglycan, Cell wall sugars	

Table 1. Phenotypic and genetic methods used for identification of bacterial strains.

identity [3]. However, cultivation of individual strains in pure form is essential to fully understand their role in health and disease thereby to carry out meaningful clinical research.

The development of 16S rRNA gene as molecular chronometer by Woese and co-workers has transformed the microbial taxonomy as the alignment of these sequences and construction of their phylogenetic trees have allowed cataloging of microbial strains and establishment of novel species [32]. The 16S rRNA gene exhibits clocklike behavior, broad phylogenetic range and appropriate size and accuracy, and these properties made this gene to the best molecular chronometer. Moreover, rRNAs are essential for protein synthesis and readily isolated from all forms of life, they are structurally and functionally conserved. They display highly variable and conserved regions to distinguish into distinct. They appear to incorporate changes in sequence very slow and do not exhibit horizontal gene transfer. This finding in combination with various PCR methods opened the door for culture-independent analyses for exact identification of microbial strains present in different microbial communities, including the uncultured bacterial species. They allowed understanding of total number of species, their richness and distribution. During the past two decades, development of high throughput tools for microbial community analysis has further improved identification process. Most of these methods include nucleic acids isolated from samples being investigated. These techniques include both nucleic acids and their PCR products. While techniques like fluorescent in situ hybridization (FISH) with fluorescently-labeled taxon-specific oligonucleotide probes and checkerboard DNA–DNA hybridization method [33] used nucleic acid, others such as random amplified polymorphic DNA (RAPD), denaturing gradient gel electrophoresis (DGGE) [34] or temperature gradient gel electrophoresis [35], terminal restriction fragment length polymorphism (T-RFLP) [36] and automated ribosomal intergenic spacer analysis [20] were carried out using PCR amplified products to analyze environmental microbial communities. Application of these techniques has revealed large number of microbial species within dental plaque with great genetic diversity. However, these techniques also showed limitations like cell lysis efficiency, nucleic acid extraction, differential amplification of target genes and differences in copy number of target genes, primer specificity and hybridization efficiency. Therefore, combining imaging tools such as the scanning electron microscope [37] and confocal laser scanning microscope [38], with molecular techniques can provide most effective identification [39].

5.2. Specific methods to discriminate oral microflora in biofilms – detection and quantification

Formation of biofilm containing multiple pathogens embedded in an extracellular polysaccharide matrix is a big threat to human health. Though biofilm formation is regulated by expression of various genes, there are multiple systems such as extracellular polysaccharides, lactones, pilin- or flagellin-like proteins, adhesins and other small molecules involved in quorum sensing and biofilm formation. Thus, considering the complexity of biofilm structure they are discriminated in qualitative and quantitative methods. The amount of EPS, types and total number of bacterial cells in biofilm must be considered as different "methods" requiring different experimental approaches. The biofilms are largely quantified using spectrophotometric and microscopic methods. The crystal violet (CV) staining method [40] is among the mostly used and also achieved by cangored method. CV staining can be performed as tube method or using microtitre plate.

5.2.1. Microtitre plate method

The microtitre plate method is most widely used method for detection of biofilm formation. It was initially developed as tissue culture plate method by Christensen et al. [40]. This method is used to test the influence of different media and addition of various sugars in media on biofilm production. Individual wells of sterile, polystyrene, 96 well-flat bottom microtitre plates were filled with 200 µl of diluted cultures in respective sterile media. They were incubated under optimal conditions required for the growth of microbes being tested. After incubation contents of wells were removed by gently tapping the plates and washed with sterile distilled water or buffer to remove free-floating bacteria. The biofilms formed by adherent mechanisms were stained with CV (0.1% w/v). Excess stain was removed by washing with deionized water and subsequently wells were air-dried. Adherent cells usually formed biofilm on all side wells and were uniformly stained with crystal violet. The crystal violet was solubilized using absolute ethanol and the quantity of biofilm quantified by measuring the OD at 595 nm. Sterile uninoculated medium is usually used as a control.

5.2.2. Tube method (TM)

This method allows qualitative assessment of biofilm formation as described by Christensen et al. [41] The medium is inoculated with loopful of culture from plates that are overnight incubated at optimal conditions. Upon incubation these tubes are decanted, washed with distilled water or PBS (pH 7.3) and air-dried. They are stained with CV (0.1%). Excess stain removed as mentioned in microtitre plate method and observed for biofilm formation. Biofilm formation was detected by a visible film lined the wall and/or bottom of the tube.

5.2.3. Congo red agar method (CRA)

This is an alternative method of screening biofilm formation by microbes [42]. Microbes being screened are grown on solid medium supplemented with 5% sucrose and Congo red. Congo red usually added as concentrated aqueous solution. Plates were inoculated and incubated under optimal conditions. While positive result was indicated by black colonies slime producers showed pink colonies.

5.3. Other qualitative straining methods to detect biofilm

5.3.1. LIVE/DEAD BacLight assay

This method is performed using a bacterial viability kit for microscopy based on the use of two different nucleic acid binding stains. Two dyes employed are green fluorescent (SYTO 9) and propidium-iodide that should be used with appropriate care. While intact cells fluoresced green with Syto9, damaged or dead cells in biofilm stains red. These stained samples are usually observed under a fluorescent microscope. The main limitation to apply this method for quantification is low quantities of the representative sample used for the total population and it does not allow tracking of individual bacteria.

5.3.2. Immunofluorescence staining

Immunoflurescent staining is used to observe biofilms under optical fluorescence microscopes and is commonly used to stain biofilms under in vivo conditions. This method employs specificity displayed by antibodies toward antigens. Usually fluorescent dye-labeled antibodies are used to fluoresce specific target molecules within a cell. This method is often used in experiments that use cell lines or tissue culture studies. Immunofluorescence is also used with other non-antibody methods by using stains like DAPI and analyzed on epifluorescence or confocal microscope. Diverse florophore molecules are used to link with antibodies. Biofilms used for image analysis using electron microscope are treated with various staining and fixing protocols using fixative or stain like glutaraldehyde, osmium tetroxide, ruthenium red etc., and observed under electron microscope. A variety of fluorescent molecules like lipophilic styryl compounds (ThermoFisher) involving plasma membrane and vesiculation was also used for biofilm detection. These water soluble and exhibit fluorescence when interact with surface of microbial cell membrane.

5.4. Metabolic assays

Biofilms can be measured by different vital or non-vital dyes that interact with metabolic products.

5.4.1. Resazurin assay

Resazurin (7-hydroxy-3H-phenoxazin-3-one-10-oxide) is a blue non-fluorescent biological dye that also known as Alamar Blue. It is used to quantify biofilms in microtiter plates as it gets converted to the pink-fluorescent resorufin upon reduction as a result of cellular metabolic activity. The resorufin can be measured spectrophotometrically and intensity of fluorescence is directly proportional to number of cells or biofilm concentration [43, 44]. However, the test is highly susceptible to bacterial respiratory efficiency and calibration of curves established with planktonic cells is much lower than signal detected in biofilm [45]. Further, this assay also reveals the presence and efficiency of antimicrobial and antibiofilm compounds [46].

5.4.2. XTT and TTC assay

Tetrazolium dyes also can be used as resazurin assay to quantify metabolically active cells in biofilm by spectrophotometric method. Tetrazolium slats like 2,3-bis (2-methoxy-4-nitro-5-sulfophenyl)-5-[(phenylamino) carbonyl]-2H-tetrazolium hydroxide (XTT) has been used to detect biofilm [47, 48] and another salt 2,3,5-triphenyl-tetrazolium chloride (TTC) also sued for the detection of biofilm [49] in microtitre plates by measuring absorbance. In fact, this method can be used to determine minimum biofilm inhibitory concentration (MBIC). Though these assays are highly sensitive and economical, the complexity and heterogeneity of biofilm structure of mature biofilm reduces the release of final products.

5.4.3. BioTimer assay

Bio Timer assay (BTA) is a biological method used to count adherent viable bacteria in bio-film life-style on any abiotic surface without manipulation of sample. BTA employs a specific reagent, phenol red that changes color from red-to-yellow based on microbial metabolism. This is specifically considering the microbes that produce diverse organic acids as their meta-bolic end products of fermenting bacteria. The time required for color change is determines the number of microbes as higher number of the organisms performs faster metabolism. Time required for initiation of color switch is correlated to the number of bacteria at time zero (N0) through a genus specific correlation described by equation $t^* = \log(1 + a/N0)/k$, where a represents metabolic product involved in color change and k is growth rate [50]. Though this technique is applied in microbiological quality analysis of foods and to evaluate antibiotic susceptibility of biofilm, is not applicable for the evaluation of multispecies biofilm.

5.5. Genetic assays to determine biofilms

Genetic assays have been used to assess the biofilm formation with focus on molecular mech-anisms involved in biofilm formation. In particular, early stage of biofilm formation including attachment to surface, which is driven by expression of various genes in different microorgan-isms. Therefore, biofilms are associated with proteins and amplification or quantification of various genes including chaperone-usher fimbriae, outer membrane proteins, poly-N acetyl glucosamine, adherent proteins and pili proteins [51–53].

5.5.1. Polymerase chain reaction (PCR)

The most important diagnostic method used in genetic techniques is Polymerase chain reaction (PCR). PCR screening is often employed to detect the genes involved in biofilm formation. The amplified products are sequenced and analyzed using various bioinfor-matics tools such as BLASTp (NCBI) to align with homologous sequences. This method allows to identify specific genetic sequences based on primer sequences used for individual bacterial species. The extracted DNA of the biofilm can be used for RAPD analysis by using specific oligonucleotide primers [54]. Amplification of genes like icaA, icaD, aap. The reaction mixture contains in general Taq polymerase enzyme, deoxynucleotides, primers, template DNA and MgCl2 in PCR buffer. The amplification is carried out in a gradient mastercycler with a program that includes initial denaturation of DNA at 95°C for 5 min. It is followed by 40 cycles of program at 94°C for 1 min, optimal temperature required for the binding of primers for 1 min, 72°C for 2 min (optimal enzyme activity and amplification) with a final extension at 72C for 5 min. Primers used in amplification of gens are as follows: icaA, 5'-AACAAGTTGAAGGCATCTCC and 5'-GATGCTTGTTTGATTCCCT [55]. Forr icaD, 5'-CCGGAGTATTTTGGATGTATTG (forward primer) and 5'-TTGAAACGCGAGACTAAATGTA (reverse primer). According to Vandecasteele et al. [56], for the detection of the aap gene, following primers were used: 5'-ATACAACTGGTGCAGATGGTTG (forward primer) and 5'-GTAGCCG TCCAAGTTTTACCAG (reverse primer). Nevertheless, PCR as such is not a suitable to quantify biofilm as it amplifies the DNA of both viable and dead cells, as well as any contamination leading to false positive results.

5.5.2. Fluorescence in situ hybridization and confocal laser scanning microscopy

Fluorescence in situ Hybridization (FISH) is a cytogenetic techniques that use fluorescent labeled oligonucleotide probes (like rRNA gene fragments) to detect microbes by hybridization of DNA with highly identical complementarity. This method allows direct visualization of species specific bacteria in a multispecies biofilm. These bacterial strains can be observed using confocal laser scanning microscopy. The technique can be modified with the samples to be observed, for example a modified version of the technique developed to identify based on peptides and termed as peptide nucleic acid-fluorescent in situ hybridization (PNA-FISH). Similarly, Flow-FISH employees flow cytometry to identify the microbes. Histo-FISH was developed to detect probiotic bacteria in gastrointestinal tract [57]. Interestingly, FISH can detect not cultivable bacteria and persister or dormant bacteria in biofilm. FISH technique is usually combined with confocal microscopy to visualize different species in a multispecies biofilm.

The aforementioned high throughput tools for microbial community analysis are largely based on PCR amplification of 16S rRNA gene sequences from microbial communities, which are relatively short, often conserved but varied enough to differentiate bacteria at species level. Although these approaches can provide us with the microbial composition within the community, unless we have genomic or other research data on those identified species, it reveals very limited information regarding what functions they might carry out within the flora.

5.6. Physical assays – biofilm imaging

5.6.1. Confocal laser scanning microscopy (CLSM)

It is a microscopy technique used in biology to study thick samples such as microbial biofilm, by processing images. Samples under investigation are stained with fluorescent dyes as mentioned in FISH so that the object can be illuminated and transformed by a photodiode in electrical signal processed by a computer. Some systems use motorized computer assisted device control for adjustment or sectioning of the biofilm and automated image acquisition. This technique often used to understand the role of EPS components, live biofilms and their in situ gene expression studies [58, 59]. The main disadvantages are semi-quantitative investigation, limited fluorescent dye usage for few stains and expensive method.

5.6.2. Mass spectrometry (MS)

A powerful analytical technique used for detection of various molecules. MALDI-TOF showed to be a strong tool for proper identification bacterial strains in biofilms. This technique utilizes the protein profile of bacterial strains for identification with a reference database. In fact, it is used for accurate identification of clinical strains in biofilms with high resistance to antibiotics [60]. In this method the object under investigation is exposed to a beam of electrons to form ions that are separated based on mass that are detected by a spectrometer and identified by their mass/charge ratios. It fulfills both qualitative and quantitative analysis of the unknown compounds. However, many steps in MS are highly invasive for the sample: high vacuum environment, aggressive chemical solvent etc. To overcome this problem,

5.6.3. Desorption-electro-spray-ionization (DESI)

This method has been proposed to overcome the disadvantages of MS like chemical solvent exposure and vacuum environment. It is carried out at atmospheric pressure and the sample is maintained under ambient conditions and can be used to for the analysis of mixed biofilms [61, 62].

5.6.4. Electron microscopy (EM) techniques

Electron microscopic technique was used to understand microbial flora in dental environment [63]. This method provide high resolution and technique is used for both scanning electron microscopy (SEM) and transmission electron microscopy (TEM). While SEM used to visualize biofilm surface TEM is used to image inner of biofilm [64]. For SEM analysis objects prepared on coverslips are washed (2–3 times) with buffer (pH 7.2) and fixed in 1% osmium tetroxide in the absence of light. Later, washed with distilled water and dehydrated in crescent concentrations of acetone baths. Upon drying, samples were mounted and analyzed on a scanning electron microscope. For TEM, the sample to be prepared as ultra-thin slices to acquire accurate images of bacterial cells and biofilms. Atomic force microscopy (AFM) is another technique used for morphological characterization. This method is used to check microbial cells in both planktonic and biofilm forms. The objective is fixed using 1 ml of modified Karnovsky fixative (containing 2% paraformaldehyde, 2% glutaraldehyde, 3% sucrose, and 0.1 M cacodylate buffer, pH 7.2) at room temperature. The analyses were performed at ambient temperature on an atomic force microscope equipped with a scanner. All images obtained were processed on specific softwares.

5.6.5. Micro-scale biogeography

Micro-scale biogeography is upcoming technique to understand the microenvironment of microbes by biofilm imaging [65]. This method also includes mimicking microenvironment including chemical ingredients and oxygen. It provides insights in understanding physiology and ecology of community their attachment with other microbes and spatial structure. Neighboring strains in physical contact play significant role in physiology such as protecting from stress conditions and secretion of metabolic end products as substrate for subsequent colonizers [66–68].

6. Metagenomics to understand complex microbial communities

The introduction and application of "metagenomics" by Jo Handelsman [69] has greatly enhanced our ability to study microbial communities including dental plaque. It includes understanding the microbial communities directly in their natural habitat using genomics approach The method do not require isolation and cultivation of any microbial strains. The basic components involved in metagenomics are PCR amplification of DNA, sequencing, bioinformatics with enhanced computational power to analyze large datasets obtained in sequencing [70]. The approach is simple and involves isolation of total DNA from sample, which is subsequently used for amplification of various genes and their subsequent analysis to gain functional and metabolic understanding [71]. Further, comparative genetics with expression microarrays and proteomics provides insights on network life style of microbes within the community such as dental plaque. Such studies provide information on potential pathogens that remained unidentified due to cultivation limitations [72].

7. Adjunctive novel technologies for biofilm study methods to complement microbial identification

7.1. Microfluidics

Miniaturization approaches to biofilm cultivation by using techniques like microfluidics studies are used to understand the natural habitat in laboratory conditions. It is performed in micro-scale channels by allowing fluid flow of growth media or chemicals with remarkable degree of control over the physical and chemical environment of microorganisms. Thus, allows manipulation of microenvironments of bacteria as these devices are made with microscopic compatible materials. It is developed as a new approach to understand cultivation method and dynamics of biofilms. It is also used as high throughput system to determine bacterial antibiotic resistance [73], cell variability in bacterial persistence, quorum sensing and chemotaxis in bacteria [74].

8. Concluding remarks

Since the initial observations of bacteria within dental plaque by Antonie van Leeuwenhoek using his primitive microscopes in 1680, our ability to identify the resident organisms in dental plaque and decipher the interactions between key components has rapidly increased. It is further increased significantly with the advent of imaging and molecular techniques during the past decade. These new techniques will have a great impact on oral and periodontal microbiology. We envision that in the future, new diagnostic tools developed with metagenomics methods would allow early detection and effective methods to combat the diseases. It also provides insights to prevent the cariogenic, endo and periodontic diseases.

Acknowledgements

We acknowledge Dr. Suresh Korpole, CSIR-Institute of Microbial Technology for valuable information on identification techniques and for useful discussions.

Conflict of interest

Authors declare there is no conflict of interest.

Author details

Vishakha Grover[1]* and Anoop Kapoor[2]

*Address all correspondence to: vishakha_grover@rediffmail.com

1 Department of Periodontology and Oral Implantology, Dr. Harvansh Singh Judge Institute of Dental Sciences and Hospital, Panjab Univeristy, Chandigarh, India

2 Department of Periodontology and Oral Implantology, Shri Sukhmani Dental College and Hospital, Derabassi, Punjab, India

References

[1] Whitman WB, Coleman DC, Wiebe WJ. Prokaryotes: The unseen majority. PNAS. 1998;**95**:6578-6583

[2] The human microbiome project consortium: Structure, function and diversity of the healthy human microbiome. Nature. 2012;**486**:207-214

[3] Dewhirst FE, Chen T, Izard J, Paster BJ, Tanner ACR, Yu W, Lashmanan A, Wade WG. The human oral microbiome. Journal of Bacteriology. 2010;**192**:5002-5017

[4] Costerton JW, Geesey GG, Cheng GK. How bacteria stick. Scientific American. 1978;**238**:86-95

[5] Marsh PD, Moter A, Devine DA. Dental palque biofilms: Communities, conflict and control. Periodontology 2000. 2011;**55**:16-35

[6] Socransky SS, Haffajee AD, Cugini MA, Smith C, Kent RL. Microbial complexes in sub-gingival plaque. Journal ofClinical Periodontology. 1998;**25**:134-144

[7] Marsh PD, Featherstone A, McKee AS, Hallsworth AS, Robinson C, Weatherell JA, New-man HN, Pitter AF. A microbiological study of early caries of approximal surfaces in schoolchildren. Journal of Dental Research. 1989;**68**:1151-1154

[8] Berezow AB, Darveau RP. Microbial shift and periodontitis. Periodontology;**2000, 55**: 36-47

[9] Mira A, Simon-Soro A, Curtis MA. Role of microbial communities in the pathogenesis of periodontal diseases and caries. Journal of Clinical Periodontology. 2017;**44**:S23-S38

[10] Darveau RP, Hajishengallis G, Curtis MA. Porphyromonas gingivalis as a potential com-munity activist for disease. Journal of Dental Research. 2012;**91**:816-820

[11] Feng Z, Weinberg A. Role of bacteria in health and disease of periodontal tissues. Periodontology 2000. 2006;**2000, 40**:50-76

[12] Frank A, Roberts FA, Darveau RP. Beneficial bacteria of the periodontium. Periodontology 2000. 2002;**2000, 30**:40-50

[13] Kolenbrander PE. Intergeneric coaggregation among human oral baceria and ecology of dental plaque. Annual Review of Microbiology. 1988;**42**:627-686

[14] Kolenbrander PE. Oral microbial communities: Biofilms, interactions, and genetic sys-tems. Annual Review of Microbiology. 2000;**54**:413-437

[15] Kolenbrander PE, Andersen RN, Blehert DS, Egland PG, Foster JS, Palmer RJJ. Com-munication among oral bacteria. Microbiology and Molecular Biology Reviews. 2002; **66**:486-505

[16] Marsh PD. Dental plaque: Biological significance of a biofilm and community life-style. Journal of Clinical Periodontology. 2005;**32**:7-15

[17] Marsh PD. Microbial ecology of dental plaque and its significance in health and disease. Advances in Dental Research. 1994;**8**:263-271

[18] Aas JA, Paster BJ, Stokes LN, Olsen I, Dewhirst FE. Defining the normal bacterial flora of the oral cavity. Journal of Clinical Microbiology. 2005;**43**:5721-5732

[19] Paster BJ, Boches SK, Galvin JL, Ericson RE, Lau CN, Levanos VA, Sahasrabudhe A, Dewhirst FE. Bacterial diversity in human subgingival plaque. Journal of Bacteriology. 2001;**183**:3770-3783

[20] Cardinale M, Brusetti L, Quatrini P, Borin S, Puglia AM, Rizzi A, Zanardini E, Sorlini C, Corselli C, Daffonchio D. Comparison of different primer sets for use in automated ribosomal intergenic spacer analysis of complex bacterial communities. Applied and Environmental Microbiology. 2004;**70**:6147-6156

[21] Domann E, Hong G, Imirzalioglu C, Turschner S, Kuhle J, Watzel C, Hain T, Hossain H, Chakraborty T. Culture-independent identification of pathogenic bacteria and

polymicrobial infections in the genitourinary tract of renal transplant recipients. Journal of Clinical Microbiology. 2003;**41**:5500-5510

[22] Dzink JL, Socransky SS, Haffajee AD. The predominant cultivable microbiota of active and inactive lesions of destructive periodontal diseases. Journal of Clinical Periodontology. 1988;**15**:316-323

[23] Hojo K, Nagaoka S, Ohshima T, Maeda N. Bacterial interactions in dental biofilm development. Journal of Dental Research. 2009;**88**:982-990

[24] Wen ZT, Yates D, Ahn S-J, Burne RA. Biofilm formation and virulence expression by *Streptococcus mutans* are altered when grown in dual-species model. BMC Microbiology. 2010;**10**:111

[25] Ford PJ, Raphael SL, Cullinan MP, Jenkins AJ, West MJ, Seymour GJ. Why should a doctor be interested in oral disease? Expert Review of Cardiovascular Therapy. 2010; **8**:1483-1493

[26] Cernohorska L, Votava M. Biofilms and their significance in medical microbiology. Epidemiologie, Mikrobiologie, Imunologie. 2002;**51**:161-164

[27] Rybtke MT, Jensen PO, Hoiby N, Givskov M, Tolker-Nielsen T, Bjarnsholt T. The implication of Pseudomonas aeruginosa biofilms in infections. Inflammation & Allergy Drug Targets. 2011;**10**:141-157

[28] Keller D, Costerton JW. Oral biofilm: Entry and immune system response. The Compendium of Continuing Education in Dentistry. 2009;**30**:24-32

[29] Cos P, Tote K, Horemans T, Maes L. Biofilms: An extra hurdle for effective antimicrobial therapy. Current Pharmaceutical Design. 2010;**16**:2279-2295

[30] Staley JT, Konopka A. Measurement of in situ activities of nonphotosynthetic microorganisms in aquatic and terrestrial habitats. Annual Review of Microbiology. 1985;**39**:321-346

[31] Turnbaugh PJ, Ley RE, Hamady M, Fraser-Liggett CM, Knight R, Gordon JI. The human microbiome project. Nature. 2007;**449**:804-810

[32] Woese CR. Bacterial evolution. Microbiological Reviews. 1987;**51**:221-271

[33] Socransky SS, Smith C, Martin L, Paster BJ, Dewhirst FE, Levin AE. "Checkerboard" DNA-DNA hybridization. BioTechniques. 1994;**17**:788-792

[34] Nakatsu C. Soil microbial community analysis using denaturing gradient gel electrophoresis. Soil Science Society of America Journal. 2007;**71, 571**:562

[35] Yoshino K, Nishigaki K, Husimi Y. Temperature sweep gel electrophoresis: A simple method to detect point mutations. Nucleic Acids Research. 1991;**19**:3153

[36] Liu W, Marsh T, Cheng H, Forney L. Characterization of microbial diversity by determining terminal restriction fragment length polymorphisms of genes encoding 16S rRNA. Applied and Environmental Microbiology. 1997;**63**:4516-4522

[37] Listgarten MA. Structure of the microbial flora associated with periodontal health and disease in man: A light and electron microscopic study. J. Periodontology 2000. 1976; **47**:1-18

[38] Netuschil L, Reich E, Unteregger G, Sculean A, Brecx M. A pilot study of confocal laser scanning microscopy for the assessment of undisturbed dental plaque vitality and topography. Archives of Oral Biology. 1998;**43**:277-285

[39] Foster JS, Kolenbrander PE. Development of a multispecies oral bacterial Community in a Saliva-Conditioned Flow Cell. Applied and Environmental Microbiology. 2004; **70**:4340-4348

[40] Christensen GD, Simpson WA, Younger JA, Baddour LM, Barrett FF, Melton DM, et al. Adherence of cogulase negative Staphylococi to plastic tissue cultures: A quantitative model for the adherence of staphylococci to medical devices. Journal of Clinical Microbiology. 1985;**22**:996-1006

[41] Christensen GD, Simpson WA, Bisno AL, Beachey EH. Adherence of slime–producing strains of *Staphylococcus epidermidis* to smooth surfaces. Infection and Immunity. 1982;**37**:318-326

[42] Freeman DJ, Falkiner FR, Keane CT. New method for detecting slime production by coagulase negative staphylococci. Journal of Clinical Pathology. 1989;**42**:872-874

[43] Peeters E, Nelis HJ, Coenye T. Comparison of multiple methods for quantification of microbial biofilms grown in microtiter plates. Journal of Microbiological Methods. 2008; **72**:157-165

[44] Tote K, Vanden Berghe D, Levecque S, et al. Evaluation of hydrogen peroxide-based disinfectants in a new resazurin microplate method for rapid efficacy testing of biocides. Journal of Applied Microbiology. 2009;**107**:606-615

[45] Sandberg ME, Schellmann D, Brunhofer G, et al. Pros and cons of using resazurin staining for quantification of viable Staphylococcus aureus biofilms in a screening assay. Journal of Microbiological Methods. 2009;**78**:104-106

[46] Van Den Driessche F, Rigole P, Brackman G, Coenye T. Optimization of resazurin-based viability staining for quantification of microbial biofilms. Journal of Microbiological Methods. 2014;**98**:31-34

[47] Ramage G, Vande Walle K, Wickes BL, Lopez-Ribot JL. Standardized method for in vitro antifungal susceptibility testing of *Candida albicans* biofilms. Antimicrobial Agents and Chemotherapy. 2001;**45**:2475-2479

[48] Koban I, Matthes R, Hubner NO, et al. Xtt assay of ex vivo saliva biofilms to test antimicrobial influences. GMS Krankenhhyg Interdiszip. 2012;**7**:Doc06

[49] Sabaeifard P, Abdi-Ali A, Soudi MR, Dinarvand R. Optimization of tetrazolium salt assay for Pseudomonas aeruginosa biofilm using microtiter plate method. Journal of Microbiological Methods. 2014;**105**:134-140

[50] Frioni AT, Natalizi M, Tendini A, Fraveto F, Pantanella F, Berlutti M, Pietropaoli D, Passeri ML, Terranova M, Rossi M, Valenti P. Biotimer assay for counting bacterial biofilm. Biophysics and Bioengineering Letters. 2010;**3**

[51] Tomaras AP, Dorsey CW, Edelmann RE, Actis LA. Attachment to and biofilm formation on abiotic surfaces by *Acinetobacter baumannii*: Involvement of a novel chaperone-usher pili assembly system. Microbiology. 2003;**149**:3473-3484

[52] Gaddy JA, Tomaras AP, Actis LA. The Acinetobacter baumannii 19606 OmpA protein plays a role in biofilm formation on abiotic surfaces and in the interaction of this pathogen with eukaryotic cells. Infection and Immunity. 2009;**77**:3150-3160

[53] Choi AH, Slamti L, Avci FY, Pier GB, Maira-Litran T. The pgaABCD locus of Acinetobacter baumannii encodes the production of poly-β-1-6-N-acetylglucosamine, which is critical for biofilm formation. Journal of Bacteriology. 2009;**191**:5953-5963

[54] Franklin RB, Taylor DR, Mills AL. Characterization of microbial communities using randomly amplified polymorphic DNA (RAPD). Journal of Microbiological Methods. 1999;**35**:225-235

[55] Tormo MA, Marti M, Valle J, Manna AC, Cheung AL, Lasa I, Penades JR. SarA is an essential positive regulator ofStaphylococcus epidermidis biofilm development. Journal of Bacteriology. 2005;**187**:2348-2356

[56] Vandecasteele SJ, Peetermans WE, Merckx RR, Rijnders BJA, Van Eldere J. Reliability of the Ica, aap and atlE genes in the discrimination between invasive, colonizing and contaminant *Staphylococcus epidermidis* isolates in the diagnosis of catheter-related infections. Clinical Microbiology and Infection. 2003;**9**:114-119

[57] Madar M, Sizova M, Czerwinski J, Hrckova G, Mudroonova D, Gancarcikova S, Popper M, Pisti J, Soltys J, Nemcova R. Histo-FISH protocol to detect bacterial compositions and biofilms formation in vivo. Beneficial Microbes. 2015;**6**:899-907

[58] Haagensen JA, Klausen M, Ernst RK, et al. Differentiation and distribution of colistin- and sodium dodecyl sulfate-tolerant cells in *Pseudomonas aeruginosa* biofilms. Journal of Bacteriology. 2007;**189**:28-37

[59] Moller S, Sternberg C, Andersen JB, et al. In situ gene expression in mixed-culture biofilms: Evidence of metabolic interactions between community members. Applied and Environmental Microbiology. 1998;**64**:721-732

[60] Gaudreau AM, Labrie J, Goetz C, Dufour S, Jacques M. Evaluation of MALDI-TOF mass spectrometry for the identification of bacteria growing as biofilms. Journal of Microbiological Methods. 2018

[61] Bhardwaj C, Moore JF, Cui Y, et al. Laser desorption VUV postionization MS imaging of a cocultured biofilm. Analytical and Bioanalytical Chemistry. 2013;**405**:6969

[62] Dean SN, Walsh C, Goodman H, van Hoek M. Analysis of mixed biofilm (*Staphylococcus aureus* and *Pseudomonas aeruginosa*) by laser ablation electrospray ionization mass spectrometry. Biofouling. 2015;**31**:151-161

[63] Listgarten MA. Structure of the microbial flora associated with periodontal health and disease in man: A light and electron microscopic study. Journal of Periodontology. 1976

[64] Richardson N, Mordan NJ, Figueiredo JA, et al. Microflora in teeth associated with apical periodontitis: A methodological observational study comparing two protocols and three microscopy techniques. International Endodontic Journal. 2009;**42**:908-921

[65] Welch JLM, Rossetti BJ, Rieken CW, Dewhirst FE, Borisy GG. Biogeography of a human oral microbiome at the micron scale. PNAS. 2016;**113**:E791-E800

[66] Diaz PI, Zilm PS, Rogers AH. Fusobacterium nucleatum supports the growth of *Porphyromonas gingivalis* in oxygenated and carbon-dioxide-depleted environments. Microbiology. 2002;**148**:467-472

[67] Traxler MF, Watrous JD, Alexandrov T, Dorrestein PC, Kolter R. Interspecies interactions stimulate diversification of the Streptomyces coelicolor secreted metabolome. MBio. 2013;**4**:e00459-13

[68] Jakubovics NS. Intermicrobial interactions as a driver for community composition and stratification of oral biofilms. Journal of Molecular Biology. 2015;**427**:3662-3675

[69] Handelsman J, Rondon MR, Brady SF, Clardy J, Goodman RM. Molecular biological access to the chemistry of unknown soil microbes: A new frontier for natural products. Chemistry & Biology. 1998;**5**:245-249

[70] Edwards RA, Rodriguez-Brito B, Wegley L, Haynes M, Breitbart M, Peterson DM, Saar MO, Alexander S, Alexander EC, Rohwer F. Using pyrosequencing to shed light on deep mine microbial ecology. BMC Genomics. 2006;**7**:57

[71] Gill SR, Pop M, DeBoy RT, Eckburg PB, Turnbaugh PJ, Samuel BS, Gordon JI, Relman DA, Fraser-Liggett CM, Nelson KE. Metagenomic analysis of the human distal gut microbiome. Science. 2006;**312**:1355-1359

[72] Kumar PS, Griffen AL, Barton JA, Paster BJ, Moeschberger ML, Leys EJ. New bacterial species associated with chronic periodontitis. Journal of Dental Research. 2003;**82**:338-344

[73] Keays MC, O'Brien M, Hussain A, Kiely PA, Dalton T. Rapid identification of antibiotic resistance using droplet microfluidics. Bioengineered. 2016;**7**:79-87

[74] Zang X-Q, Li Z-Y, Zhang X-Y, Jiand L, Ren N-Q, Sun K. Advances in bacteria chemotaxis on microfluidic devices. Chinese Journal of Analytical Chemistry. 2017;**45**:1734-1744

2

Periodontal Disease and Autoimmunity: What We Have Learned from Microbiome Studies in Rheumatology

Zoe Rutter-Locher, Nicholas Fuggle, Marco Orlandi,
Francesco D'Aiuto and Nidhi Sofat

Abstract

The oral cavity is home to vast populations of commensal microbial organisms which constitute the 'healthy oral microbiome.' Periodontitis is a destructive, infectious, inflammatory condition affecting the gums. Initially, a biofilm structure develops, causing localized inflammation. This biofilm is then colonized by certain anaerobic bacteria, including the 'red complex' organisms. There is an increasing interest in the communication between these organisms and host immune surveillance, a dialog which may plays an important role in the development of autoimmune diseases. Studies have shown an association between periodontitis and other inflammatory conditions including rheumatoid arthritis, psoriatic arthritis, ankylosing spondylitis and systemic lupus. The advent of accessible 16S ribosomal sequencing has led to exciting developments in the characterization of the human microbiome and the ability to study this interaction in more detail. The transmucosal communication between periodontitis and host immunity may provide avenues of discovery regarding the etiology and progression of rheumatic diseases.

Keywords: *Porphyromonas gingivalis*, gums, biofilm, periodontal membrane, microbiome, rheumatology, rheumatoid arthritis, psoriatic arthritis, ankylosing spondylitis, systemic lupus erythematosus, osteoarthritis

1. Introduction

It is known that the human body is covered with microbes. Until recently, many of these have been thought of as indolent, 'commensal' organisms, living in harmony with the host and thought of little relevance. If we consider that a single human being consists of approximately 1 trillion human cells but 10 trillion bacterial cells and, at a genetic level, 20,000 human genes but between 2 and 20 million bacterial genes, the indolence of these bacteria has to be questioned. There is therefore increasing interest in the roles played by these microorganisms on host immunology and physiology.

The oral mucosa is home to vast populations of these 'commensal' microbial organisms. It is therefore an arena which is ripe for communication between foreign organisms and host immune surveillance, a dialog which may play an important role in the development of autoimmune diseases.

The thrust of this chapter is to provide an update on the current literature regarding the role of microbiota in rheumatological conditions including rheumatoid arthritis, psoriatic arthritis, ankylosing spondylitis, osteoarthritis and systemic lupus.

2. The human microbiome

The term 'microbiome' refers to the sum of bacterial communities that colonize a particular area [1]. In humans, this includes almost any surface, for example, the skin, gut, airways, genitourinary tract and oral cavity. It is estimated that the human body is comprised of 1 trillion human cells [1], with genetic material accounting for approximately 20,000 human genes [2]. The bacteria which colonize the human body are estimated to contribute a further 20 trillion cells and between 2 and 20 million bacterial genes [1]. This does not include estimates of fungi and viruses which inhabit the human corpus. This had led to conjecture that a human is not simply 'an organism' but rather 'a superorganism' comprised of multiple separate organisms. Whether this is the case or not, it is certainly conceivable that the microorganisms that colonize the various niche environments of the human body contribute to physiology, biochemistry and immunity.

Study of the bacterial microbiome was previously limited by culture-dependent techniques which are limited in their ability to identify beyond the most prevalent organisms or that are amenable to culture in the media available. However, there have been exciting developments in the characterization of the human microbiome with the relatively recent advent of accessible 16S ribosomal sequencing.

Prokaryotic cells contain 70S ribosomes which consist of larger 50S and smaller 30S subunits [3]. The latter is comprised of 22 ribonucleoproteins and 16S ribosomal RNA. Due to the slow rate of evolution and highly conserved primer binding sites, 16S ribosomal RNA has been developed as a tool for phylogenetic studies [4]. With developments in the processes of RNA extraction, amplification with 16S rRNA primer and high-throughput sequencing, this has become an increasingly available method of bacterial identification, providing proportionally quantitative data on all bacteria in a sample. Identification libraries are growing and initiatives including the human microbiome project (HMP) [5] in the USA and metagenomics of the human intestinal tract (MetaHIT) [2] in Europe aim to catalogue the microbiomic constituents of the human body in health and disease. Of course, in order to identify changes in the microbiome related to disease, the spectrum of normality must first be established.

The human microbiome represents a previously unexplored arena which may provide discoveries relating the etiology, progression and management of human disease. However, it must be recognized that the horizons of human-microorganism interaction are vast and include bacterial proteomics, metabolomics, not to mention the human virome. Much endeavor is required to delineate the role played by these organisms in human diseases, including rheumatoid arthritis and periodontitis.

3. Periodontitis and the oral microbiome

3.1. Periodontitis

The periodontium is made up of the gingiva and the underlying attachment tissues. Gingivitis is a reversible form of gingival inflammation characterized by redness, swelling and bleeding. Periodontitis occurs once the inflammation extends to the deeper tissues including the periodontal ligament and alveolar bone. The loss of periodontal attachment and bone produces deepening of the gingival sulcus (periodontal pocket) and progressive loosening of teeth eventually leading to their loss [6].

The prevalence of periodontitis varies internationally; however, approximately 10–15% of the global adult population are affected by the condition [7]. The etiology is multifactorial and is composed of genetic predisposition, bacterial dysbiosis associated with a specific local and systemic host response and environmental factors [8] Although there is a genetic element to periodontitis, it is usually polygenic and so difficult to predict. Known risk factors include smoking, age, diabetes mellitus, educational level, gender and immunological diseases (e.g., HIV) [7, 9].

Plaque-induced periodontitis is the most common presentation. Initially, a biofilm structure develops which causes localized inflammation in the form of gingivitis. This biofilm is then colonized by anaerobic bacteria which causes further inflammation and neutrophilic activation. Matrix metalloproteinases are spilled, leading to tissue destruction, exacerbating the attachment loss and deepening the periodontal pocket. These results in further anaerobic colonization, soft tissue destruction, alveolar bone loss and ultimately tooth loss [8].

Management of periodontitis is aimed at excellent oral hygiene with twice-daily brushing of teeth and use of interdental brush and flossing. Plaque removal with scaling and debridement can be used to prevent excessive buildup of plaque. Low-dose doxycycline can inhibit matrix metalloproteinases such as collagenase and therefore reduce tissue damage. In severe cases and nonresolving gingival inflammation, there are surgical options which could allow for some regeneration of the lost soft and hard tissues [8].

3.2. The oral microbiome

The oral microbiome is composed of the microorganisms found in the oral cavity, or as defined by Joshua Lederberg 'the ecological community of commensal, symbiotic, and pathogenic microorganisms that literally share our body space '[10]. Although about 280 species have been cultured, it is estimated that they make up less than half of the bacterial species present in the oral cavity and the true number is likely to be between 500 and 700 [11, 12].

The advent of next generation sequencing has allowed the development of the human microbiome project. Findings suggest that although each individual body site is colonized by a characteristic microbiome, it is the individual who is colonized which is the primary factor affecting the bacterial makeup [11]. In the mouth, there are three distinct bacterial communities: the buccal mucosa, gingivae and hard palate forming one; the saliva, tongue, tonsils and throat forming another; and lastly the supra- and subgingival plaque [13].

Ninety-six percent of the bacterial community of the mouth is the phyla *Firmicutes, Bacteroidetes, Proteobacteria, Actinobacteria, Spirochaetes* and *Fusobacteria* [11, 14]. The composition of bacteria in 'healthy' and 'diseased' sites in the mouth is shown in **Table 1**.

Of these bacteria, there is the most evidence that *Porphyromonas gingivalis* has a key role to play in the pathogenesis of periodontitis and that with 'accessory pathogens' it alters the host immune response [8]. For example, *P. gingivalis* has specifically been implicated in blocking complement activation and inhibiting complement function [9].

'Healthy' sites; more gram-positive organisms	Dental caries	Gingivitis; gram-positive aerobes, facultative anaerobes, gram negatives	Periodontitis; gram-negative and anaerobic organisms
Actinomyces	*Streptococcus mutans*	*Actinomyces*	*Porphyromonas gingivalis**
Streptocci	*Streptococcus sobrinus*	*Streptococci*	*Porphyromonas endodontalis*
Veillonella	*Actinomyces*	*Treponema*	*Tannerella forsythia**
Granulicatella	*Lactobacillus acidophilus*	*Synergistetes*	*Treponema denticola**
Corynebacterium	*Bifidobacterium*		*Aggregatibacter actinomycetemcomitans**
Fusobacterium	*Propionibacterium*		*Anaeroglobus geminatus*
Gamella	*Veillonella*		*Eubacterium saphenum*
Rothia			*Filifactor alocis*
Porphyromonas			*Prevotella denticola*
Prevotella			*Prevotella nigrescens*
Staphylococcus			*Fusobacterium nucleatum*
Lactobacterium			
Haemophilis			
Peptostreptococcus			

*Red-complex organisms implicated in periodontitis [11–14].

Table 1. Selection of bacteria found in oral microbiome in health and disease.

3.3. Measures of periodontitis

In order to carry out high-quality studies investigating the association of periodontitis with other conditions, it is imperative to have valid and reliable measures of periodontitis.

There are a number of measures, shown in **Table 2**, which have been developed, looking at both gingivitis severity and periodontal disease [15, 16].

These measures have significant limitations. Multiple confounders such as age, smoking and immunosuppressant therapy can make them very difficult to interpret [7, 17]. Some measures under- or overestimate periodontal disease as they are affected by gum recession alone. However, the most significant limitation is that there is no single gold standard definition of a threshold for a diagnosis of 'periodontitis'. Most studies use varying thresholds which has a significant impact on prevalence rates and means studies need to be compared with caution [18].

	Measure	Definition	Method	Characteristic
Gingivitis	Bleeding on probing (BOP)	Bleeding of gingiva on gentle probing	Bleeding within 10 seconds, following gentle probing of gingival crevice	Assessment of gingivitis
	Bleeding index	BOP, calculated as an index	Number of sites BOP, divided by the total number of available sites multiplied by 100	Assessment of gingivitis
	Loe and Sillness Gingival index	Degree of gingival inflammation, characterized by erythema, hypertrophy and bleeding	Degree of inflammation given score out of four. The scores of four areas of the tooth are averaged	Assessment of gingivitis
Periodontitis	Missing teeth	Number of missing teeth	Count missing teeth	Crude, may be due to reasons other than periodontal disease
	Alveolar bone loss	Loss of the bone which supports the teeth	Periapical radiograph	Associated with tooth loss secondary to periodontitis
	Probing depth (PD)	Depth of the periodontal pocket	Measure the distance from the gingival margin to the base of the pocket	Measure of current periodontitis
	Clinical attachment level (CAL)	Measurement of the position of the soft tissue in relation to the cementoenamel junction (CEJ)	Calculated using the probing depth and the level of the gingival margin	Measure of cumulative periodontal disease

Table 2. Gingivitis and periodontal disease clinical measures [15, 16].

4. Periodontitis and systemic inflammation

The interest in the systemic inflammatory profile of patients affected by periodontitis has risen in the last 30 years to investigate the plausibility of the hypothesis that periodontal infection might have an impact on the systemic health. Particularly, the effect of periodontitis on the cardiovascular system but more recently a large spectrum of conditions such as neurodegenerative diseases, diabetes mellitus and rheumatoid arthritis, has been investigated. All these diseases are characterized by an increased systemic inflammatory profile, and periodontitis could contribute to their onset and progression by elevating pro-inflammatory markers. Consistent evidence from observational studies has suggested that severe periodontitis is associated with increased serum levels of C-reactive protein (CRP), moderate leukocytosis, as well as increased serum levels of interleukin-1 (IL-1) and IL-6 [19–23]. Furthermore, elevated serum levels of CRP have been associated with presence of keystone periodontal pathogens [24].

A recent systematic review confirmed a weighted mean difference of 1.56 mg/l ($p < 0.00001$) of CRP levels between cases with periodontitis and controls [25]. Further, the review reported on data from six intervention studies, concluding that periodontal treatment produced a 0.50 mg/l (95% CI 0.08–0.93) ($p < 0.02$) reduction of CRP serum levels. A recent meta-analysis on the effects of periodontal therapy and systemic inflammation reported a 0.23-mg/l reduction in CRP levels after treatment ($-0.231; p = 0.000$) [26]. Interestingly, a further analysis confirmed that the anti-inflammatory effect of periodontal treatment was more evident in clinical trials involving patients with periodontitis and other comorbidities like diabetes [27]. Individuals with periodontitis also show increased serum concentration of IL-6 and TNF-α compared to controls. Intervention trials reported inconclusive results on the effect of periodontal treatment on serum levels of these markers [28].

Different plausible mechanisms by which periodontitis could cause an increase in systemic inflammatory levels have been suggested. Firstly, multiple studies have reported the production of inflammatory cytokines in the periodontal pocket [29] and it has been postulated that these mediators could reach the bloodstream leaking from the inflamed periodontal lesions. Some of these mediators (i.e., IL-6) could have an effect on distant tissues and organs such as the liver, triggering an acute-phase response. However, for the time being, there is a limited evidence supporting this mechanism [30].

Secondly, bacteria colonizing the periodontal pockets and/or their by-products have been detected in the peripheral circulation [31]. A disruption of the subgingival epithelium could lead to short-lived bacteremia. This could trigger an immune response as well as allow bacteria to directly impact on the vasculature or distant organs (like the liver or kidney). In support of this hypothesis, periodontal bacteria DNA [32] and viable pathogens [33] have been detected in human atherosclerotic plaques. Thirdly, several antibodies induced by periodontal pathogens might trigger a molecular mimicry with cross-reactive antibodies recognizing host antigens.

Lastly, periodontitis and other comorbidities such as cardiovascular diseases and diabetes, share many common risk factors, including obesity and smoking [34, 35] which both have an effect on the systemic inflammatory profile [36]. This might account for a spurious association between periodontitis and systemic inflammation. However, the majority of the observational and experimental evidence available seems to support the concept that periodontitis could independently contribute to systemic levels of different inflammatory mediators and that periodontal treatment could result in their reduction. The systemic low-grade inflammation generated by periodontal infection might represent the link between periodontitis and systemic conditions [37, 38].

5. Periodontitis and rheumatoid arthritis

5.1. Rheumatoid arthritis

Rheumatoid arthritis (RA) is an autoimmune disease characterized by joint inflammation and destruction with extra-articular features including rheumatoid nodules, pulmonary disease, vasculitis and neuro-inflammation [39]. It can lead to chronic disability, early mortality, systemic complications and high socioeconomic burden on society as a whole [40]. The prevalence of RA is 0.5–1.0% [13] with apparent variation according to latitude and urban/rural habitation [41, 42].

It is currently classified according to the 2010 American College of Rheumatology/European League against rheumatism criteria by joint involvement, positive serology for rheumatoid factor or anti-citrullinated protein antibodies (ACPA), raised acute-phase reactants and the duration of symptoms [43]. Treatment regimens traditionally include corticosteroid to induce remission used in combination with maintenance of disease-modifying antirheumatic drugs, though have been much improved by the intervention of biologic agents.

5.2. Pathogenesis of rheumatoid arthritis

The exact etiology of RA is unknown; however, it is thought to be secondary to an interaction between genetic attributes and environmental exposures.

Indeed, genetic studies in twins have estimated approximately 60% heritability of rheumatoid arthritis [44]. Genetic polymorphisms including HLA-DRB1 [45] are implicated. However, other susceptibility alleles including genes involved in the differentiation of T cells, selection of antigens and peptide affinity have been identified by genome-wide association studies.

In terms of environmental insults, smoking has long been associated with RA [46] as have social factors including lower socioeconomic class and education but other areas of interest include silica, exogenous infections, periodontitis and the microbiota of mouth, gut and lung [47].

Autoantibodies to the Fc portion of immunoglobulin are known as rheumatoid factor and antibodies that are known to form against citrullinated proteins are called anti-citrullinated protein antibody (ACPA) or anti-cyclic citrullinated peptide (anti-CCP) antibodies. If either of these are present, they confer 'seropositivity,' which is seen in 70–80% of patients [48]. In addition to forming an element of the diagnostic criteria [43], seropositivity is also associated with more aggressive disease and with the earlier development of erosions. Rheumatoid factor is limited in diagnostic application by low specificity; however, ACPA is 95–98% specific [49].

ACPA has been shown to be present in RA patient sera up to a decade prior to the development of the disease [50] although the amount of ACPA and inflammatory cytokine levels rise sharply a few months before the synovitis presents [51]. It is therefore hypothesized that as well as citrullination of endogenous proteins, a second inflammatory 'hit' is required to stimulate the development of RA. Citrullinated proteins are also associated with other environmental factors such as smoking and pathological conditions including periodontitis.

Peptidyl arginine deiminase (PAD) causes the posttranslational modification of arginine to citrulline. It is hypothesized that this citrullination leads to amino acid chains being recognized as autoantigens, which leads to the development of autoantibodies and the subsequent autoimmune damage that is the signature for rheumatoid arthritis. PAD is produced by human cells, for example, in the lung; however, it is also produced by the microbe *P. gingivalis* [52].

Mucosal surfaces provide a rich opportunity for cross-talk between the immune system and the microorganisms which inhabit them. It is supposed that these microbes are not simply left unattended and indolent, but are held in a constant state of tension by physiological barriers (mucus and immunoglobulin A), epithelial tight junctions, innate immune surveillance (by macrophages and dendritic cells) and adaptive immune response.

The mucosal-joint axis hypothesis is supported by the fact that 20% of chronic inflammatory bowel disease patients develop an enteropathic arthropathy and that reactive arthritis can develop in response to chlamydial and dysenteric organism. A possible mechanism is therefore that disruption in pathogenic-commensal bacterial balance at the mucosal surface leads to innate activation and pro-inflammatory cytokine release, leading to a lasting adaptive immune response. If we then consider that some bacterial epitopes are shared with cartilage [53], it is possible that the adaptive immunity, in response to transmucosal exposure to a microorganism, could lead to sustained autoimmunity.

5.3. *P. gingivalis* and rheumatoid arthritis

PAD production by *P. gingivalis*, an anaerobic prokaryote, has been demonstrated in vitro. Due to this organism's role in the development of periodontal disease and the association of rheumatoid arthritis with periodontitis, it has been hypothesized that *P. gingivalis* provides a causal link between periodontal disease, citrullination and RA [54].

The temporal nature of this association is a point of conjecture, though it has been shown that non-RA (as defined by the American College of Rheumatology (ACR) criteria) patients with risk factors for the development of RA such as first-degree relatives and ACPA positivity had a higher concentration of anti-*P. gingivalis* antibodies [55]. This finding suggests that *P. gingivalis* (one of the 'red complex' organisms) appears prior to the development of rheumatoid arthritis in an 'at risk' population. Indeed, an etiological role of *P. gingivalis* is implicated by the recent finding that anti-*P. gingivalis* antibodies are significantly higher in RA cases compared to controls and, similar to ACPA, are present in sera years before the onset of symptoms of inflammatory arthropathy [56].

In addition to an etiological role, there is longitudinal evidence to suggest that *P. gingivalis* PAD may attenuate response to biologic Disease-modifying anti rheumatic drugs [57].

Together, these elements suggest a role for this organism in various aspects of rheumatoid disease and pronounce *P. gingivalis* as a viable avenue for further research.

5.4. Periodontitis in rheumatoid arthritis

Epidemiological studies have shown a strong association between periodontitis and RA [58, 59], though these have been hampered by their cross-sectional nature, variability in definition of periodontitis and dental endpoints, the extent of oral examination and the limited RA information collected. However, despite the above, there remains a significant amount of robust evidence to support the association between periodontitis and RA including a recent meta-analysis of 17 studies and over 150,000 participants, found a significant association between RA and periodontitis with a relative risk of 1.13 (95% CI 1.04–1.23, $p = 0.006$) compared to healthy controls [60].

Shared risk factors, including cigarette smoke, provide possible confounders; however, an increased risk of periodontitis has been demonstrated in a nonsmoking RA group [61], and a comparison of periodontitis in osteoarthritis versus RA demonstrated that RA patients were twice as likely to have moderate to severe periodontitis independent of smoking, age or sex [62]. In addition, there is evidence to suggest that periodontitis responds to RA treatment [63].

5.5. Oral microbiome in rheumatoid arthritis

The association of periodontitis and *P. gingivalis* with rheumatoid arthritis has led to a great deal of interest in the oral microbiome in rheumatoid disease. Indeed, oral bacterial DNA and antibodies to *P. gingivalis, T. forsythia* and *P. intermedia* have been demonstrated in synovial fluid and the site of inflammation in rheumatoid arthritis [64]. It is also interesting that the medications with an antibacterial action against these species (including levofloxacin and clarithromycin) seem to have a beneficial effect in RA [65].

Animal studies have demonstrated a possible role periodontal bacteria in inflammatory arthritis. In a murine model of collagen-induced arthritis, oral infection with bacteria associated with periodontitis in humans developed exacerbated signs of inflammatory arthropathy, raised levels of matrix metalloproteinase 3 and histological evidence of active arthritis [66].

A study by Scher and colleagues used 16S ribosomal RNA sequencing to investigate oral microbiota from the subgingival plaque in patients with new-onset, Disease-modifying anti rheumatic drug naïve rheumatoid arthritis [67]. They found significantly higher levels of *Prevotella* and *Leptotrichia* species in the new-onset RA group compared to controls, which was robust to adjustment for periodontal disease status. In addition, *Streptococcus* and *Corynebacterium* genera were reduced in the new-onset RA group compared to healthy controls. They also investigated a chronic RA (Disease-modifying anti rheumatic drug treated) group and found higher levels of red complex bacteria in the new-onset RA group compared to the established disease group. These findings illustrate the changes in subgingival microbiota over time, and further work is required to delineate any independent roles of these changes in the microbial landscape.

Investigations of the oral microbiome are potentially hampered by the site of sampling as the oral microbiome varies depending on the region sampled. The gingival sulcus, tooth surface, hard and soft palate, saliva and tonsils are home to significantly different compositions of bacterial populations at a baseline. With the addition of the increased expertise required to acquire samples, there are far fewer studies investigating the oral microbiome than the gut microbiome in RA.

5.6. Gut microbiome in rheumatoid arthritis

The gut microbiome is the most densely populated microbial environment in the human body and is the most extensively studied. The benefit of extensive investigation is that the spectrum of the bacterial constituents of a 'normal' gut microbiome is more clearly defined [68] than in the oral cavity.

Disruption of the gut microbiome has been demonstrated in patients with rheumatoid arthritis compared to controls [69], and preceding work in animal models has highlighted possible etiological mechanisms of action.

For example, manipulating the gut microbiome by instilling segmented filamentous bacteria into the small intestine of mice induces CD4 T cells which produce the pro-inflammatory cytokine IL-17 in the intestinal lamina propria [70]. The experimental creation of small bowel bacterial overgrowth leads to reactivation of resolved arthritis in a rat model [71]. The resultant proposed hypothesis is that bacterial overgrowth leads to systemic, transmucosal absorption of Lipopolysaccharide which deposits in the liver and joints, leading to an inflammatory response.

Subtraction of microbiota as well as addition can lead to a pro-inflammatory phenotype, as in an adjuvant-induced arthritis, rat model, gnotobiotic (germ-free) rats demonstrated significantly greater joint inflammation than those with normal gut microbiota [72].

Analysis of the fecal microbiome of patients with rheumatoid arthritis found that haemophilus species were significantly reduced and lactobacillus species were significantly increased [69]. This study also showed that the intestinal dysbiosis was attenuated by Disease-modifying anti rheumatic drugs. *Prevotella copri* is raised in new-onset RA [73] and correlated with shared epitope genes, drawing attention to the organism as a potential environmental trigger for the development of RA.

The rapidly engorging literature regarding the gut microbiome and rheumatoid arthritis acts as encouragement to investigate other mucosal surfaces, and, with the marked associations with periodontitis and oral bacteria, the oral microbiome is a viable candidate for investigation.

5.7. Potential interventions

In addition studies to delineate the role of the microbiome in the etiology and progression of RA, it is worth considering the possible therapeutic interventions which could be developed.

Antibiotic administration is an apparent start, and doxycycline (which was historically used to treat RA) when used in conjunction with methotrexate has been shown to outperform methotrexate alone [74]. In patients with mild-to-moderate RA, minocycline was shown to significantly improve joint swelling, tenderness and erythrocyte sedimentation rate in a placebo-controlled trial [75]. However, the use of broad spectrum antibiotics introduces the risk of depleting all elements of the microbiome and opening the door to hostile organism invasion.

Other postulated interventions include probiotics, fecal microbiota transplant [64], harnessing bacterial secretions and single-target approaches to modify bacterial composition and by-products. Although they are exciting opportunities for research, these approaches are still in relative infancy.

5.8. Conclusion

There are strong data to support the association between rheumatoid arthritis, periodontitis and *P. gingivalis*. The role of mucosal immunity in the development of autoimmunity has been demonstrated extensively in the gut, and similar pathogenic processes could occur in the oral mucosa, though further investigation is required to clarify the role played by the oral microbiome in RA.

6. Periodontitis and ankylosing spondylitis

6.1. Ankylosing spondylitis

Ankylosing spondylitis (AS) is a chronic inflammatory condition primarily affecting the spine and sacroiliac joints. It is characterized by inflammatory back pain caused by enthesitis, bone erosion and new bone formation. Clinical features also include peripheral arthritis, anterior uveitis and rarely lung fibrosis, heart block and aortic regurgitation [76].

The overall prevalence of AS is between 0.1 and 1.4% with most cases coming from Europe [77]. Onset occurs young with 80% of patients presenting before the age of 30 and less than 5% present after the age of 45. Men are 2–3 times more commonly affected than women [77].

The diagnosis of AS is based on clinical features and presence of sacroiliitis on X-ray or MRI [78]. Treatment options are still limited, and emphasis is placed on physiotherapy and nonsteroidal anti-inflammatory medications, with anti-TNF therapy reserved for those who experience a persistently high level of disease activity. However, these have many potential side effects [78] and further understanding of the etiology of AS is needed in order to develop other treatment options.

6.2. Pathogenesis of ankylosing spondylitis

More than 90% of the risk of developing ankylosing spondylitis is determined genetically [79]. An important contribution of this is from human leucocyte antigen B27 (HLA-B27), a class 1 surface antigen encoded by MHC which has a role in presenting antigens to CD8 T cells. HLA B-27 is present in 90–95% of patients with AS, and the risk of developing AS in

HLA-B27-positive individuals is 2–5%. This is increased to 15–20% in HLA-B27-positive first-degree relative of AS patients [77].

The remainder of the risk comes from environmental factors. There is already substantial evidence to support a role of bacteria in the pathogenesis of AS. Reactive arthritis, another subtype of spondyloarthropathy, is triggered by genitourinary infections or enteritis caused by gram-negative enterobacteria. It is believed that the persistence of microbial antigens in the synovium of these patients contributes to the propagation of inflammation [77]. The possible role of these bacteria in the pathogenesis of AS is highlighted by the fact that 10–20% of HLA B27-positive patients with reactive arthritis develop the full clinical picture of ankylosing spondylitis [80]. Furthermore, 54% of HLA B27-positive patients with Crohn's disease develop ankylosing spondylitis, possibly due to the inflammatory processes in the gut allowing interaction of the gut bacteria and immune system [81]. TNF-alpha and T cell response is thought to be an important driver of inflammation in AS.

6.3. Periodontitis and ankylosing spondylitis

The similarities in the pathogenesis of ankylosing spondylitis and periodontitis have led to the hypothesis that periodontitis may allow oral bacteria access to the immune system and perpetuate inflammatory processes in those patients with genetic susceptibility. HLA A9 and B15, both associated with susceptibility to AS, may also be a susceptibility factor in aggressive periodontitis [82]. In particular, T lymphocyte-driven inflammation certainly plays a role in periodontitis [83] as well as in AS [84]. Interleukin (IL)-2, IL-6 and TNF-α are all raised in AS [85] as well as being implicated in periodontitis [86]. In fact, anti-TNF therapy in AS patients leads to a significant improvement in periodontal disease markers [87].

Ratz et al. performed a meta-analysis in 2015 of 6 studies comparing periodontitis measures in cases of AS and controls, and ranging in size between 90 and 40,926 participants [18]. All studies showed a positive correlation between AS and periodontitis severity, but only two showed statistical significance. On meta-analysis, the risk of developing AS in those with periodontitis was almost double with an overall odds ratio of 1.85 (CI 1.72–1.98). Despite no significant difference in probing depth and Clinical attachment level (CAL), there was a significant association in Bleeding on probing (BOP) with those with AS ($p = 0.0005$) [18].

Other studies since have looked further at the association between spondyloarthropathies, of which AS is a subtype, and periodontitis. In a group of 30 patients with spondyloarthropathy of which 8 had a diagnosis of AS, those patients with more than 5 years of evolution of disease had significantly worse periodontal disease [88]. In contrast, another group found that in 79 spondyloarthropathy patients, of which 19 had AS, levels of insertion loss were lower compared to the control group [89]. The association with *P. gingivalis* is still not certain, with contrasting findings that antibody titers were higher and lower in AS compared to controls [89, 90]

Recently, the oral microbiome has been studied in patients with axial spondyloarthritis. Patients were matched for age, gender and ethnicity to healthy controls. Interestingly, although patients had significantly greater prevalence of periodontitis (PPD $\geq$ 4 mm at $\geq$4 sites), a higher plaque index and higher mean bleeding on probing [91], there was no difference in either community structure or in diversity of organisms in the plaque bacterial communities analyzed. However, it is important to note that the small sample size in this study made it unlikely that any small effect size would be measured and so further larger studies are warranted to investigate this.

6.4. Conclusion

Overall, evidence does suggest an association between periodontitis and AS. When small studies were combined in meta-analysis, a significant odds ratio was calculated. Shared pathogenic mechanisms may explain some of this association, but the details of the underlying processes remain largely unknown.

7. Periodontitis and psoriatic arthritis

7.1. Psoriatic arthritis

Psoriatic arthritis (PsA) is an inflammatory arthritis associated with the presence of psoriasis, usually prior to joint involvement. Ninety-five percent are a peripheral arthritis, usually involving more than five joints in an asymmetrical pattern. The spine and sacroiliac joints are also affected in about 5% of patients [92].

Psoriatic arthritis is uncommon in the general population affecting <1%. However, it occurs in up to 30% of patients with psoriasis. It occurs equally in men and women and most commonly in those between 30 and 50 years of age [93].

Diagnosis is made clinically by the presence of inflammatory joint pain, personal or family history of psoriasis and typical X-ray findings. The treatment can be subdivided firstly into the treatment of psoriasis and secondly into the treatment of arthritis with Non-steroidal anti-inflammatory drugs, disease-modifying anti rheumatic drugs and biologics [94]. Again, the treatment options for PsA are limited and further understanding of disease etiology may lead to alternative treatments.

7.2. Pathogenesis of psoriatic arthritis

Similarly to the other seronegative spondyloarthropathies, psoriatic arthritis is thought to be caused by an environmental trigger in a genetically primed individual. Indeed, about 15% of first-degree relatives of a patient with psoriatic arthritis will also be affected and studies have elucidated genetic variants [93]. The most important of these are on the human leucocyte antigen 1 (HLA-1) which is involved in presenting antigens to CD8 T cells. Variants such as HLA-Cw6, HLA-B27 and HLA-B39 are associated with specific phenotypes of PsA. These variants highlight that psoriatic arthritis is not just a subset of psoriasis and provide important clues as to the pathogenesis of PsA in which the CD8 T cell plays a key role [93].

It is hypothesized that the molecules encoded by these HLA variants may recognize self-antigens in the synovium and enthesis. However, the true pathogenesis is likely to be more complex as T cell expanded clones in the synovial tissue of patients with psoriatic arthritis lack common motifs to explain a single trigger. Fitzgerald and Winchester propose that in fact CD8 T cells are stimulated through NK receptors which respond to molecules produced in inflammation and stress [93]. In support of this, both physical trauma and immunization with rubella vaccine have been shown to proceed development of psoriatic arthritis. Stimulation of the inflammatory response leads to infiltration of T cells and cytokines including TNF-alpha, Il-1, IL-6, IL-12, IL-15, IL-17, IL-18 and IF-γ in the synovium and ultimately to the clinical finding of synovitis [93]

7.3. Periodontitis and psoriatic arthritis

The characteristic lymphocytic infiltration of the joint with activated T cells and thus with the secretion of the pro-inflammatory cytokines IL-1 and TNF-α potentiates abnormal bone remodeling and the activation of matrix metalloproteinases in PsA. Interestingly, chronic periodontitis has a similar cytokine profile which has led to research investigating the relationship between them.

In 2013, Ustun et al. compared the periodontal status of 51 patients with PsA to that of healthy controls. Clinical attachment level, the gold standard measure of periodontitis severity and past disease activity, was significantly greater in those with PsA ($p = 0.037$). Although not statistically significant, probing depth was greater in those with PsA [95]. In another study, probing depth was statistically greater in patients with PsA [96]. A much larger Danish nationwide cohort study including 6428 patients with PsA found that incidence rates of periodontitis were significantly greater in patients with PsA compared to reference population. Of note, periodontitis rates were also greater in patients with PsA compared to psoriasis alone [97].

One cause for this may be the trapping of oral bacterial DNAs in synovial fluid. Mean number of oral bacterial species is significantly higher in both sera and synovial fluid of PsA patients, and periodontitis-associated species *P. gingivalis* and *Prevotella nigrescens* have been exclusively detected in PsA sera and synovial fluid [98].

A systematic review in 2016 presented 10 studies which all showed an association between psoriasis and periodontitis [99]. Eight of these, with between 33 and 115,365 cases, found measures of periodontitis including probing depth and CAL were increased in those with psoriasis compared to controls [95, 100–106]. A large population cohort study concluded that self-reported alveolar bone loss and loss of teeth increased risk of subsequent psoriasis [104]. Furthermore, these studies concluded that the presence of psoriasis was associated with greater severity of periodontitis.

7.4. Conclusion

Although there are still a limited number of studies, those which have been carried out provide strong evidence for an association between PsA and periodontitis. Importantly, they also highlight the distinct association of PsA, rather than psoriasis, with periodontitis.

8. Periodontitis and systemic lupus erythematosus

8.1. Systemic lupus erythematosus

Systemic lupus erythematosus (SLE) is a multi-systemic, chronic inflammatory condition which primarily affects connective tissues and is associated with specific serological signatures. Clinical features are extremely varied but common features include facial rash, oral ulcers, photosensitivity and nonerosive and nondeforming arthritis. Almost all body systems can be affected including renal, neurological, cardiac, respiratory, ophthalmic, gastrointestinal and hematological.

The estimated prevalence of SLE in the USA is 51/100,000, with females being affected 9 times more commonly than males. It is more common in people from Afro-Caribbean and Latin American decent. Most diagnosis is between the ages of 16–55 years with about 30% diagnosed younger than 16 or older than 55 years [107].

Diagnosis is based on clinical assessment and laboratory measures. Antibody tests including ANA, Anti-ds DNA and Anti-Sm may aid diagnosis but need to be used in the context of the clinical presentation [107].

Treatment for SLE depends on clinical presentation and disease activity, but the backbone is immunosuppression. However, given that the major cause of mortality in SLE is infection and malignancy which have both been attributed to long-term immunosuppression, there is a need to further understand disease etiology and find ways to prevent disease initiation and progression.

8.2. Pathogenesis of systemic lupus erythematosus

SLE occurs in genetically susceptible individuals, in whom an inflammatory response is triggered by a secondary stimulus. There is a strong genetic predisposition, and siblings of patients with SLE are 30 times more likely to have SLE than the general population [107]. Certain genetic variants which alter the inflammatory process and lead to impaired clearance of immunoglobulins have been implicated. Estrogen-driven stimulation of humeral activity may at least in part explain the female predominance [108]. Known environmental factors include UV light, demethylating drugs and infections such as EBV virus. These lead to the initiation of apoptosis and impaired clearance of cells. The nucleic acids are transferred to endosomal sensors, leading to the activation of endosomal toll-like receptors (TLRs) and dendritic cells which produce IFN alpha. These inflammatory mediators activate the inflammatory cascade, immune complex production and vascular damage. Immune complexes cause tissue destruction by deposition in tissues [109].

8.3. Periodontitis and systemic lupus erythematosus

Several case reports have suggested that patients with SLE have a greater severity of periodontitis [110–114]. The similar mechanisms of tissue destruction for periodontitis and SLE could explain a potential association. Polymorphisms in the Fcγ receptor leading to impaired clearing of immune complexes have already been implicated in susceptibility to both periodontitis and SLE [115]. The inflammatory cytokine profile is similar in periodontitis and SLE. For example, IL-18 levels are increased in patients with SLE and correlate with SLE disease activity index (SLEDAI) [116], while there is a significant correlation between IL-18 levels and periodontal parameters [116]. Interestingly, higher levels of IF-γ, IL 10, IL-17, IL-1β and IL-14 found in healthy patients with periodontitis are also present in patients with SLE even in the absence of periodontitis [117]

TLRs which modulate the inflammatory response to microorganisms in periodontal disease have also been implicated in SLE. Activation of TLRs which respond to specific pathogen-associated molecular patterns (PAMPs) such as Lipopolysaccharide produced by bacteria, triggers cell signaling pathways and release of pro-inflammatory cytokines. The overexpression of TLR-4 leads to autoimmune lupus and is essential for the production of anti-DsDNA antibodies found in SLE [108]. Therefore, the influence of the microorganisms in periodontal disease may affect the expression of TLRs in SLE and stimulate the autoimmune process.

Periodontitis is common in patients with SLE, with frequency varying between 60 and 93.8% [113, 118]. One Japanese study found that the frequency of periodontitis in SLE patients was 70% as compared to 30% in the general population [115].

Cross-sectional studies have found that periodontitis is more common in SLE than in controls [119–125]. A comparison of periodontal status in 105 SLE patients and geographically matched samples of the Adult Dental Health Survey in the UK found that, with adjustments for age and sex, patients with SLE were significantly more likely to have periodontitis with an OR 7.25 (95% CI 3.84–13.68) [121]. In another study, SLE patients had a significant 1.69-fold increased odds (CI 1.37–3.25) of having periodontitis defined by CAL > 3 mm [125]. These findings have been replicated in juvenile SLE patients where periodontal parameters were significantly higher than in controls [122]. Interestingly, SLE disease activity as measured by SLEDAI index correlates with periodontal condition and is a significant predictor of periodontitis [125, 126].

Three further studies have found nonsignificant findings that periodontitis is more prevalent in SLE patients [119, 123, 121]. The lack of statistical significance may be due to small sample size, use of immunosuppressants which can affect periodontal disease activity, and age. In fact, one study did highlight the fact that although there was no statistical difference in periodontal status, SLE cases were significantly younger than controls and so one could conclude that periodontitis is premature in SLE patients [120]. A study which did not find that periodontitis is more prevalent in SLE patients may have been due to the use of anti-inflammatory agents and the fact that controls were skewed to being older than cases [127].

No differences in bacterial species have been found in SLE patients compared to controls when specific periodontitis-associated bacteria have been examined [116] However, there have been no studies to date which have sequenced the oral microbiome in SLE patients.

Nonsurgical treatment of periodontitis in patients with SLE significantly improves both periodontitis measures and SLE disease activity index (SLEDAI) at 3 months [128]. This suggests treatment of periodontitis leads to a reduction in SLE disease activity and periodontitis may be an important factor in maintaining the inflammatory process in SLE.

8.4. Conclusion

There are some very compelling biological arguments including the shared pathogenesis and specifically a possible role of TLRs which could explain the link between periodontitis and SLE. To date, the evidence from case control studies suggesting an association is promising. However, further work with larger studies and identification of the oral microbiome in SLE patients is required to explain the role of periodontitis both in the initiation and in the maintenance of the inflammatory process in SLE.

9. Periodontitis and osteoarthritis

Osteoarthritis (OA) is a chronic degenerative condition of the joints characterized by cartilage loss, bone remodeling and periarticular muscle weakness. In contrast to RA, PsA, AS and SLE, there is not thought to be a primary inflammatory element in the disease process in OA though, as a patient group, they are considered to be good controls for the inflammatory arthropathies due to a similar demography [129, 54].

Osteoarthritis is extremely common, affecting more than 10% of people over the age of 45 [130]. Diagnosis is made on clinical symptoms and signs, and typical X-ray findings can be helpful although not required.

OA usually occurs due to chronic stress on the joint but can be accelerated by trauma, infection, crystal deposition and inflammatory arthritidies. Interestingly physical factors alone are not responsible for the development of OA. In fact, family history is a significant predictor of disease development and genome-wide association studies have identified multiple significant loci associated with OA [131].

There are elements of oral microbial flora that are of interest. A recent study has demonstrated the presence of periodontal bacteria in the joints of patients following joint replacement that may play a role in loosening and replacement failure [132]. However, compared to RA, the risk of periodontitis is significantly lower in OA [62] and no association has been found between OA and mild, moderate or severe periodontitis [133].

10. Conclusion

The advent of 16S sequencing techniques has allowed further study of the interaction between the oral microbiome and inflammatory arthritidies. It is clear that periodontitis is associated with systemic inflammation. The underlying mechanisms for this are less clear but may be due to the interaction of microbes with the immune system in the periodontal pocket or as a result of bacteremia. There is strong evidence to suggest an association between periodontitis and rheumatoid arthritis with PAD producing *P. gingivalis*, having a key role in this interaction. There is also accumulating evidence for other inflammatory arthritidies including ankylosing spondylitis, psoriatic arthritis and systemic lupus erythematosus. Common pathogenic mechanisms may explain this, but details of these interaction still need to be elucidated. Studies have been hampered by different measures of periodontitis, small sample size, multiple confounders and their cross-sectional nature. Further longitudinal studies which address these issues are needed. In the future, there may be a role for antibiotics, probiotics or interventions, targeting specific bacteria in these autoimmune conditions.

Author details

Zoe Rutter-Locher[1*†], Nicholas Fuggle[2†], Marco Orlandi[3], Francesco D'Aiuto[3] and Nidhi Sofat[1]

*Address all correspondence to: Zrutter-locher@nhs.net

1 Musculoskeletal Research Group, Institute of Infection and Immunity, St George's University of London, London, UK

2 MRC Lifecourse Epidemiology Unit, University of Southampton, UK

3 Unit of Periodontology, UCL Eastman Dental Institute, London, UK

† These authors contributed equally

References

[1] Turnbaugh PJ, Ley RE, Hamady M, Fraser-Liggett CM, Knight R, Gordon JI. The human microbiome project. Nature [Internet]. 2007 [cited 2017 Mar 6];**449**(7164):804-810. Available from: http://www.ncbi.nlm.nih.gov/pubmed/17943116

[2] Qin J, Li R, Raes J, Arumugam M, Burgdorf KS, Manichanh C, et al. A human gut microbial gene catalogue established by metagenomic sequencing. Nature [Internet]. 2010 [cited 2017 Mar 6];**464**(7285):59-65. Available from: http://www.nature.com/doifinder/10.1038/nature08821

[3] Maguire BA, Zimmermann RA. The ribosome in focus. Cell [Internet]. 2001 [cited 2017 Mar 6];**104**(6):813-816. Available from: http://www.ncbi.nlm.nih.gov/pubmed/11290319

[4] Kuczynski J, Lauber CL, Walters WA, Parfrey LW, Clemente JC, Gevers D, et al. Experimental and analytical tools for studying the human microbiome. Nature Reviews Genetics [Internet]. 2011 [cited 2017 Mar 6];**13**(1):47-58. Available from: http://www.nature.com/doifinder/10.1038/nrg3129

[5] Peterson J, Garges S, Giovanni M, McInnes P, Wang L, Schloss JA, et al. The NIH Human Microbiome Project. Genome Research [Internet]. 2009 [cited 2017 Mar 6];**19**(12):2317-2323. Available from: http://www.ncbi.nlm.nih.gov/pubmed/19819907

[6] Williams RC. Periodontal disease. The New England Journal of Medicine. 1990;**322**:373-382. Downloaded from nejm.org ST Georg Univ

[7] Dye BA. Global periodontal disease epidemiology. Periodontology 2000. 2012;**58**(1):10-25

[8] Hajishengallis G. Periodontitis: From microbial immune subversion to systemic inflammation. Nature reviews. Immunology. 2015;**15**:30-44

[9] Schmidt J, Jentsch H, Stingu C-S, Sack U. General immune status and oral microbiology in patients with different forms of periodontitis and healthy control subjects. PLoS One. 2014;**9**(10):e109187

[10] McCray LJAT. 'Ome sweet 'omics- a genealogial treasury of words. Scientist. 2001;**15**:8-10

[11] Dewhirst FE, Chen T, Izard J, Paster BJ, Tanner ACR, Yu W-H, et al. The human oral microbiome. Journal of Bacteriology [Internet]. 2010 [cited 2017 Jan 31];**192**(19):5002-5017. Available from: http://www.ncbi.nlm.nih.gov/pubmed/20656903

[12] Zarco MF, Vess TJ, Ginsburg GS. The oral microbiome in health and disease and the potential impact on personalized dental medicine. Oral Dis. 2012;**18**(2):109-120

[13] Wade WG. The oral microbiome in health and disease. Pharmacological Research. 2013;**69**(1):137-143

[14] Alcaraz LD, Belda-Ferre P, Cabrera-Rubio R, Romero H, Simón-Soro Á, Pignatelli M, et al. Identifying a healthy oral microbiome through metagenomics. Clinical Microbiology and Infection. 2012;**18**(Suppl. 4):54-57

[15] Armitage GC. Development of a classification system for periodontal diseases and conditions. Annals of Periodontology. 1999;**4**(1):1-6

[16] Jacob S. Measuring periodontitis in population studies: A literature review Medição de periodontite em estudos populacionais: uma revisão de literatura. Revista Odonto Ciência. 2011;**26**(4):346-354

[17] Chi AC, Neville BW, Krayer JW, Gonsalves WC. Oral Manifestations of systemic disease. American Family Physician2010;**82**(11):1381-1388

[18] Ratz T, Dean LE, Atzeni F, Reeks C, Macfarlane GJ, Macfarlane TV. A possible link between ankylosing spondylitis and periodontitis: A systematic review and meta-analysis. Rheumatology (Oxford) [Internet]. 2015 [cited 2016 Nov 21];**54**(3):500-510. Available from: http://www.ncbi.nlm.nih.gov/pubmed/25213130

[19] Kweider M, Lowe GDO, Murray GD, Kinane DF, McGowan DA. Dental disease, fibrinogen and white cell count; links with myocardial infarction? Scottish Medical Journal [Internet]. 1993 [cited 2017 Mar 6];**38**(3):73-74. Available from: http://www.ncbi.nlm.nih.gov/pubmed/8356427

[20] Ebersole JL, Machen RL, Steffen MJ, Willmann DE. Systemic acute-phase reactants, C-reactive protein and haptoglobin, in adult periodontitis. Clinical & Experimental Immunology [Internet]. 1997 Feb [cited 2017 Mar 6];**107**(2):347-352. Available from: http://www.ncbi.nlm.nih.gov/pubmed/9030874

[21] Loos BG, Craandijk J, Hoek FJ, Dillen PMEW, Velden U Van Der. Elevation of systemic markers related to cardiovascular diseases in the peripheral blood of periodontitis patients. Journal of Periodontology [Internet]. 2000 [cited 2017 Mar 6];71(10):1528-1534. Available from: http://www.ncbi.nlm.nih.gov/pubmed/11063384

[22] Slade GD, Offenbacher S, Beck JD, Heiss G, Pankow JS. Acute-phase inflammatory response to periodontal disease in the US population. Journal of Dental Research [Internet]. 2000 [cited 2017 Mar 6];79(1):49-57. Available from: http://www.ncbi.nlm.nih.gov/pubmed/10690660

[23] Hutter JW, van der Velden U, Varoufaki A, Huffels RA, Hoek FJ, Loos BG. Lower numbers of erythrocytes and lower levels of hemoglobin in periodontitis patients compared to control subjects. Journal of Clinical Periodontology [Internet]. 2001 [cited 2017 Mar 6];28(10):930-936. Available from: http://www.ncbi.nlm.nih.gov/pubmed/11686811

[24] Noack B, Genco RJ, Trevisan M, Grossi S, Zambon JJ, Nardin E De. Periodontal infections contribute to elevated systemic c-reactive protein level. Journal of Periodontology [Internet]. 2001 [cited 2017 Mar 6];72(9):1221-1227. Available from: http://www.ncbi.nlm.nih.gov/pubmed/11577954

[25] Paraskevas S, Huizinga JD, Loos BG. A systematic review and meta-analyses on C-reactive protein in relation to periodontitis. Journal of Clinical Periodontology [Internet]. 2008 [cited 2017 Mar 6];35(4):277-290. Available from: http://www.ncbi.nlm.nih.gov/pubmed/18294231

[26] Freitas COT de, Gomes-Filho IS, Naves RC, Nogueira Filho G da R, Cruz SS da, Santos CA de ST, et al. Influence of periodontal therapy on C-reactive protein level: A systematic review and meta-analysis. Journal of Applied Oral Science [Internet]. 2012 [cited 2017 Mar 6];20(1):1-8. Available from: http://www.ncbi.nlm.nih.gov/pubmed/22437670

[27] Teeuw WJ, Slot DE, Susanto H, Gerdes VEA, Abbas F, D'Aiuto F, et al. Treatment of periodontitis improves the atherosclerotic profile: A systematic review and meta-analysis. Journal of Clinical Periodontology [Internet]. 2014 [cited 2017 Mar 6];41(1):70-79. Available from: http://www.ncbi.nlm.nih.gov/pubmed/24111886

[28] D'Aiuto F, Orlandi M, Gunsolley JC. Evidence that periodontal treatment improves biomarkers and CVD outcomes. Journal of Periodontology [Internet]. 2013 [cited 2017 Mar 6];40:S85–S105. Available from: http://www.ncbi.nlm.nih.gov/pubmed/23627337

[29] Preshaw PM, Taylor JJ. How has research into cytokine interactions and their role in driving immune responses impacted our understanding of periodontitis? Journal of Clinical Periodontology [Internet]. 2011 [cited 2017 Mar 6];38:60-84. Available from: http://www.ncbi.nlm.nih.gov/pubmed/21323705

[30] Teles R, Wang C-Y. Mechanisms involved in the association between peridontal diseases and cardiovascular disease. Oral Diseases [Internet]. 2011 [cited 2017 Mar 6];17(5):450-461. Available from: http://www.ncbi.nlm.nih.gov/pubmed/21223455

[31] Kinane DF, Riggio MP, Walker KF, MacKenzie D, Shearer B. Bacteraemia following peri-odontal procedures. Journal of Clinical Periodontology [Internet]. 2005 [cited 2017 Mar 6];**32**(7):708-13. Available from: http://www.ncbi.nlm.nih.gov/pubmed/15966875

[32] Haraszthy VI, Zambon JJ, Trevisan M, Zeid M, Genco RJ. Identification of periodon-tal pathogens in atheromatous plaques. Journal of Periodontology [Internet]. 2000 [cited 2017 Mar 6];**71**(10):1554-1560. Available from: http://www.ncbi.nlm.nih.gov/pubmed/11063387

[33] Kozarov EV, Dorn BR, Shelburne CE, Dunn WA, Progulske-Fox A. Human atherosclerotic plaque contains viable invasive actinobacillus actinomycetemcomitans and *Porphyromonas gingivalis*. Arteriosclerosis, Thrombosis, and Vascular Biolog [Internet]. 2005 [cited 2017 Mar 6];**25**(3):e17–e18. Available from: http://www.ncbi.nlm.nih.gov/pubmed/15662025

[34] Bergström J, Minenna L, Farina R, Scabbia A, Trombelli L, Hart A, et al. Periodontitis and smoking: An evidence-based appraisal. Journal of Evidence-Based Dental Practice [Internet]. 2006 [cited 2017 Mar 6];**6**(1):33-41. Available from: http://www.ncbi.nlm.nih.gov/pubmed/17138394

[35] Leone A, Landini L, Picano E. Modifying cardiovascular risk factors: Epidemiology and characteristics of smoking-related cardiovascular diseases. Current Pharmaceutical Design [Internet]. 2010 [cited 2017 Mar 6];**16**(23):2504-2509. Available from: http://www.ncbi.nlm.nih.gov/pubmed/20550498

[36] Ritchie CS. Obesity and periodontal disease. Periodontology 2000 [Internet]. 2007 [cited 2017 Mar 6];**44**(1):154-163. Available from: http://www.ncbi.nlm.nih.gov/pubmed/17474931

[37] D'Aiuto F, Parkar M, Nibali L, Suvan J, Lessem J, Tonetti MS. Periodontal infections cause changes in traditional and novel cardiovascular risk factors: Results from a ran-domized controlled clinical trial. American Heart Journal [Internet]. 2006 [cited 2017 Mar 6];**151**(5):977-984. Available from: http://www.ncbi.nlm.nih.gov/pubmed/16644317

[38] Pussinen PJ, Tuomisto K, Jousilahti P, Havulinna AS, Sundvall J, Salomaa V. Endotoxemia, immune response to periodontal pathogens, and systemic inflammation associate with incident cardiovascular disease events. Arteriosclerosis, Thrombosis, and Vascular Biology [Internet]. 2007 [cited 2017 Mar 6];**27**(6):1433-1439. Available from: http://www.ncbi.nlm.nih.gov/pubmed/17363692

[39] Fuggle NR, Howe FA, Allen RL, Sofat N. New insights into the impact of neuro-inflam-mation in rheumatoid arthritis. Frontiers in Neuroscience [Internet]. 2014 [cited 2017 Feb 23];**8**:357. Available from: http://www.ncbi.nlm.nih.gov/pubmed/25414636

[40] McInnes IB, Schett G. The pathogenesis of rheumatoid arthritis. The New England Journal of Medicine. 2011;**365**(23):2205-2219.

[41] Alamanos Y, Voulgari PV., Drosos AA. Incidence and prevalence of rheumatoid arthri-tis, based on the 1987 American College of Rheumatology criteria: A systematic review. Seminars in Arthritis and Rheumatism [Internet]. 2006 [cited 2017 Feb 23];**36**(3):182-188. Available from: http://www.ncbi.nlm.nih.gov/pubmed/17045630

[42] Silman AJ, Pearson JE. Epidemiology and genetics of rheumatoid arthritis. Arthritis Research [Internet]. 2002 [cited 2017 Feb 23];**4**(Suppl 3):S265. Available from: http://www.ncbi.nlm.nih.gov/pubmed/12110146

[43] Aletaha D, Neogi T, Silman AJ, Funovits J, Felson DT, Bingham CO, et al. 2010 rheumatoid arthritis classification criteria: An American College of Rheumatology/European League Against Rheumatism collaborative initiative. Annals of the Rheumatic Diseases [Internet]. 2010 [cited 2017 Feb 23];**69**(9):1580-1588. Available from: http://www.ncbi.nlm.nih.gov/pubmed/20699241

[44] MacGregor AJ, Snieder H, Rigby AS, Koskenvuo M, Kaprio J, Aho K, et al. Characterizing the quantitative genetic contribution to rheumatoid arthritis using data from twins. Arthritis & Rheumatism [Internet]. 2000 Jan [cited 2017 Feb 23];**43**(1):30-37. Available from: http://www.ncbi.nlm.nih.gov/pubmed/10643697

[45] Kallberg H, Padyukov L, Plenge RM, Ronnelid J, Gregersen PK, van der Helm-van Mil AHM, et al. Gene-gene and gene-environment interactions involving HLA-DRB1, PTPN22, and smoking in two subsets of rheumatoid arthritis. The American Journal of Human Genetics. 2007;**80**(5):867-875.

[46] Hutchinson D, Moots R. Cigarette smoking and severity of rheumatoid arthritis. Rheumatology (Oxford). 2001;**40**(12):1426-1427.

[47] Smolen JS, Aletaha D, McInnes IB. Rheumatoid arthritis. Lancet [Internet]. 2016 [cited 2017 Feb 23];**388**(10055):2023-2038. Available from: http://www.ncbi.nlm.nih.gov/pubmed/27156434

[48] El-Gabalawy H. The preclinical stages of RA: Lessons from human studies and animal models. Best Practice & Research: Clinical Rheumatology. 2009;**23**(1):49-58.

[49] Avouac J, Gossec L, Dougados M. Diagnostic and predictive value of anti-cyclic citrullinated protein antibodies in rheumatoid arthritis: A systematic literature review. Annals of the Rheumatic Diseases. 2006;**65**(7):845-851.

[50] Nielen MMJ, van Schaardenburg D, Reesink HW, van de Stadt RJ, van der Horst-Bruinsma IE, de Koning MHMT, et al. Specific autoantibodies precede the symptoms of rheumatoid arthritis: A study of serial measurements in blood donors. Arthritis & Rheumatism. 2004;**50**(2):380-386.

[51] Sokolove J, Bromberg R, Deane KD, Lahey LJ, Derber LA, Chandra PE, et al. Autoantibody epitope spreading in the pre-clinical phase predicts progression to rheumatoid arthritis. PLoS One. 2012;**7**(5):e35296.

[52] Sofat N, Wait R, Robertson SD, Baines DL, Baker EH. Interaction between extracellular matrix molecules and microbial pathogens: Evidence for the missing link in autoimmunity with rheumatoid arthritis as a disease model. Frontiers in Microbiology. 2014;**5**:783

[53] Van den Broek MF, Van de Putte LB, Van den Berg WB. Crohn's disease associated with arthritis: A possible role for cross-reactivity between gut bacteria and cartilage in

the pathogenesis of arthritis. Arthritis & Rheumatism [Internet]. 1988 [cited 2017 Feb 23];**31**(8):1077-1079. Available from: http://www.ncbi.nlm.nih.gov/pubmed/3408509

[54] Mikuls TR, Payne JB, Yu F, Thiele GM, Reynolds RJ, Cannon GW, et al. Periodontitis and *Porphyromonas gingivalis* in patients with rheumatoid arthritis. Arthritis & Rheumatology (Hoboken, NJ). 2014;**66**(5):1090-100

[55] Mikuls TR, Thiele GM, Deane KD, Payne JB, O'dell JR, Yu F, et al. *Porphyromonas gingivalis* and disease-related autoantibodies in individuals at increased risk of rheumatoid arthritis. Arthritis & Rheumatology. 2012;**64**(11):3522-3530

[56] Johansson L, Sherina N, Kharlamova N, Potempa B, Larsson B, Israelsson L, et al. Concentration of antibodies against *Porphyromonas gingivalis* is increased before the onset of symptoms of rheumatoid arthritis. Arthritis Research & Therapy [Internet]. 2016 [cited 2017 Feb 23];**18**(1):201. Available from: http://arthritis-research.biomedcentral.com/articles/10.1186/s13075-016-1100-4

[57] Kobayashi T, Ito S, Yasuda K, Kuroda T, Yamamoto K, Sugita N, et al. The combined genotypes of stimulatory and inhibitory fcγ receptors associated with systemic lupus erythematosus and periodontitis in Japanese adults. Journal of Periodontology [Internet]. 2007 [cited 2016 Nov 16];**78**(3):467-474. Available from: http://www.joponline.org/doi/10.1902/jop.2007.060194

[58] Persson GR. Rheumatoid arthritis and periodontitis—inflammatory and infectious connections. Review of the literature. Journal of Oral Microbiology. 2012;**4**:11829

[59] Demmer RT, Molitor JA, Jacobs DR, Michalowicz BS. Periodontal disease, tooth loss and incident rheumatoid arthritis: results from the First National Health and Nutrition Examination Survey and its epidemiological follow-up study. Journal of Clinical Periodontology. 2011;**38**(11):998-1006.

[60] Arleevskaya MI, Korotkova M, Renaudineau Y, Sofat N, Fuggle NR, Smith TO, et al. Hand to mouth: A systematic review and meta-analysis of the association between rheumatoid arthritis and periodontitis. Frontiers in Immunology. 2016;**7**:80.

[61] Potikuri D, Dannana KC, Kanchinadam S, Agrawal S, Kancharla A, Rajasekhar L, et al. Periodontal disease is significantly higher in non-smoking treatment-naive rheumatoid arthritis patients: results from a case-control study. Annals of the Rheumatic Diseases. 2012;**71**(9):1541-1544.

[62] Dissick A, Redman RS, Jones M, Rangan B V., Reimold A, Griffiths GR, et al. Association of periodontitis with rheumatoid arthritis: A pilot study. Journal of Periodontology [Internet]. 2010 [cited 2017 Feb 22];**81**(2):223-230. Available from: http://www.ncbi.nlm.nih.gov/pubmed/20151800

[63] Assuma R, Oates T, Cochran D, Amar S, Graves DT. IL-1 and TNF antagonists inhibit the inflammatory response and bone loss in experimental periodontitis. The Journal of Immunology. 1998;**160**(1):403-409

[64] Jethwa H, Abraham S; The evidence for microbiome manipulation in inflammatory arthritis. Rheumatology (Oxford) 2016; 275, 53, 263 kew374. doi: 10.1093/rheumatology/kew374

[65] Ogrendik M. Periodontal pathogens are likely to be responsible for the development of ankylosing spondylitis. Current Rheumatology Reviews. 2015;11(1):47-49

[66] Chukkapalli S, Rivera-Kweh M, Gehlot P, Velsko I, Bhattacharyya I, Calise SJ, et al. Periodontal bacterial colonization in synovial tissues exacerbates collagen-induced arthritis in B10.RIII mice. Arthritis Research & Therapy [Internet]. 2016 [cited 2017 Feb 23];18(1):161. Available from: http://www.ncbi.nlm.nih.gov/pubmed/27405639

[67] Scher JU, Ubeda C, Equinda M, Khanin R, Buischi Y, Viale A, et al. Periodontal disease and the oral microbiota in new-onset rheumatoid arthritis. Arthritis & Rheumatism. 2012;64(10):3083-3094.

[68] González A, Vázquez-Baeza Y, Knight R. SnapShot: The human microbiome. Cell [Internet]. 2014 [cited 2017 Feb 23];158(3):690-690.e1. Available from: http://www.ncbi.nlm.nih.gov/pubmed/25083877

[69] Zhang X, Zhang D, Jia H, Feng Q, Wang D, Liang D, et al. The oral and gut microbiomes are perturbed in rheumatoid arthritis and partly normalized after treatment. Nature Medicine [Internet]. 2015;21(8):895-905. Available from: http://www.ncbi.nlm.nih.gov/pubmed/26214836\nhttp://www.nature.com/nm/journal/v21/n8/full/nm.3914.html?WT.ec_id=NM-201508&spMailingID=49267143&spUserID=ODM2MjM4OTIwNA S2&spJobID=741033692&spReportId=NzQxMDMzNjkyS0

[70] Ivanov II, Atarashi K, Manel N, Brodie EL, Shima T, Karaoz U, et al. Induction of intestinal Th17 cells by segmented filamentous bacteria. Cell [Internet]. 2009 [cited 2017 Feb 23];139(3):485-498. Available from: http://www.ncbi.nlm.nih.gov/pubmed/19836068

[71] Lichtman SN, Wang J, Sartor RB, Zhang C, Bender D, Dalldorf FG, et al. Reactivation of arthritis induced by small bowel bacterial overgrowth in rats: Role of cytokines, bacteria, and bacterial polymers. Infection and Immunity [Internet]. 1995 [cited 2017 Feb 23];63(6):2295-2301. Available from: http://www.ncbi.nlm.nih.gov/pubmed/7768612

[72] Kohashi O, Kuwata J, Umehara K, Uemura F, Takahashi T, Ozawa A. Susceptibility to adjuvant-induced arthritis among germfree, specific-pathogen-free, and conventional rats. Infection and Immunity [Internet]. 1979 [cited 2017 Feb 23];26(3):791-794. Available from: http://www.ncbi.nlm.nih.gov/pubmed/160888

[73] Nakayama J, Watanabe K, Jiang J, Matsuda K, Chao S-H, Haryono P, et al. Diversity in gut bacterial community of school-age children in Asia. Scientific Reports [Internet]. 2015 [cited 2017 Feb 23];5:8397. Available from: http://www.nature.com/articles/srep08397

[74] O'Dell JR, Elliott JR, Mallek JA, Mikuls TR, Weaver CA, Glickstein S, et al. Treatment of early seropositive rheumatoid arthritis: Doxycycline plus methotrexate versus methotrexate alone. Arthritis & Rheumatism [Internet]. 2006 [cited 2017 Feb 23];54(2):621-627. Available from: http://www.ncbi.nlm.nih.gov/pubmed/16447240

[75] Tilley BC, Alarcón GS, Heyse SP, Trentham DE, Neuner R, Kaplan DA, et al. Minocycline in rheumatoid arthritis. A 48-week, double-blind, placebo-controlled trial. MIRA Trial Group. Annals of Internal Medicine [Internet]. 1995 [cited 2017 Feb 23];**122**(2):81-89. Available from: http://www.ncbi.nlm.nih.gov/pubmed/7993000

[76] Tam L-S, Gu J, Yu D. Pathogenesis of ankylosing spondylitis. Nature Reviews Rheumatology [Internet]. 2010 [cited 2017 Jan 26];**6**(7):399-405. Available from: http://www.ncbi.nlm.nih.gov/pubmed/20517295

[77] Braun J, Sieper J. Ankylosing spondylitis. Lancet. 2007;**369**:1379-1390. www.thelancet.com

[78] Taurog JD, Chhabra A, Colbert RA. Ankylosing spondylitis and axial spondyloarthritis. The New England Journal of Medicine. 2016;**26374**:2563-2574.

[79] Reveille JD. The genetic basis of ankylosing spondylitis. Current Opinion in Rheumatology [Internet]. 2006 [cited 2017 Jan 26];**18**(4):332-341. Available from: http://www.ncbi.nlm.nih.gov/pubmed/16763451

[80] Leirisalo-Repo M, Helenius P, Hannu T, Lehtinen A, Kreula J, Taavitsainen M, et al. Long-term prognosis of reactive salmonella arthritis. Annals of the Rheumatic Diseases [Internet]. 1997 [cited 2017 Jan 26];**56**(9):516-520. Available from: http://www.ncbi.nlm.nih.gov/pubmed/9370874

[81] Purrmann J, Zeidler H, Bertrams J, Juli E, Cleveland S, Berges W, et al. HLA antigens in ankylosing spondylitis associated with Crohn's disease. Increased frequency of the HLA phenotype B27,B44. The Journal of Rheumatology [Internet]. 1988 [cited 2017 Jan 26];**15**(11):1658-1661. Available from: http://www.ncbi.nlm.nih.gov/pubmed/3266250

[82] Stein JM, Machulla HKG, Smeets R, Lampert F, Reichert S. Human leukocyte antigen polymorphism in chronic and aggressive periodontitis among Caucasians: A meta-analysis. Journal of Clinical Periodontology [Internet]. 2008 [cited 2017 Jan 26];**35**(3):183-192. Available from: http://doi.wiley.com/10.1111/j.1600-051X.2007.01189.x

[83] Bartold PM, Marshall RI, Haynes DR. Periodontitis and rheumatoid arthritis: A review. Journal of Periodontology. 2005;**76**(11 Suppl):2066-2074.

[84] Sieper J, Braun J, Rudwaleit M, Boonen A, Zink A. Ankylosing spondylitis: an overview. Annals of the Rheumatic Diseases [Internet]. 2002 [cited 2017 Jan 26];**61**(Suppl 3):iii8–iii18. Available from: http://www.ncbi.nlm.nih.gov/pubmed/12381506

[85] Bal A, Unlu E, Bahar G, Aydog E, Eksioglu E, Yorgancioglu R. Comparison of serum IL-1 beta, sIL-2R, IL-6, and TNF-alpha levels with disease activity parameters in ankylosing spondylitis. Clinical Rheumatology. 2007;**26**(2):211-215.

[86] Pischon N, Pischon T, Kröger J, Gülmez E, Kleber B-M, Bernimoulin J-P, et al. Association among rheumatoid arthritis, oral hygiene, and periodontitis. Journal of Periodontology. 2008;**79**(6):979-986.

[87] Fabri GMC, Pereira RMR, Savioli C, Saad CGS, de Moraes JCB, Siqueira JTT, et al. Periodontitis response to anti-TNF therapy in ankylosing spondylitis. JCR Journal of

Clinical Rheumatology [Internet]. 2015 [cited 2016 Nov 21];**21**(7):341-345. Available from: http://content.wkhealth.com/linkback/openurl?sid=WKPTLP:landingpage &an=00124743-201510000-00002

[88] Londoño J, Romero-Sánchez C, Bautista-Molano W, Segura S, Cortes-Muñoz A, Castillo D, et al. AB0569 Association between periodontal condition with disease duration and activity in colombian patients with spondyloarthritis. Annals of the Rheumatic Diseases [Internet]. 2013 [cited 2016 Nov 21];**72**(Suppl 3):A963.2–A963. Available from: http://ard. bmj.com/lookup/doi/10.1136/annrheumdis-2013-eular.2891

[89] Giraldo Q S, Romero-sanchez C, Bautista-Molano W, Bello-Gualtero JM, De-Avila J, Chila ML, et al. AB0675 is the periodontal clinical and microbiological condition in spondyloarthritis similar than rheumatoid arthritis? Annals of the Rheumatic Diseases. 2016;**75**(Suppl 2):1135-1136.

[90] Rueda JC, Bautista-Molano W, Avila J De, Bello-Gualtero JM, Castillo DM, Lafaurie GI, et al. FRI0422 periodontal disease in spondyloarthritis subtypes. Is there a difference? Annals of the Rheumatic Diseases. 2016;**75**(Suppl 2):588-588.

[91] Stebbings SM, Bisanz JE, Suppiah P, Thomson WM, Milne T, Yeoh N, et al. The oral microbiome of patients with axial spondyloarthritis compared to healthy individuals. PeerJ. 2016;**4**:e2095

[92] Gilliland WR. Arthritis associated with psoriasis and other skin conditions. In: West SG, editor. Rheumatology Secrets. 3rd ed. Philadelphia: Elsevier Mosby; 2015. pp. 284-288.

[93] FitzGerald O, Winchester R. Psoriatic arthritis: from pathogenesis to therapy. Arthritis Research & Therapy [Internet]. 2009 [cited 2017 Feb 14];**11**(1):214. Available from: http:// arthritis-research.biomedcentral.com/articles/10.1186/ar2580

[94] Gossec L, Coates LC, de Wit M, Kavanaugh A, Ramiro S, Mease PJ, et al. Management of psoriatic arthritis in 2016: A comparison of EULAR and GRAPPA recommenda-tions. Nature Reviews Rheumatology [Internet]. 2016 [cited 2017 Feb 22];**12**(12):743-750. Available from: http://www.nature.com/doifinder/10.1038/nrrheum.2016.183

[95] Üstün K, Sezer U, Kısacık B, Şenyurt SZ, Özdemir EÇ, Kimyon G, et al. Periodontal dis-ease in patients with psoriatic arthritis. Inflammation. 2013;**36**(3):665-669

[96] Mayer Y, Elimelech R, Balbir-Gurman A, Braun-Moscovici Y, Machtei EE. Periodontal condition of patients with autoimmune diseases and the effect of anti-tumor necrosis factor-a therapy. Journal of Periodontology. 2013;**84**(2):136-142

[97] Egeberg A, Mallbris L, Gislason G, Hansen PR, Mrowietz U. Risk of periodontitis in patients with psoriasis and psoriatic arthritis. Journal of the European Academy of Dermatology and Venereology [Internet]. 2017 [cited 2016 Nov 21]; **31**(2):288-293. Available from: http://doi.wiley.com/10.1111/jdv.13814

[98] Moen K, Brun JG, Valen M, Skartveit L, Eribe EKR, Olsen I, et al. Synovial inflammation in active rheumatoid arthritis and psoriatic arthritis facilitates trapping of a variety of oral bacterial DNAs. Clinical and Experimental Rheumatology. 2006;**24**(6):656-663.

[99] Monson CA, Porfirio G, Riera R, Tweed JA, Petri V, Atallah ÁN. Periodontal aspects for psoriasis: A systematic review. Clinical Research in Dermatology: Open Access. 2016 [cited 2017 Jan 24]; 3(1):1-8. Available from: www.symbiosisonlinepublishing.com

[100] Preus HR, Khanifam P, Kolltveit K, Mørk C, Gjermo P. Periodontitis in psoriasis patients. A blinded, case-controlled study. Acta Odontologica Scandinavica [Internet]. 2010 [cited 2017 Feb 14];68(3):165-170. Available from: http://www.tandfonline.com/doi/full/10.3109/00016350903583678

[101] Kathariya R, Pradeep AR. Chronic plaque psoriasis and plaque-induced chronic periodontitis; is there any association: A cross-sectional study. Journal of Periodontology & Implant Dentistry [Internet]. 2011 [cited 2017 Feb 14];3(1):13-20. Available from: http://dentistry.tbzmed.ac.ir/jpid

[102] Keller JJ, Lin H-C. The effects of chronic periodontitis and its treatment on the subsequent risk of psoriasis. British Journal of Dermatology [Internet]. 2012 [cited 2017 Feb 14];167(6): 1338-1344. Available from: http://doi.wiley.com/10.1111/j.1365-2133.2012.11126.x

[103] Lazaridou E, Tsikrikoni A, Fotiadou C, Kyrmanidou E, Vakirlis E, Giannopoulou C, et al. Association of chronic plaque psoriasis and severe periodontitis: A hospital based case-control study. Journal of the European Academy of Dermatology and Venereology [Internet]. 2013;27(8):967-972. Available from: http://www.ncbi.nlm.nih.gov/pubmed/22703187

[104] Nakib S, Han J, Li T, et al. Periodontal disease and risk of psoriasis among nurses in the United States. Acta Odontologica Scandinavica. 2013;71(6):1423-1429

[105] Skudutyte-Rysstad R, Slevolden EM, Hansen BF, Sandvik L, Preus HR. Association between moderate to severe psoriasis and periodontitis in a Scandinavian population. BMC Oral health. 2014; Volume 14, Number 1, Page 1

[106] Sharma A, Raman A, Pradeep A. Association of chronic periodontitis and psoriasis: periodontal status with severity of psoriasis. Oral Diseases [Internet]. 2015 [cited 2017 Feb 14];21(3):314-319. Available from: http://doi.wiley.com/10.1111/odi.12271

[107] Bertsias G, Cervera R, Boumpas DT, Espinosa G, D'cruz D. Learning objectives: Systemic lupus erythematosus: Pathogenesis and clinical features. Eular On-line Course on Rheumatic Diseases -module n°17. 2009. Available online; [http://www.eular-online-course.org/sample_chapter/module17.pdf]

[108] Marques CPC, Maor Y, De Andrade MS, Rodrigues VP, Benatti BB. Possible evidence of systemic lupus erythematosus and periodontal disease association mediated by Toll-like receptors 2 and 4. Clinical & Experimental Immunology. 2016;183(2):187-192

[109] Tsokos GC. Mechanisms of disease systemic lupus erythematosus. The New England Journal of Medicine. 2011;36522365(1):2110-2121.

[110] Jaworski CP, Koudelka BM, Roth NA, Marshall KJ. Acute necrotizing ulcerative gingivitis in a case of systemic lupus erythematosus. Journal of Oral and Maxillofacial Surgery. 1985;43:43-46.

[111] Meyer U, Kleinheinz J, Gaubitz M, Schulz M, Weingart D, Joos U. Oral manifestations in patients with systemic lupus erythematosus. Mund Kiefer Gesichtschir [Internet]. 1997 [cited 2016 Nov 16];1(2):90-94. Available from: http://www.ncbi.nlm.nih.gov/pubmed/9410618

[112] Nagler RM, Lorber M, Ben-Arieh Y, Laufer D, Pollack S. Generalized periodontal involvement in a young patient with systemic lupus erythematosus. Lupus [Internet]. 1999;8(9):770-772. Available from: http://www.ncbi.nlm.nih.gov/pubmed/10602452

[113] Rhodus NL, Johnson DK. The prevalence of oral manifestations of systemic lupus erythematosus. Quintessence International [Internet]. 1990 [cited 2016 Nov 17];21(6):461-465. Available from: http://www.ncbi.nlm.nih.gov/pubmed/2243950

[114] Vogel RI. Periodontal disease associated with amegakaryocytic thrombocytopenia in systemic lupus erythematosus. Journal of Periodontology [Internet]. 1981 [cited 2016 Nov 17];52(1):20-23. Available from: http://www.joponline.org/doi/10.1902/jop.1981.52.1.20

[115] Kobayashi T, Ito S, Yamamoto K, Hasegawa H, Sugita N, Kuroda T, et al. Risk of periodontitis in systemic lupus erythematosus is associated with Fcγ receptor polymorphisms. Journal of Periodontology [Internet]. 2003 [cited 2016 Nov 16];74(3):378-384. Available from: http://www.joponline.org/doi/10.1902/jop.2003.74.3.378

[116] Areas A, Braga F, Miranda LA, Fischer RG, Figueredo CM, Miceli V, et al. Increased IL-18 serum levels in patients with juvenile systemic lupus erythematosus. Acta Reumatológica Portuguesa [Internet]. 2007;32(4):397-398. Available from: http://www.ncbi.nlm.nih.gov/pubmed/18159210

[117] Marques CPC, Victor EC, Franco MM, Fernandes JMC, Maor Y, de Andrade MS, et al. Salivary levels of inflammatory cytokines and their association to periodontal disease in systemic lupus erythematosus patients. A case-control study. Cytokine. 2016;85:165-170.

[118] Novo E, Garcia-MacGregor E, Viera N, Chaparro N, Crozzoli Y. Periodontitis and anti-neutrophil cytoplasmic antibodies in systemic lupus erythematosus and rheumatoid arthritis: A comparative study. Journal of Periodontology [Internet]. 1999 [cited 2016 Nov 16];70(2):185-188. Available from: http://www.joponline.org/doi/10.1902/jop.1999.70.2.185

[119] Al-Mutairi K, Al-Zahrani M, Bahlas S, Kayal R, Zawawi K. Periodontal findings in systemic lupus erythematosus patients and healthy controls. Saudi Medical Journal. 2015;36(4):463-468

[120] Calderaro DC, Ferreira GA, Dias Corrêa J, Maria S, Mendonça S, Silva T, et al. Is chronic periodontitis premature in systemic lupus erythematosus patients? Clinical Rheumatology. 2017;36:713-718

[121] de Pablo P, Dewan K, Dietrich T, Chapple I, Gordon C. AB0603 periodontal disease is common in patients with systemic lupus erythemathosus. Annals of the Rheumatic Diseases [Internet]. 2015 [cited 2016 Nov 16];74(Suppl 2):1101.2-1101. Available from: http://ard.bmj.com/lookup/doi/10.1136/annrheumdis-2015-eular.6245

[122] Fernandes EG, Savioli C, Siqueira JT, Silva CA. Oral health and the masticatory system in juvenile systemic lupus erythematosus. Lupus [Internet]. 2007;**16**(9):713-719. Available from: http://ovidsp.ovid.com/ovidweb.cgi?T=JS&PAGE=reference&D=emed 8&NEWS=N&AN=2007485131

[123] Meyer U, Kleinheinz J, Handschel J, Kruse-Losler B, Weingart D, Joos U. Oral findings in three different groups of immunocompromised patients. Journal of Oral Pathology & Medicine [Internet]. 2000 [cited 2016 Nov 17];**29**(4):153-158. Available from: http://doi.wiley.com/10.1034/j.1600-0714.2000.290402.x

[124] Wang C-Y, Chyuan I-T, Wang Y-L, Kuo MY-P, Chang C-W, Wu K-J, et al. β2-Glycoprotein I-dependent anti-cardiolipin antibodies associated with periodontitis in patients with systemic lupus erythematosus. Journal of Periodontology [Internet]. 2015;**86**(8):995-1004. Available from: http://www.ncbi.nlm.nih.gov/pubmed/25817824

[125] Zhang Q, Yin R, Fu T, Zhang L, Li L, Gu Z. Periodontal disease in patients with systemic lupus erythematosus. In 2016. Available from: http://ovidsp.tx.ovid.com/sp-3.22.1b/ovidweb.cgi?&S=PCLHFPJKPODDDNDKNCHKMFOBGPPFAA00&Abstract=S.sh.36%7c3%7c1

[126] De Araújo L, Sales R, Vassalo S, Das M, Afonso G, Chaves M, et al. Periodontal disease and systemic lupus erythematosus activity. Revised Interdisciplinary Estud Exp. 2009;(1):14-20.

[127] Mutlu S, Richards A, Maddison P, Scully C. Gingival and periodontal health in systemic lupus erythematosus. Community Dent Oral Epidemiol [Internet]. 1993 [cited 2016 Nov 17];**21**(3):158-161. Available from: http://doi.wiley.com/10.1111/j.1600-0528.1993.tb00742.x

[128] Fabbri C, Fuller R, Bonfa E, Guedes LK, D'Alleva PS, Borba EF. Periodontitis treatment improves systemic lupus erythematosus response to immunosuppressive therapy. Clinical Rheumatology [Internet]. 2014;**33**(4):505-509. Available from: http://www.ncbi.nlm.nih.gov/pubmed/24415114

[129] Coburn BW, Sayles HR, Payne JB, Redman RS, Markt JC, Beatty MW, et al. Performance of self-reported measures for periodontitis in rheumatoid arthritis and osteoarthritis. Journal of Periodontology. 2015;**86**(1):16-26.

[130] Bedson J, Jordan K, Croft P. The prevalence and history of knee osteoarthritis in general practice: a case-control study. Family Practice [Internet]. 2004 [cited 2017 Feb 17];**22**(1):103-108. Available from: http://www.ncbi.nlm.nih.gov/pubmed/15640302

[131] arcOGEN Consortium, arcOGEN Collaborators, Zeggini E, Panoutsopoulou K, Southam L, Rayner NW, et al. Identification of new susceptibility loci for osteoarthritis (arcOGEN): A genome-wide association study. Lancet [Internet]. 2012 [cited 2017 Feb 17];**380**(9844):815-823. Available from: http://www.ncbi.nlm.nih.gov/pubmed/22763110

[132] Ehrlich GD, Hu FZ, Sotereanos N, Sewicke J, Parvizi J, Nara PL, et al. What role do periodontal pathogens play in osteoarthritis and periprosthetic joint infections of the knee? Journal of Applied Biomaterials & Functional Materials. 2014;**12**(1):13-20.

[133] Kandati; SUSKEI. Osteoarthritis and periodontal disease—is there an association? In: 142nd APHA Annual Meeting and Exposition 2014; 2014.

3

Influence of the Oral Microbiome on General Health

Zvi G. Loewy, Shoshana Galbut, Ephraim Loewy and
David A. Felton

Abstract

The prevalence of edentulism is common worldwide. While improvements in access to healthcare and dental care are reducing the prevalence rate of edentulism, the rapidly growing number of elderly as a percent of the global population will sustain a need for denture therapy for the foreseeable future. While denture use has positive impacts on the quality of life, their use is associated with some problems and risks. Denture stomatitis, a chronic infection-related inflammatory disorder of the oral mucosa, is extremely common and has been reported to occur in up to two-thirds of denture wearers. Importantly, epidemiology studies have shown edentulism and denture wearing, while not proven as causative factors, to be associated with significant increases in risk for serious systemic diseases, such as chronic obstructive pulmonary disease (COPD), cardiovascular diseases, diabetes, and arthritic disorders. A common linkage across these diseases is an association between increased risk for the disease and chronic inflammation. The nature of surface properties and porosity of denture materials contributes to the attachment of microorganisms and the establishment and growth of the adherent biofilm. Hence, proper denture cleansing is critical in maintaining oral hygiene and general health and perhaps to reduce the risk factors for systemic disease.

Keywords: *Candida*, biofilm, stomatitis, chronic obstructive pulmonary disease, edentulism

1. Introduction

Loss of natural dentition and use of removable dental prostheses is extremely common worldwide. While improved global access to oral care is decreasing the incidence of partial and complete edentulism, the prevalence of edentulism remains high and, among the elderly, can exceed 50% in many countries. Furthermore, over the next few years, the global population of elderly individuals will dramatically increase, and this will require the ongoing management of edentulism, at least for the foreseeable future. Edentulism adversely impacts nutrition and quality of life. For example, edentulism is associated with decreased masticatory performance, and this limits the types of food which individuals can chew and eat; furthermore, edentulous individuals report limiting their social function due to negative perceptions related to self-appearance and/or embarrassment and discomfort when eating in social settings.

Restoring dentition by use of an appropriate prosthesis is the treatment approach to edentulism. Denture prostheses can significantly improve masticatory performance, but their impact on changing and improving dietary habits is much less clear. Similarly, dentures can positively impact quality of life regarding appearance and social function, but limitations related to functional improvement often remain. Finally, denture wearing can uniquely impact oral health. Denture surfaces rapidly develop a complex biofilm of bacteria, yeasts and other microorganisms, which can contribute to oral mucosal pathologies. For example, denture stomatitis, a chronic inflammatory disorder, is one of the most common adverse conditions associated with denture use and is associated with contamination of denture surfaces and the underlying oral mucosa by *Candida albicans*, an opportunistic yeast pathogen. Hence, appropriate denture hygiene is beginning to be recognized as critical for maintenance of oral health and perhaps has a role in reducing risk of systemic disease as well. More recently, the potential that denture contamination may also impact systemic disease has been hypothesized and is an ongoing area of research.

This review provides an update of recent developments related to edentulism and denture use. The summary initially focuses on the demographics of edentulism and denture use and potential relationships between edentulism and increased risk of comorbid disease. Current understanding of the role of the denture biofilm as a contributory factor to disease risk is discussed, as are the relationships between biofilm formation and denture materials. Finally, the critical importance of denture cleansing to control the formation of the denture biofilm is summarized with a focus on approaches which can help maintain oral health and potentially reduce risk for systemic disease.

2. Results and discussion

2.1. Demographics and risk of comorbidities

Edentulism and use of dentures is very common among the elderly. This is of critical importance, as the elderly represent a dramatically increasing segment of the world population. In 2000, only 6% of the global population was estimated to be 65 years of age or older. In contrast, by 2030, the percentage of the world population who are at least 65 years of age is estimated to double to 12%, with the largest increases occurring in North America, Europe, Asia and South America [1]. Similarly, in 1998, the World Health Organization reported 390 million people worldwide to be >65 years of age and estimated that this would double by 2025 [2]. Hence, the rapid growth of the elderly as a percentage of the world population will outpace changes in oral health management designed to reduce edentulism and will sustain a significant incidence of edentulism, the need for denture prostheses, and the requirement to manage the oral and systemic health of denture wearers.

The global prevalence of edentulism varies widely across countries. Current estimates range from 12 to 15% in Hong Kong, India, and several European countries to >60% reported in a survey of residents from Botucatu, Brazil [3, 4]. In the USA, the prevalence of edentulism is estimated to be 36% based on a national population-based survey (NHANEs III) [5]. This survey also reported that the prevalence of edentulism increased with age. In a separate population-based study, Felton reported that 26% of the US population between the ages of 65 and 74 are completely edentulous [6]. A report summarizing data from a 2003 population-based survey conducted in Canada illustrated the dramatic association between increased denture usage with increasing age among both men and women [7]. Similarly, 32 and 59% of residents of Botucatu, Brazil, aged 60–64 are reported to use complete lower and upper dentures, respectively. This increases to 52 and 82%, among those ≥75 years of age [3]. In general, the prevalence of edentulism is generally shown to be positively associated with having lower income or socio-economic status, lower education, and in some countries living in rural areas [8–14].

There are also well-demonstrated relationships between edentulism, denture wearing, poor oral health and increased risk of systemic disease. While associations between denture use and some oral diseases, such as denture stomatitis, are well known and have been widely reported and reviewed in the literature, associations between edentulism, denture use, and their potential to increase the risk for non-oral systemic diseases are less well understood. In a review, Felton reported increased risk for several systemic diseases, including asthma (odds ratio [OR] was 10.52), coronary arterial plaque (OR was 2.32), rheumatoid arthritis (OR was 2.27), diabetes (OR was 1.82), and various cancers (OR was 1.54–2.85) to be associated with edentulism [6]. A study conducted in Thailand among patients wearing either removable complete or removable partial dentures demonstrated a correlation between the presence of oral mucosal lesions or denture-related lesions with several different systemic conditions. In this study, denture patients were found to have significant comorbidities, including bone and joint disorders (26.5% of complete denture wearers), hypertension (23.2%), diabetes (19.4%), cardiovascular disease (8.4%), as well as other illnesses [15]. The study did not, however, include a reference or control group of dentate individuals. Thus, odds ratios for any increase in risk among denture users cannot be determined. Overall, there appears to be an association for significant increases of risk of comorbid disease among denture wearers; however, whether these relationships are causal or casual remains unknown.

2.2. Structure/function relationships between denture material and microbial adhesion

Two factors associated with denture structure and material, surface roughness and the presence of surface pores within the material matrices appear to be the major material-related factors which are associated with microbial adhesion. Both surface roughness and porosity provide mechanisms for the attachment of various microorganisms, and this can promote their colonization within the denture biofilm, which develops on the denture surface. The biofilm is a complex matrix of various microorganisms [16]. In addition, some of the biofilm micro-organisms can colonize within pores which open on the denture surface and hence penetrate into the material matrix. Colonization of these microscopic pores is of critical importance, as common denture cleaning approaches, such as brushing or the use of various antimicrobial rinse products, may be less able to access these sites and remove or kill these organisms. Hence, the microbes which reside within the pore structures may serve as a reservoir of resid-ual organisms which can lead to rapid regeneration of the biofilm following surface cleaning.

2.3. Early colonizer: *Streptococcus oralis*

Different dental materials, such as acrylic, porcelain, and hydroxyapatite, have differing sur-face roughness; however, denture acrylic, which is the most commonly used denture mate-rial, has the highest level of surface roughness. Even smooth acrylic has a surface roughness approximately fourfold greater than that of smooth porcelain [17]. Charman et al. demon-strated more extensive in vitro colonization by *Streptococcus oralis*, an early colonizer which initiates the formation of denture biofilm, on rough (surface Ra 1.14 μm) versus smooth sur-face (Ra 0.07 μm) denture acrylic [18]. This supports the concept that an increase in roughness of the acrylic surface or other denture materials would promote more rapid establishment of the biofilm.

2.4. Denture biofilm composition

Denture biofilms are complex matrices containing many microorganisms. Using molecular biology approaches, Sachdeo et al. and Campos et al. characterized the microbiota in the oral cavities of healthy denture wearers as well as in denture stomatitis populations [19, 20]. As reported by Campos et al., a total of 82 bacterial species were identified in both the healthy subjects and the patients with denture stomatitis. Twenty-nine bacterial species were pres-ent exclusively in patients with denture stomatitis, and 26 species were detected only in the healthy subjects.

Using scanning electron microscopy, Glass et al. recently published images which exemplify the microbial complexity of these biofilms [21]. These images show a range of different micro-organisms inhabiting the biofilm matrix and even penetrating into the pores of the denture acrylic [21]. In what may be the first study of its kind, these authors further characterized the biofilm population, identifying potential pathogens and disease-causing microorganisms. Biofilm samples isolated from the dentures of 51 individuals living in different regions of the USA were obtained. Techniques allowing the differential growth of specific microorganisms identified 916 unique microbial isolates from these dentures, of which 711, 67, 125, and 13 were aerobic bacteria, anaerobic bacteria, yeasts, and amoebae, respectively. Interestingly, no two dentures harbored the same microbiota; in addition, no association between biofilm composition and denture cleanliness could be demonstrated [21]. Hence, the microbiology of denture biofilms is complex. Biofilms occur on both complete dentures and partial dentures. Since the potential involvement of the biofilm in the disease is determined by the composi-tion of the organisms contained within the biofilm, controlling and limiting the growth of this matrix by stringent and appropriate cleaning of dentures are critical.

2.5. Oral microbiome and systemic disease

Oral bacteria have been implicated in bacterial endocarditis, aspiration pneumonia, gastrointestinal infection, and chronic obstructive pulmonary disease. Dentures provide a reservoir for microorganisms associated with these infections, in particular respiratory and systemic opportunistic pathogens. As such, they may present an environment for antibiotic-resistant bacteria [22]. Because dentures on occasion may spend time in non-hygienic environmental conditions, non-resident oral microorganisms including *Streptococcus pneumoniae, Haemophilus influenzae, Klebsiella* spp., *Pseudomonas* spp., and *Staphylococci* including MRSA strains have been isolated [23, 24]. The continuous aspiration of microorganisms from denture plaque exposes patients to the risks of infection and the role of dentures may be significant [25].

It is not our purpose in this chapter to provide an extensive review of our knowledge and understanding of denture stomatitis, which has been broadly and extensively reviewed by others [26–36]. Denture stomatitis is a common disorder, occurring in up to 65% of denture wearers. It is characterized by a chronic inflammation of the oral mucosa, most often on mucosal areas which lie beneath the denture base. While denture stomatitis was originally considered to be, at least in part, a traumatic disorder due to poorly fitting dentures, it is now recognized as an inflammatory disorder. If there is any causative role of traumatic injury from poor-fitting dentures in denture stomatitis, it is minor. Emerging evidence suggests that ill-fitting may be a risk factor for the development of oral cancer [37]. The degree of inflammation varies and for diagnostic purposes is graded by using the well-established three-point Newton score [38]. Importantly, regardless of the severity of the inflammatory score, patients with denture stomatitis may be symptomatic or asymptomatic.

2.6. *Candida albicans* association with denture stomatitis

Denture biofilm has a role in denture stomatitis as there is a clear association between the occurrence of denture stomatitis and the presence of *Candida albicans* colonizing both denture materials and the oral mucosa. Indeed, *C. albicans* has been reported to have a selective affinity for colonizing biofilms formed on denture acrylic, with about fourfold greater biomass within biofilms on this substrate as compared to hydroxyapatite [17]. In the pathogenesis of denture stomatitis, *C. albicans* is considered an opportunistic pathogen. While *C. albicans* manifests a significantly greater presence on denture surfaces of patients with denture stomatitis, a clear causal relationship for *C. albicans* as the primary infectious agent responsible for development of this disorder has not been demonstrated. Hence, our current understanding is that *C. albicans* infection is not the single cause of denture stomatitis but has an association with the disorder and may have a role in increasing the likelihood of, or sustaining the associated, oral mucosal inflammation. Denture-related factors associated with denture stomatitis include poor denture cleanliness and hygiene, age of dentures, and continual denture wearing [28, 34, 39–41]. All of these have been reported to significantly increase the risk of denture stomatitis. All of these factors also promote formation of the adherent biofilm on the denture surfaces and hence provide conditions which increase the likelihood of the presence of *C. albicans*. Typical treatment strategies include efforts to improve denture cleanliness and oral hygiene among patients, which can also include replacing old dentures with new prosthetic devices as well as treatment with topical or oral antifungal agents. In general, treatments can eradicate fungal infection and reduce inflammation, but stomatitis rapidly recurs once treatment is halted unless there has been a successful concomitant effort to clean and subsequently maintain the cleanliness of patients' dentures.

2.7. The importance of denture cleansing in reducing microbial biofilms and disease risk

The development of denture adherent biofilm provides the opportunity for colonization of a wide range of pathogenic and opportunistic pathogenic microbial organisms. Since the microbiota may contribute to both oral and systemic infectious disease, maximizing their eradication from the denture surfaces during routine denture cleansing could be of critical importance in improving the health of denture wearers. A number of studies evaluating different denture cleanser methods on bacterial survival have been reported [42]. These studies suggest that differences between denture cleaning methods exist and that there are simple approaches which can potentially maximize eradication of contaminating pathogens from denture surfaces.

Brushing dentures with standard toothpastes remains the most common approach to denture cleaning; however, this is inadequate. Combining brushing and use of a soaking cleanser is superior for killing bacteria and removing the adherent biofilm and plaque [30, 31, 33]. Furthermore, toothpastes generally contain abrasive components, and cleaning dentures by brushing with dentifrices has been shown to increase surface roughness [43]. Increased roughness of denture surfaces has been shown to increase adherence of microorganisms and development of the adherent biofilm. In addition, others have reported a positive correlation between denture surface roughness and colonization with C. albicans [44, 45]. Hence, the method used to clean dentures may be important in controlling future microbial adherence. Use of denture cleansers which can effectively eradicate or remove microbial contaminants and disrupt the denture biofilm without the use of abrasive cleansers may offer significant benefits for denture wearers.

A study by Li et al. reported differences in eradication of C. albicans biofilms when evaluated by different denture cleansing methods [46]. The study compared several popular denture cleansing products used in China including (a) soaking with Kyoshin denture cleanser tablet (Kyoshin Company Ltd., Japan); (b) brushing with Colgate Cavity Protection toothpaste (Colgate, NY, USA); (c) brushing with Bamboo Salt & UDCA toothpaste (LG, Beijing, China); (d) brushing with Yunnan Baiyao toothpaste (Yunnan Baiyao Group Co., Kumming, Yunnan, China); (e) brushing with Zhonghua Aloe toothpaste (Unilever, Heifei, Anhui, China); (f) soaking with Polident denture cleanser (GSK, Brentford, UK); and (g) soaking with sodium bicarbonate (0.5 g, Neptunus, Fuzhou, Fujian, China). Compared to the control (PBS) and all other treatments, only Polident, which combined soaking with a commercial denture cleanser and brushing using the same solution, resulted in almost complete removal, or eradication, of C. albicans from the denture acrylic disks. Furthermore, no significant regrowth of C. albicans was noted over a subsequent 24-h incubation following treatment with Polident. In comparison, the other procedures resulted in some reduction in C. albicans; however, rapid regrowth and reestablishment of C. albicans and the denture biofilm were observed within 6–24 h.

Lee et al. evaluated six different cleaning methods for dentures including (a) mechanical—brushing with Colgate Extra Clean toothpaste (Colgate-Palmolive, Guangzhou, China); (b) chemical—soaking with a Polident denture cleanser (GSK, Dublin, Ireland); (c) combined chemical and mechanical; (d) chemical—soaking in a commercial chlorhexidine gluconate mouthwash (Parmason Shining, Taipei, Taiwan); (e) UV irradiation (ADH Health Products, Seoul, Korea); and (f) soaking in water [47]. Compared to the control (water), brushing, soaking with a denture cleanser, and the combination mechanical-chemical method were found to be superior to soaking in a commercial mouthwash or irradiation with UV light [47].

In 2009, the American College of Prosthodontists convened a task force to establish evidence-based guidelines for the care and maintenance of dentures. Based upon a review of several hundred abstracts and articles, the recommendation put forth by the task force for effective denture cleaning was daily soaking and brushing with an effective, non-abrasive denture cleanser [48].

3. Conclusions

The relationships between oral and systemic health are complex. As illustrated in **Figure 1**, various societal factors, such as attitudes, beliefs, education and income, and behavioral factors such as oral hygiene, diet, general health maintenance, and engaging in high-risk activities, contribute to oral health. Specifically, these factors will impact dental caries and the development of periodontal disease. While not addressed specifically in this review, periodontal disease is associated with a chronic inflammatory condition and has been shown to have a relationship for increasing risk and contributing to the development of chronic systemic disorders, including cardiovascular disease, stroke, diabetes, renal disease, and respiratory diseases. This review has focused on the health impacts of edentulism and denture wearing and how we can control and improve adverse risks associated with denture wearing. Eventual tooth loss and the requirement for denture prostheses are generally considered an outcome of dental caries. The use of removable dentures, whether complete or partial dentures, is associated with changes in eating and social habits and alterations in the microbiota (or oral ecology). It is well established that the sustained presence of novel pathogenic and opportunistic pathogens in the denture biofilm, especially *C. albicans*, clearly contributes to an increased risk for denture wearers to develop denture stomatitis. In addition, the range of pathogens which colonizes denture surfaces also appears to contribute to increasing the risk for several systemic diseases. The risk potential appears to be related to the potential for these pathogens to support chronic systemic inflammation.

Hence, there is a critical need for the education of both professionals and denture patients on the importance of maintaining denture hygiene and the most appropriate and effective means for doing so. Recent studies have demonstrated differences between denture cleansing methods on removal of surface-contaminating microorganisms. In general, the use of a commercial denture cleanser appears to provide better removal and eradication of microorganisms from the denture surface and also slows the rate for regrowth of specific organisms on the dentures. The effects of denture cleansers combined with brushing using the cleaning solution appear to exceed that of brushing with an abrasive dentifrice alone.

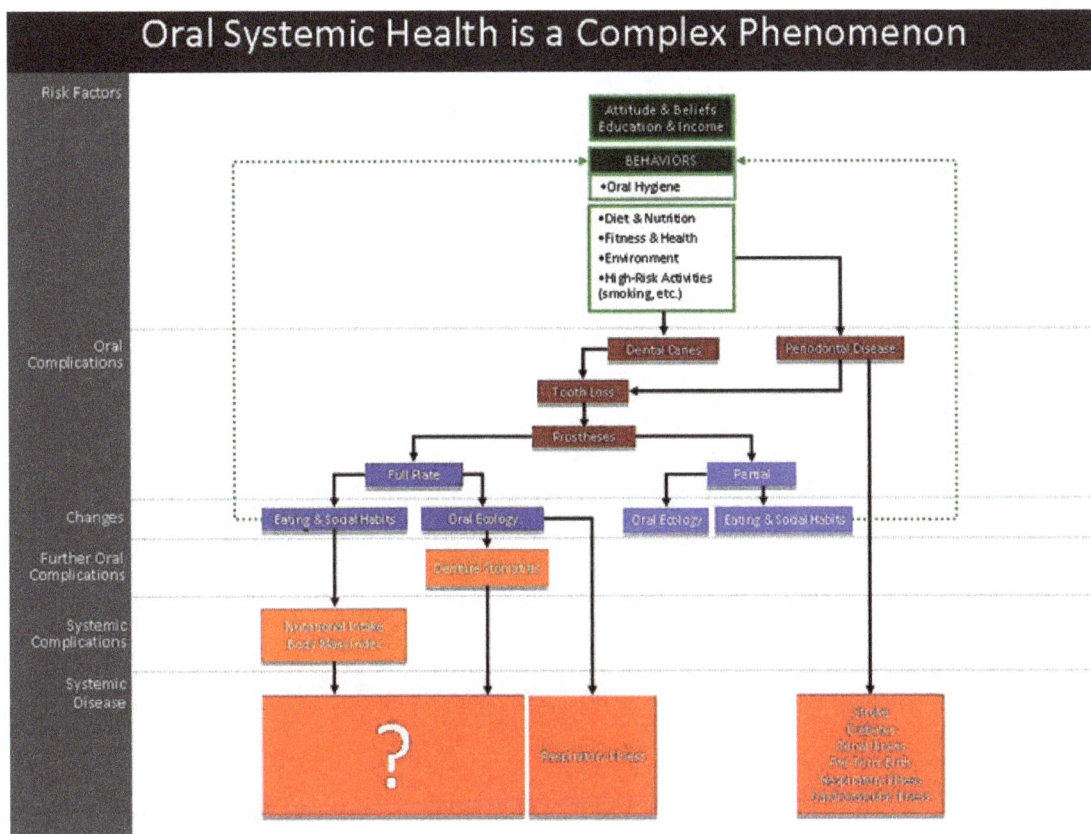

Figure 1. The oral and systemic health linkage has been pioneered by evaluating the relationship between periodontal disease and systemic diseases including diabetes, cardiovascular and stroke as summarized on the right side of this chart. Oral and systemic health as it relates specifically to the denture wearer is summarized on the left side of the chart. Initial systemic targets have included stomatitis and respiratory disease.

In summary, the age distribution of the world population is changing. Over the next 1–2 decades, there will be a significant increase in the number of elderly individuals worldwide. In many countries, this will be associated with a significant increase in the percent of their respective populations who are edentulous and who will rely on denture prostheses. There is an association between denture wearing and adverse impact on systemic health. This may become more profound with the ongoing demographic population shift we are experiencing. Improving hygienic maintenance of dentures, especially among the growing population of elderly, may reduce their risk of developing systemic disease. Furthermore, relatively simple approaches, such as the regular use of denture cleansers to clean dentures, may greatly improve denture hygiene, reduce accumulation of denture biofilm and plaque, and reduce chronic inflammatory conditions which can contribute to oral disorders, such as denture stomatitis and various systemic diseases.

Acknowledgements

The authors thank Chaya Weiss for expert assistance in the preparation of this manuscript.

Conflict of interest

The authors of this manuscript have no conflict of interest with the subject matter of this chapter.

Author details

Zvi G. Loewy[1]*, Shoshana Galbut[2], Ephraim Loewy[3] and David A. Felton[4]

*Address all correspondence to: zvi.loewy@touro.edu

1 Touro College of Pharmacy, New York Medical College, New York, NY, USA

2 Lander College for Women, Touro College, New York, NY, USA

3 University of Maryland School of Dentistry, Baltimore, Maryland, USA

4 University of Mississippi School of Dentistry, Jackson, MS, USA

References

[1] Jones JA, Orner MB, Spiro A III, et al. Tooth loss and dentures: Patients' perspectives. International Dental Journal. 2003;**53**(5 Supplement):337-334. DOI: 10.1111/j.1875-595X.2003.tb00906.x

[2] Data from World Health Organization Epidemiological Survey on Population Trends. 2018. Available from: www.who.int

[3] de Silveira Moreira R, Nico LS, Tomita NE. Oral health conditions among the elderly in southeastern Sao Paolo state. Journal of Applied Oral Science. 2009;**17**(3):170-178. DOI: 10.1590/S1678-77572009000300008

[4] Muller F, Naharro M, Carlsson GE. What are the prevalence and incidence of tooth loss in the adult and elderly population in Europe? Clinical Oral Implants Research. 2007;**18**(Suppl 3):2-14. DOI: 10.1111/j.1600-0501.2007.01459.x

[5] Nowjack-Raymer RE, Sheiham A. Association of edentulism and diet and nutrition in US adults. Journal of Dental Research. 2003;**82**(2):123-126. DOI: 10.1177/154405910308200209

[6] Felton DA. Edentulism and comorbid factors. Journal of Prosthodontics. 2009;**18**:88-96. DOI: 10.1111/j.1532-849X.2009.00437.x

[7] Millar WJ, Locker D. Edentulism and denture use. Health Reports. 2005;**17**(1):55-58

[8] Eklund SA, Burt BA. Risk factors for total tooth loss in the United States; longitudinal analysis of national data. Journal of Public Health Dentistry. 1994;**54**:5-14. DOI: 10.1111/j.1752-7325.1994.tb01173.x

[9]   Palmqvist S, Soderfelt B, Arnbjerg D. Explanatory models for total edentulousness, pres-
      ence of removable dentures, and complete dental arches in a Swedish population. Acta
      Odontologica Scandinavica. 1992;**50**:133-139. DOI: 10.3109/00016359209012756

[10] Marcus SE, Kaste LM, Brown LJ. Prevalence and demographic correlates of tooth loss
      among the elderly in the United States. Special Care in Dentistry. 1994;**5414**:123-127.
      DOI: 10.1111/j.1754-4505.1994.tb01117.x

[11] Uneil L, Sodervfeldt B, Halling A, et al. Explanatory models for oral health expressed
      as number of remaining teeth in an adult population. Community Dental Health.
      1998;**15**:155-161

[12] Dolan TA, Gilbert GH, Duncan RP, et al. Risk indicators for edentulism, partial tooth
      loss and prosthetic status among black and white middle-aged and older adults.
      Community Dentistry and Oral Epidemiology. 2001;**29**:329-340. DOI: 10.1111/j.
      1600-0528.2001.290502.x

[13] Tuominen R, Rajala M, Paunio I. The association between edentulousness and the acces-
      sibility and availability of dentists. Community Dental Health. 1984;**1**:201-206

[14] Bouma J, van de Poel F, Schaub RM, et al: Differences in total tooth extraction between an
      urban and rural area in the Netherlands. Community Dentistry and Oral Epidemiology.
      1987;**15**:301-305. DOI: 10.1111/j.1600-0528.1986.tb01528.x

[15] Jainkittivong A, Aneksuk V, Langlais RP. Oral mucosal lesions in denture wearers.
      Gerodontology. 2010;**27**:26-32. DOI: 10.1111/j.1741-2358.2009.00289.x

[16] von Fraunhofer JA, Loewy ZG. Factors involved in microbial colonization of oral pros-
      theses. General Dentistry. 2009;**57**(2):136-143

[17] Li L, Finnegan MB, Ozkan S, et al. In vitro study of biofilm formation and effective-
      ness of antimicrobial treatment on various dental material surfaces. Molecular Oral
      Microbiology. 2010;**25**:384-390. DOI: 10.1111/j.2041-1014.2010.00586.x

[18] Charman KM, Fernandez P, Loewy Z, et al. Attachment of *Streptococcus oralis* on acrylic
      substrates of varying roughness. Letters in Applied Microbiology. 2009;**48**:472-477. DOI:
      10.1111/j.1472-765X.2008.02551.x

[19] Sachdeo A, Haffajee AD, Socransky SS. Biofilms in the edentulous oral cavity. Journal of
      Prostodontics. 2008;**17**:348-356. DOI: 10.1111/j.1532-849X.2008.00301.x

[20] Campos MS, Marchini L, Bernardes LAS, et al. Biofilm microbial communities of
      denture stomatitis. Oral Microbiology Immunology. 2008;**23**:419-424. DOI: 10.1111/j.
      1399-302X.2008.00445.x

[21] Glass RT, Conrad RS, Bullard JW, et al. Evaluation of microbial flora found in previously
      worn prostheses from the northeast and southwest regions of the United States. The
      Journal of Prosthetic Dentistry. 2010;**103**:384-389. DOI: 10.1016/S0022-3913(10)60083-2

[22] Coulthwaite L, Verran J. Potential pathogenic aspects of denture plaque. British Journal
      of Biomedical Science. 2007;**64**:180-189. DOI: 10.1080/09674845.2007.11732784

[23] Sumi Y, Miura H, Sunakawa M, Michiwaki Y, Sakagami N. Colonization of denture plaque by respiratory pathogens in dependent elderly. Gerodontology. 2002;**19**:25-29. DOI: 10.1111/j.1741-2358.2002.00025.x

[24] Rossi T, Laine J, Eerola E, Kotilainen P, Pettonen R. Denture carriage of methicillin resistant *Staphylococcus aureus*. Lancet. 1995;**345**:1577. DOI: 10.1016/S0140-6736(95)91129-4

[25] Coulthwaite L, Verran J. Denture plaque: A neglected biofilm. In: Allison D, Verran J, Spratt D, Upton M, Pratten J, Mcbain A, editors. Biofilms: Persistence and Ubiquity. The Biofilm Club: Manchester; 2005. pp. 311-321

[26] Budtz-Jorgensen E, Bertram U. Denture stomatitis. I. The etiology in relation to trauma and infection. Acta Odontologica Scandinavica. 1970;**28**:71-92. DOI: 10.3109/00016357009033133

[27] Budtz-Jorgensen E. The significance of *Candida albicans* in denture stomatitis. Scandinavian Journal of Dental Research. 1974;**82**:151-190. DOI: 10.1111/j.1600-0722.1974.tb00378.x

[28] Budtz-Jorgensen. Oral mucosal lesions associated with the wearing of removable dentures. Journal of Oral Pathology. 1981;**10**:65-80. DOI: 10.1111/j.1600-0714.1981.tb01251.x

[29] Arendorf TM, Walker DM. Denture stomatitis: A review. Journal of Oral Rehabilitation. 1987;**14**:217-227. DOI: 10.1111/j.1365-2842.1987.tb00713.x

[30] Lombardi T, Budtz-Jorgensen E. Treatment of denture-induced stomatitis: A review. European Journal of Prosthodontics and Restorative Dentistry. 1993;**2**(1):17-22

[31] Webb BC, Thomas CJ, Willcox MDP, et al. Candida-associated denture stomatitis. Aetiology and management. A review. Part 1. Factors influencing distribution of *Candida* species in the oral cavity. Australian Dental Journal. 1998;**43**(1):45-50. DOI: 10.1111/j.1834-7819.1998.tb00152.x

[32] Webb BC, Thomas CJ, Willcox MDP, et al. Candida-associated denture stomatitis. Aetiology and management. A review. Part 2. Oral diseases caused by *Candida* species. Australian Dental Journal. 1998;**43**(3):160-166. DOI: 10.1111/j.1834-7819.1998.tb00157.x

[33] Webb BC, Thomas CJ, Willcox MDP, et al. Candida-associated denture stomatitis. Aetiology and management. A review. Part 3. Treatment of oral candidosis. Australian Dental Journal. 1998;**43**(4):244-249. DOI: 10.1111/j.1834-7819.1998.tb00172.x

[34] Figueiral MH, Azul A, Pinto E, et al. Denture-related stomatitis: Identification of aetiological and predisposing factors–A large cohort. Journal of Oral Rehabilitation. 2007;**34**:448-455. DOI: 10.1111/j.1365-2842.2007.01709.x

[35] Pereira-Cenci T, Del Bel Cury AA, Crielaard W, et al. Development of Candida-associated denture stomatitis: New insights. Journal of Applied Oral Science. 2008;**16**(2):86-94. DOI: 10.1590/S1678-77572008000200002

[36] Gendreau L, Loewy Z. Epidemiology and etiology of denture stomatitis. Journal of Prostodontics. 2011;**20**:251-260. DOI: 10.1111/j.1532-849X.2011.00698.x

[37] Manoharan S, Nagaraja V, Eslick GD. Ill-fitting dentures and oral cancer: A meta-analysis. Oral Oncology. 2014;**50**(11):1058-1061. DOI: 10.1016/j.oraloncology.2014.08.002

[38] Newton AV. Denture sore mouth. British Dental Journal. 1962;**112**:357-360

[39] Kulak-Ozkan Y, Kazazoglu E, Arikan A. Oral hygiene habits, denture cleanliness, presence of yeasts and stomatitis in elderly people. Journal of Oral Rehabilitation. 2002;**29**:300-304. DOI: 10.1046/j.1365-2842.2002.00816.x

[40] Shulman JD, Rivera-Hidalgo F, Beach MM. Risk factors associated with denture stomatitis in the United States. Journal of Oral Pathology & Medicine. 2005;**34**:340-347. DOI: 10.1111/j.1600-0714.2005.00287.x

[41] Wilson J. The aetiology, diagnosis, and management of denture stomatitis. British Dental Journal. 1998;**185**(8):380-384. DOI: 10.1038/sj.bdj.4809821

[42] Paranhos HF, Silva-Lovato CH, de Souza RF, et al. Effect of three methods for cleaning dentures on biofilms formed in vitro on acrylic resin. Journal of Prosthodontics. 2009;**18**:427-431. DOI: 10.1111/j.1532-849X.2009.00450.x

[43] Goldstein GR, Lerner T. The effect of toothbrushing on hybrid composite resin. The Journal of Prosthetic Dentistry. 1991;**66**:498-500. DOI: 10.1016/0022-3913(91)90511-T

[44] Radford DR, Sweet SP, Challacombe SJ, et al. Adherence of *Candida albicans* to denture-base materials with different surface finishes. Journal of Dentistry. 1998;**26**:577-583

[45] Verran J, Maryan CJ. Retention of *Candida albicans* on acrylic resin and silicone of different surface topography. The Journal of Prosthetic Dentistry. 1997;**77**:535-539. DOI: 10.1016/S0022-3913(97)70148-3

[46] Li L-N, Kim Y, Shu Y, et al. Effect of various methods for cleaning *C. albicans* biofilms formed on denture acrylic resin in vitro. International Journal of Oral Medicine. 2010;**37**:157-168

[47] Lee H-E, Li C-Y, Chang H-W, et al. Effects of different denture cleaning methods to remove *Candida albicans* from acrylic resin denture based material. Journal of Dental Science. 2011;**6**:216-220. DOI: 10.1016/j.jds.2011.09.006

[48] Felton D, Cooper L, Duqum I, et al. Evidence-based guidelines for the care and maintenance of complete dentures. Journal of the American Dental Association (Chicago, IL). 2011:1S-19S. DOI: 10.1111/j.1532-849X.2010.00683.x

4

Immunopathogenesis of Chronic Periodontitis

Ana Maria Sell, Josiane Bazzo de Alencar,
Jeane Eliete Laguila Visentainer and
Cleverson de Oliveira e Silva

Abstract

Periodontitis is a chronic inflammatory condition characterized by destruction of non-mineralized and mineralized connective tissues. The pathogenesis of periodontitis involves a complex interplay between periodontopathogens and the host immunity, greatly influenced by genetic and environmental factors. Failure in the inflammation resolving mechanism leads to establishment of a chronic inflammatory process, resulting in the progressive destruction of bone and soft tissue. The aim of this chapter is to summarize the role of innate and specific immune response involved in pathogenesis of periodontitis. Cells and inflammatory mediators, those participating in inflammatory process of the ligamentous supporting structure and in resorption of alveolar bone, will be presented.

Keywords: periodontal diseases, immune response, cytokines, chemokines, immune cells

1. Introduction

Periodontitis is one of the most common and a complex infectious disease of the oral cavity. Studies suggest that up to 60% of the population is affected by the common form of the disease, termed chronic periodontitis. Periodontitis is a multifactorial disease, with participation of bacterial, environmental, and host factors. The disease is characterized by an inflammatory response to commensal and pathogenic oral bacteria. Due to bacterial infection, gingival tissues become inflamed, characterizing gingivitis, and if left untreated, periodontal supporting tissues can be slowly destroyed by the action of the inflammatory process, which characterizes periodontitis. In the course of periodontitis, teeth lose their ligamentous supporting structure to the alveolar bone, the alveolar bone is resorbed, and the teeth become mobile. In its severe form, it may lead to tooth loss.

There are two major forms of periodontitis, chronic periodontitis (CP) and aggressive periodontitis (AP). CP is a slowly progressing disease, which can be categorized as mild/early, moderate or severe based on clinical criteria, such as probing pocket depth (PPD) and clinical attachment loss (CAL). AP occurs in 1–3% of the population and is characterized by rapid rate of disease progression in an otherwise clinically healthy patient, absence of large accumulations of plaque, and familial inheritance.

Traditional and fundamental procedures for diagnosis of periodontitis include visual examination, tactile sensation, PPD, CAL, plaque index, bleeding on probing, and radiographic assessment of alveolar bone loss. Periodontal bleeding reveals the ulcerated area of subgingival tissue, whereas probing depth reveals the extent of the area of tissue covered by subgingival biofilm. Although different estimates for quantification of the area of periodontal injury have been reported in the literature, the inflammatory challenge of periodontal disease usually consists of an affected area of 15–72 cm^2 [1].

Bacteria have been considered to be the initiating factors to trigger periodontitis. Especially, Gram-negative anaerobic bacteria including *Porphyromonas gingivalis* (*P. gingivalis*) and *Aggregatibacter actinomycetemcomitans* (*A. actinomycetemcomitans*) have been strongly implicated in disease. Localized aggressive periodontitis is associated with *A. actinomycetemcomitans*, while generalized forms of chronic disease involve *P. gingivalis*, and also *Tannerella forsythia*, *Prevotella intermedia*, *Treponema denticola*, and *Fusobacterium nucleatum* (*F. nucleatum*) [2]. *P. gingivalis* has been implicated to be one of the most important periodontal pathogens, and its important features in mediated CP include the ability to adhere to and invade host cells, to disseminate through host cells and tissues, and to subvert host immunological defense mechanisms. The cell wall components of *P. gingivalis*, especially lipopolysaccharide (LPS), can cause direct destruction of periodontal tissues and trigger a wide range of immune responses, including the production of proinflammatory cytokines, antiinflammatory cytokines and chemokines, which might be important in periodontitis development [3]. A distinct systemic response was observed among different strains of *P. gingivalis in vivo*: strains that induced expression of high levels of IL-4 were shown to induce alveolar bone loss, whereas strain that increased IL-10 did not significantly promote bone resorption in mice [4].

Current evidence supports the importance of several factors increasing onset and progression of periodontal diseases, including smoking, diabetes, hormonal changes, and osteoporosis. Other potential interactions with periodontal disease are those involving obesity, adverse pregnancy outcomes, cardiovascular diseases, psychosocial factors and socioeconomic status [5].

In this way, the aim of this chapter is to summarize the role of innate and specific immune response involved in pathogenesis of chronic periodontitis. The neutrophils, monocytes/macrophages, and T and B lymphocytes and inflammatory mediators, including cytokines, those participating in inflammatory process of the ligamentous supporting structure and in resorption of alveolar bone, will be discussed.

2. Immunopathogenesis of chronic periodontitis

The host response during periodontitis involves the innate and adaptive immune system, leading to chronic inflammation and progressive destruction of tooth-supporting tissues. The pathogenesis of periodontal disease involves a complex interplay between periodonto-pathogens and the host immunity, greatly influenced by genetic and environmental factors (as smoking). Dental plaque is necessary, but not sufficient for disease, where an exacerbated, poorly specific and effective inflammatory response is mounted. Failure in the inflammation resolving mechanism leads to establishment of a chronic inflammatory process, resulting in the destruction of bone and soft tissue.

The host inflammatory response is mediated mainly by neutrophils, monocytes/macrophages, and T and B lymphocytes. Neutrophils are the first cells to arrive at the inflammatory infiltrate. The innate response involves the recognition of microbial components by Toll-like receptors (TLRs) expressed by host cells in the infected microenvironment. When the resolution of inflammation is not achieved, antigen-presenting cells are activated by bacterial products and interact with naïve T helper cells (Th0), driving their differentiation into several subsets, such as Th1, Th2, Th17, and Treg. T lymphocytes are central to adaptive immunity and provide help for B cells to generate specific antibodies. T cell receptor recognition of peptide antigen in the context of major histocompatibility complex can result in CD4 T cells activation. Activated Th0 may differentiate into either Th1 lymphocytes expressing Interleukin (IL)-2, interferon-gamma (IFN-γ), and tumor necrosis factor-alpha (TNF-α); or Th2 lymphocytes, expressing IL-4, IL-5, and IL-13; or Th17 expressing IL-17A, IL-17F, IL-21, and IL-22. Activated and effec-tor T cells may become memory T cells. T regulatory (Treg) cells are responsible for mecha-nisms of tolerance: the T cells CD4$^+$ CD25$^+$ have been shown to be higher in periodontitis than gingivitis, suggesting the importance of immunoregulation in periodontitis.

2.1. The innate immune response

The innate immune response constitutes the first line of defense and is able to recognize non-self microorganisms trigging immune response to eliminate them.

Unlike adaptive immunity, innate immunity does not recognize every possible antigen. Instead, it recognizes a few highly conserved structures present in many different microorgan-isms such as LPS, peptidoglycans, bacterial DNA, double-strand RNA, N-formylmethionine found in bacterial proteins, the sugar mannose and proteases (named pathogen-associated molecular patterns, PAMPs). The defense cells have pattern-recognition receptors (PPRs) for these PAMPs and trigger immediate response against the microorganism. PPRs are found on inflammatory cells and on periodontal tissue resident cells, such as epithelial cells (ECs), gingival fibroblasts (GFs), periodontal ligament fibroblast (PDLF), dendritic cells (DCs), and osteoblasts (OBs). These receptors include TLRs, nucleotide-binding oligomerization domain (NOD) proteins, cluster of differentiation 14 (CD14), complement receptor-3, lectins, and scavenger receptors. PAMPs can also be recognized by a series of soluble pattern-recognition receptors in the blood that function as opsonins and initiate the complement pathways.

After bacterial challenge, the resident cells recognize PAMPS, via TLRs, and initiate an orchestrated signaling events resulting in the production of proinflammatory cytokines and chemokines, and recruitment of inflammatory cells. The TLR4 has been shown to specifically recognize LPS from gram-negative bacteria. Cytokines, such as tumor necrosis factor-α (TNF-α), interleukin (IL)-1β and IL-6, within periodontal lesions, orchestrate the cascade of destructive events that occur in the periodontal tissues. These events include the production of inflammatory enzymes and mediators (such as matrix metalloproteinases and prostaglandins), and osteoclast recruitment, and differentiation through receptor activator of nuclear factor-$\kappa\beta$ ligand (RANKL)-dependent and -independent pathways resulting in irreversible hard and soft tissue damage and in chronic periodontitis.

These cells involved in innate response and molecular factors involved in the local inflammatory reaction will be discussed later.

2.1.1. Cells involved in innate immune response

2.1.1.1. Neutrophils and monocytes/macrophages

Neutrophils, also called polymorphonuclear leukocytes (PMN), are one of the first responders of inflammatory cells to migrate toward the site of periodontal inflammation. The nucleus of neutrophils is segmented into three to five lobules, and the cytoplasm contains granules of two types: specific granules which are filled with enzymes such as lysozyme, collagenase, and elastase; and azurophilic granules which are lysosomes containing microbicidal substances as enzymes, defensins and cathelecidins. After periodontal pathogens successfully overcome epithelial barriers and invade soft tissues, signals from bacteria and gingival epithelial cells, human mesenchymal stem cells, connective fibroblast, and resident macrophages induce the production of cytokines and chemokines by the gingival epithelium. The chemoattractant molecules (such as IL-8 and IL-1β, and serum-derived plaque activated C5a) increase the expression of adhesion molecules, the permeability of gingival capillaries, and the migration of neutrophils through the junctional epithelium and into the gingival sulcus [6].

The interaction between the oral microbiota and neutrophils is a key determinant of oral health status. Neutrophils form a "wall" between the junctional epithelium and the pathogen-rich dental plaque providing a robust secretory structure (reactive oxygen species [ROS] and bactericidal proteins) and a phagocytic apparatus. However, this protection is not without cost because neutrophils from periodontitis patients are hyperreactive and contribute to tissue destruction: ROS and the enzymes released by cytoplasmic granules degrade the structural elements of tissue cells and extracellular matrix and cause tissue damage [7, 8]. A recently discovered innate defense strategy of neutrophils is the release of DNA to the extracellular environment, where the web-like DNA threads trap and kill microorganisms by means of DNA-bound antimicrobial proteins and peptides. These neutrophil extracellular traps (NETs) are also known to arise in periodontal tissues and purulent pockets. NETs represent a host defense mechanism but may also cause host tissue injury [9]. On the other hand, alterations in neutrophils function result in an acute, severe, and generalized clinical phenotype of periodontitis. These alterations can involve different functions, such as adhesion capabilities, chemotaxis response, and phagocytic function [10]. Added to this, neutrophils with normal functions in individuals with alterations in the IL-8 production and/or mutations in Duffy antigen receptor chemokines (DARC) expression on erythrocytes predispose those individuals to periodontitis [11]. It occurs because adsorption of IL-8 onto erythrocytes by DARC leads to an increased recruitment of leukocytes from the blood to the tissue compared to individuals without DARC on the erythrocytes.

Monocytes/macrophages belong to mononuclear phagocytes system. They are also important innate immune cells at infection sites in patients with CP. These cells produce large amounts of proinflammatory cytokines, antiinflammatory cytokines, and chemokines, including TNF-α, IL-1β, IL-8, and IL-10. These chemokines produced by these cells attract neutrophils; however, neutrophils also produce chemokines, which attract macrophages to inflamed periodontal site. Thus, a crosstalk exists between these innate cells. Macrophages are important in triggering the specific immune response serving as antigen-present cells that display antigens to and activate T lymphocytes. Added, monocytes/macrophages can differentiate into osteoclasts [12].

2.1.1.2. Fibroblasts

Periodontal ligament fibroblast (PDLF) and gingival fibroblasts (GF) are the main cells of the soft connective tissue. In conjunction with infiltrating inflammatory cells, GFs take part in the inflammatory process in the periodontium and contribute to the disease persistence. After microorganisms breach the epithelial barrier, these cells produce cytokines and degradation molecules. Expression of matrix metalloproteinases (MMPs) became accentuated. Fibroblasts from periodontitis patients expressed higher mRNA of IL-1β, IL-6, and TIMP-3 and lower mRNA of IL-4 [13]. PDFL also produces IL-8, TNF-α, macrophage inflammatory protein (MIP)-1 alpha, and receptor activator of nuclear factor-$\kappa\beta$ ligand (RANKL), which are regulators on inflammation and alveolar bone loss. When in cell-cell contact with osteoclast precursors, PDFL upregulated osteoclastogenesis-related genes and significantly increased the number of osteoclast-like cells [14].

2.1.1.3. Dendritic cells

Dendritic cells (DCs) are the most important antigen-present cells for activating naïve T cells. These cells function in both innate and adaptive immune responses and are a link between these two components of host defense. They are part of myeloid lineage and arise from the same monocyte precursor. DCs have long membrane projections and phagocytic capabilities. Similar to macrophages, they express receptors that recognize bacteria and respond by secreting cytokines. They produce IL-12 and IL-18 that consequently promote interferon-gamma (INF-γ) secretion by natural killer (NK) cells and latter by T cells. In response to activation by microorganism, conventional DCs become mobile, migrate to lymph nodes, and display antigens to T lymphocytes.

2.1.2. Molecular factors involved in the local inflammatory reaction

In the innate immune response, the bacterial activation of resident cells culminates in a production of proinflammatory cytokines involved in periodontal immunopathogenesis. In order to eliminate the bacteria, the inflammatory process is triggered; however, the inflammation culminates in periodontal tissue lesions and alveolar bone resorption [15].

2.1.2.1. Toll-like receptors (TLRs)

TLRs play an important role in the recognition of pathogens. TLRs are a family of trans-membrane proteins expressed by immunologically competent cells. They recognize and bind to PAMPs derived from bacterial plaque. TLRs are evolutionarily conserved proteins with a highly conserved intracellular toll-interleukin receptor (TIR) domain involved in protein-protein interaction and signaling activation. The extracellular domain, with leucin-rich repeats (LRRs) is related to ligand recognition. LRR motifs vary among TLRs. After PAMPs recognizing, TLRs initiate the activation of several transcription factors including nuclear factor-kappa B (NF-κB) and activator protein 1 (AP-1) through the mitogen-activated protein kinase (MAK) cascade. NF-κB is a key transcription factor complex that appears to play a critical role in the regulation of an acute inflammation. NF-κB enters the nucleus of the cell and induces expression of proinflammatory mediators including adhesion molecules (ICAM-1, VCAM-1, and E-selectin), enzymes (COX-2, 5-LO, CPLA, and iNOS), cytokines (IL-1, TNF, IL-6, GM, and G-CSF), and chemokines (IL-8, RANTES, MCP-1, eotaxin, and MIP-1κ). An increase in the recruitment of leukocytes is generated [16, 17].

TLR-2, 3, 4 and 9 are much expressed in gingival tissues of periodontitis patients, and TLR-2 and TLR-4 expressions are increased in severe disease states, suggesting that these receptors have an increased capacity to signal and influence downstream cytokine expression. TLR-4 is present on antigen presenting cells, fibroblasts, and keratinocytes of gingival epithelium. TLR4 has been shown to specifically recognize LPS from gram-negative bacteria and thus recognize PAMPs of periodontopathogens such as *P. gingivalis, A. actinomycetemcomitans,* and *V. parvula.* Tool-like receptor-4 acts in cooperation with its coreceptors CD14 protein and MD-2 complex, as well as TLR4 adaptor proteins such as myeloid differentiation primary response gene 88 (MyD88) playing an important role in maintenance of periodontal healthy. However, over production of proinflammatory cytokines due to chronic stimulation of TLRs may lead to tissue damage. LPS-triggered TLR4 activation leads to an increased secretion of proinflammatory cytokines, mediators and matrix metalloproteinases (MMPs) from a variety of cells including monocytes, macrophages, neutrophils, lymphocytes, and gingival fibro-blasts. Repeated stimulations of these receptors may also lead to development of tolerance to bacterial products. TLR-2 engagement has been shown to trigger production of proinflammatory and antiinflammatory cytokines [18, 19].

CD14 is a myeloid differentiation marker found primarily on monocytes and macrophages, although low levels are also found on neutrophils and endothelial cells. CD14 is a coreceptor for LPS. The CD14 gene is located on chromosome 5q31.3 and encodes two forms of protein: one is anchored to the membrane glycosylphosphatidylinositol (mCD14) and is a 55-kDa gly-coprotein, and another is a soluble form (sCD14) found in body fluids. CD14 lacks the trans-membrane domain and is unable to transmit LPS signaling. The major function of CD14 is to serve as an initial receptor for LPS and facilitate the binding of LPS to TLR4/MD-2 complex. In addition, CD14 also recognizes other PAMPS such as lipoteichoic acid. Proinflammatory and antiinflammatory effect of CD14 has been shown indicating dual roles in response to Gram-negative bacteria [20, 21].

2.1.2.2. Matrix metalloproteinases (MMPs)

The matrix metalloproteinases (MMPs) are a structural and functional family of zinc-dependent extracellular proteinases, which are responsible for the remodeling and degradation of tissue extracellular matrix (ECM), including collagens, elastins, gelatin, matrix glycoproteins, and proteoglycans. To date, at least 26 members of MMPs have been identified and they are grouped according to their structural properties and substrate specificity in collagenases (MMP-1, -8, -13, -14), gelatinases (MMP-2 and -9), stromelysins, matrilysins, and membrane type matrix metalloproteinases. The balance between MMPs and their endogenous inhibitors (tissue inhibitor of matrix metalloproteinases, TIMPs) controls the MMP activity. MMPs play an important role in tissue degradation observed in periodontitis, and elevated levels of MMP-1, -2, -3, -8, and -9 have been detected in gingival crevicular fluid, peri-implant sulcular fluid, and gingival tissue of periodontitis patients. MMP-1 is produced by periodontal resident cells and is considered as central in the physiological remodeling of extracellular matrix in wound healing. MMP-8, mainly produced by neutrophils, is associated to periodontal collagen destruction and represents the major collagenase in gingival and crevicular fluids; its levels can differentiate periodontitis from gingivitis and healthy sites. MMP-9 has been associated with collagen breakdown and periodontal inflammation. MMP-13 is little or not expressed on normal tissues, but its upregulation has been involved in periodontitis progression and bone loss. MMPs can be released or activated during periodontal disease by proinflammatory cytokines, as TNF-α and IL-1β, reactive oxygen species, and proteases; IL-18 may be related to be involved in the regulation of MMPs [22–24].

2.1.2.3. Cytokines

The resident cells and migrating cells release cytokines during inflammatory response involving in chronic periodontitis. Endothelial cells and GF produce IL-8, a chemokine that is neutrophils chemoattractant and that increase the monocytes adhesion. Neutrophils (the migrant cells) and PDLF produce IL-1, IL-6, and TNF-α. GF also produces IL-6 and TNF-α. PDLF and also bacterial antigens could promote the expression of the RANKL by the osteoblasts. DC IL-12p40, IL-18, IL-6, and TGF-β (transforming growth factor beta) act as antigen-present cells to T lymphocytes. The role of this cytokines will be described later.

After this initial primary response, activation of T cells by APCs initiates the adaptive response. Subsequently, the effector mechanisms of innate immunity are improved by adaptive immunity involving an efficient loop for microbial clearance. Chronic periodontal inflammation perpetuates and amplifies itself through numerous autocrine and paracrine loops of cytokines, acting on cells within the periodontal tissue.

2.2. The adaptive immune response

When the resolution of inflammation is not achieved, adaptive immune response is initiated. Therefore, APCs are activated by bacterial products and interact with naïve T helper cells (CD4 T cells, Th0: CD45RA+), driving their differentiation into several subsets (CD45RO+), such as Th1, Th2, Th17, and Treg. Adaptive immune cells and their cytokines have important participation in pathogenesis of the chronic periodontitis, including the resolution of infection, tissue damages, and osteolytic process.

2.2.1. T cell subsets enrolled in the pathogenesis of CP

For a long time, periodontitis lesions were conceptually defined based on a Th1/Th2 paradigm. Currently, Th1 and Th2 responses, added to the Th17 subset, have been related to the disease progression and bone resorption. T cell lymphocytes (CTLs) are primarily involved in the cell-mediated immunity. CTLs were named because their precursors, which arise in the bone marrow, migrate and mature in the thymus. The two major T cell subsets are CD4 (T helper) and CD8 CTLs, which express a highly diverse and clonally distributed antigen receptor called the αβ receptor. Both effector cells usually express surface protein indicative of recent activation, such CD25, a component of the receptor for the T cell growth factor IL-2. Th cells express surface molecules as CD40 ligand (CD154) [25].

2.2.1.1. T-helper 1 (Th1 cells)

Th1 cells are generated under the influence of interleukin-12 and/or interferon-γ (INF-γ) signaling that leads to the activation of the transcription factor T-bet. In diseased gingival tissues, Th1 cells have been predominant. Activated Th1 cells secret INF-γ, present in high levels in human and experimental periodontal lesions. INF-γ is associated to onset and progression of lesions. Besides, INF-γ stimulates osteoclast formation and bone loss via antigen-driven T cell activation or through the chemoattraction of RANKL cells. Also, INF-γ can contribute to the migration of CD4/80+ cells, monocyte/macrophage-like phenotypes, a potential osteoclast precursor subpopulation [26, 27].

2.2.1.2. T-helper 2 (Th2 cells)

Th2 cells are generated under the influence of interleukin-4 and the activation of the transcription factor GATA-3. IL-4 secreted by Th2 exhibits antiinflammatory and suppressive properties related to the induction of IL-10 and suppression of Th1 response. In pathogenesis of periodontitis, it can be associated with the ability to inhibit the production of tissue degrading factors such as MMPs and the major osteoclastogenic factor RANKL. Therefore, IL-4 could attenuate the soft and mineralized tissue destruction. However, IL-4 levels were found lower in crevicular fluid from periodontitis patients.

Added to this fact, Th2 cells could be related to B cell function and humoral immunity in the periodontal lesion. B cells seem to contribute to periodontal disease development since B cell deletion prevented alveolar bone loss in mice after infection with *P. gingivalis* and because

the majorly of B cells in periodontal lesions are RANKL+ [28]. IgG is the more frequent antibody class present in the gingival crevicular fluid and gingiva of patients with periodontitis;
therefore, IgA and IgM are also found. IgM and IgG classes were related to autoimmunity in
periodontitis where high titers of anticollagen type I, antifibronectin and antilaminin were
found [26, 27].

2.2.1.3. T-helper 17 (Th17 cells)

Th17 cells are generated under the influence of IL-6/IL-21/IL-23/TGF-β and the activation
of the transcription factor RORγT. After TGF-β and IL-6 driver Th17, IL-23 amplifies the
phenotype. Th17 cells have been linked to the development of pathological inflammatory
disorders. Cytokines secreted by Th17, such as IL-17 and IL-22 are crucial for host protection against many extracellular pathogens. Furthermore, IL-17 contributes to innate and specific immunity by recruiting inflammatory cells and immobilizing macrophages in inflamed
tissue. The consequence is an abundance of other inflammatory cytokines as IL-1β and TNF-
α, and RANKL. Th17 cells have been linked to several autoimmune disorders and are also
linked to the development of pathological inflammatory disorders, and their presence was
demonstrated in the gingival tissue from patients with periodontitis [29, 30].

2.2.1.4. T regulatory cells (Treg cells)

Treg cells are generated under the influence of IL-10/TGF-β and the activation of the transcription factor forkhead box P3 (FOXp3). They also expressed as a αβ antigen receptor. Treg
cells specifically regulate the activation, proliferation, and effectuating functions of activated
T cells. There are two types of Treg: (i) endogenous or natural (Treg), which are derived
from the thymus and control autoreactivity; (ii) adaptive or induced (aTreg or iTreg), which
regulate responses upon antigenic exposure in the periphery. In noninflammatory tissues,
they are in resting state. The cytokines TGF-β, IL-10, and cytotoxic T lymphocyte-associated
molecule 4 (CTLA-4) are supposed to mediate the suppressive activity in peripheral tissues
and attenuate periodontal diseases progression and protect the bone resorption. Treg cells are
shown to attenuate RANKL expression by other activated T cells. Treg cells were identified
in periodontal tissues; however, deficiency of Treg cells was observed in periodontitis [31].

Another subset of Treg cells includes the Tcreg. In animal models and under noninflammatory conditions, murine osteoclasts can recruit naïve CD8 T-cells and activate these T-cells to
induce CD25 and FoxP3 (Tcreg). Tcreg can potently and directly suppress bone resorption by
osteoclasts. The activation of CD8 T cells by osteoclasts also induced the cytokines IL-2, IL-6,
IL-10, and interferon (IFN-c). Individually, these cytokines can activate or suppress osteoclast
resorption [32].

2.2.1.5. T CD8 cells

After naïve cells are activated, they became larger and proliferate, and are called lympho-
blasts. Some of these cells differentiate into CD8 CTLs. CD8 cells have cytoplasmic granules
filled with proteins that, when released, kill the cells that the CDLs recognize. They are also

called cytotoxic T cells. In an animal models, which allow investigating the stages of periodontitis, CD8 T cell knockout mice showed no significant change in bone loss after infection with *P. gingivalis* [33].

The activated T helper subsets, their produced cytokines and their general functions are summarized in **Table 1**.

2.2.2. The adaptive immunity in the pathogenesis of chronic periodontitis

Adaptive immune responses to most immunogens can begin only after the immunogen has been captured, processed, and presented by an APC to naïve T helper cells. The reason of this is that T cells only recognize immunogens that are bound to major histocompatiblity complex (MHC) proteins on the surfaces of other cells. There are two different classes of MHC proteins. Class I MHC proteins are expressed virtually in all somatic cell types and are used to present substances to CD8 T cells. Class II MHC proteins, on the other hand, are expressed only by macrophages, dendritic cells and a few other APCs, and are necessary for antigen presentation to T helper cells. The interaction of APC-T cells is dependent on other membrane receptors. The TCR complex confers specificity because it contains the antigen-specific receptor. The interaction is enhanced through coreceptors including CD27, CD28, CD40 ligand, or inhibited by coinhibitor receptors such as CTLA4, programmed cell death protein (PD1), and CD28 induced costimulator (ICOS) [25].

	Stimulating cytokines	Differentiated T cells subsets and respective transcriptional factors (italic)	Produced cytokines *	Regulatory cytokines	Host defense	General roles in diseases
Naive TCD4 T cells	IL-12 IL-18 INF-γ	T_H1 *T-bet, STAT1, STAT4*	INF-γ LTA RANKL	IL-4 IL-10, TGF-β	Intracellular pathogens	Tissue damage associated with chronic infections
	IL-2 IL-4	T_H2 *GATA-3, STAT6*	IL-4 IL-15 IL-13	INF-γ TGF-β	Extracellular pathogens Humoral immunity	Allergic diseases Autoimmune diseases
	IL-6 TGF-β	T_H2 *2AHR*	IL-22	TGF-β	Extracellular pathogens	
	IL-6 TGF-β IL-21	T_H17 *RORγT, STAT3*		IL-2 IL-4 IL-27 INF-γ	Homeostasis at mucosal sites/ inflammation	Organ-specific autoimmunity

*The cytokines produced by these T cells subsets determine their effector functions and roles in diseases. The cytokines also participate in development and expansion of the respective subsets.

Table 1. T cell subsets differentiation and general functions in immune response.

The acquired immune response is known to be important for periodontal disease development. Specific microbial components activate APCs, such as DC, and both migrate to local lymph nodes. In APC, immunogen become enclosed within membrane-lined vesicles in the cytoplasm and within these vesicles, undergo a series of alterations called antigen processing and a limited number of the resulting peptides are noncovalently associated to MHC class II proteins, and transported to APC surface, where it is detected by CD4 T cells. After specific antigen recognition, activation phase is initiated by the sequences of events induced in lymphocytes. The Th0 differentiation is dependent of the local cytokine milieu. Then, the CTL proliferate, leading to expansion of the clones of antigen-specific CTL and the amplification of the response. The pattern of cytokines expressed determines subsequent polarization of a distinct antigen-specific CTL response. Next, CTL differentiates to cells that function to eliminate foreign antigens: some T cells (CD4) differentiate into cells T helper subsets, that activate phagocytes to kill intracellular antigens, or in others T cells (CD8) that directly lyses cells that are producing foreign antigens, and also B cells, which transform to plasma cells that secreted specific antibodies. The effector phase is the stage that leads to antigen elimination. In this phase, inflammatory response is amplified after recruitment of specific and nonspecific effector cells (lymphocytes, macrophages, neutrophils) and their soluble products (lymphokines, monokines, complement, kinines, arachidonic acid derivates, mast cells—basophile products).

Characteristic markers of Th1, Th2, Th17 and Treg cell subsets have all been described in diseased periodontal tissues. Therefore, the exact crosstalk that occurs among Th cytokines in periodontal disease and its impact on disease outcome is still to be determined. However, it is clear that Th cells are essential for periodontal destruction because the absence of B cells does not impede LPS-induced bone resorption.

There are tissue resident memory cells within the oral mucosa. When compared with primary immune response, the recall of memory is faster and shows fewer requirements for antigen presentation by MHC and costimulation. In gingival tissues, IL-15 is found in abundance and seen to be responsible for the survival and proliferation of memory cells.

2.3. Cytokines in the pathogenesis of chronic periodontitis

Cytokines are low molecular weight water-soluble glycoprotein secreted by hematopoietic and nonhematopoietic cells in response to infection, and they are important key molecules and signal mediators in the pathogenesis of periodontitis. The cytokines involved in immunopathology of periodontal disease act in a highly complex coordinated network and play role in the maintenance of specific leucocytes on periodontal tissue, in the osteoclastogenesis activation and stimulation of bone resorption. Several of the cytokines have been demonstrated to serve either as proinflammatory (IL-1, IL-12, IL-17, IL-18, TNF-α) or antiinflammatory (IL-4, IL-10) mediators of the inflammatory process [34].

2.3.1. Interleukin-1 (IL-1)

IL-1 is a potent proinflammatory mediator and bone-resorbing cytokine formerly known as the osteoclast-activating factor. The *IL1* gene cluster is located on chromosome 2q13–q21 (https://www.ncbi.nlm.nih.gov/gene/3553) [35]. In the IL-1 superfamily members, two ago-nists and one antagonist members are highlighted: IL-1α and IL-1β (proinflammatory cyto-kines), and IL-1/IL-receptor antagonist (antiinflammatory cytokine). Between them, IL-1β is the most studied due its role in immunoinflammatory diseases. IL-1β, even as IL-1α, is able to bind and activate interleukin-1 receptors resulting in the recruitment of several intracellu-lar adapter molecules, including MyD88, NFκB, AP-1, and mitogen activated protein kinase (MAPks). This interaction leads to transcription of genes of intercellular adhesion molecule-1 (ICAM-1) that incites the innate immune response, and genes of lymphocyte function associ-ated antigen-1 (LFA-1) that culminates in a greater migration of leukocytes in tissue direction. Once secreted, IL-1 may activate lymphocytes, incite macrophage chemotaxis and prostaglan-din production, and stimulate osteoclastic resorption of bone [36, 37].

In periodontitis, IL-1 is detected in the periodontal tissue and in the gingival crevicular fluid and is important in the metabolism of collagen, in bone destruction, and other inflam-matory processes. IL-1β is secreted mainly by macrophages and resident cells. IL-1 could mediate the gingival and periodontal tissue destruction and bone resorption by different ways: (i) IL-1β and IL-1α stimulate the release of lysosomal enzymes such as metallopro-teinase which degrades the extracellular matrix; (ii) IL-1β stimulates the production of prostaglandin E2 (PGE2) by fibroblasts and osteoblasts (OB). PGE2 stimulates bone resorp-tion mediated by RANKL expression in OB; and (iii) IL-1β enhances RANKL expression on OB [38–40].

2.3.2. Tumor necrosis factor: alpha (TNF-α)

TNF-α is a very potent proinflammatory cytokine with a pleotropic effect on both immune and skeletal systems. It is encoded by *TNF* gene located on chromosome 6 (https://www.ncbi.nlm.nih.gov/gene/7124) [41] and is primary produced by activated T cells, monocytes/macro-phages, and fibroblasts during inflammation. It is expressed as a transmembrane protein with 26 kDa or as a soluble TNF form with 17 kDa. When binding in the TNF receptors, TNF-RI of 55-kDa or TNF-RII of 75-kDa, the intracellular signaling pathways are activated via c-Jun, NF-kB, and calcium signaling leading to biological cellular response of inflammation. This response includes: (i) increase of adhesion molecules for leukocytes, as ICAM-1 and E-selectin; (ii) recruitment of leukocytes; (iii) increase of vascular permeability; (iv) increase the produc-tion of metalloproteinase and proinflammatory cytokines; and (v) osteoclasts differentiation dependent and independent of RANKL. The inappropriate or excessive TNF-α production can be harmful to tissue [42, 43].

TNF-α was detected in higher levels in saliva and crevicular fluid of patients with periodontal disease and its role and contribution to inflammation, loss of connective tissue attachment, and alveolar bone resorption has been well documented [44].

2.3.3. Interleukin-6 (IL-6)

IL-6 is a pleiotropic cytokine not only exerting immunological effect but also functioning in hematopoiesis, bone metabolism, and tissue regeneration. The human *IL6* gene is located in the short arm of chromosome 7 (7p21; https://www.ncbi.nlm.nih.gov/gene/3569) [45]. IL-6 is a cytokine produced by T cells, B cells, monocytes/macrophages, endothelial cells, GF, OB and, periodontal ligament cells. It has multifunctional properties and is secreted in response to bacterial LPS or IL-1β and TNF-α stimulus. The IL-6 binding receptor (IL-6R) is located in membrane of cells and dimerizes with two gp130 subunits when IL-6 binds. Besides this, there is also a soluble form of receptor, and both receptors when activated are able to promote biological effects into the cells. IL-6 in promoting inflammation, it can also be involved in the regulation of tissue destruction. IL-6 induces the production of inhibitors of MMPs, suppresses IL-1β and TNF-α expression, and induces IL-1 receptor antagonist. Another positive point that favors the reduction of tissue damage is that IL-6 can stimulate fibroblasts to produce collagen and glycosaminoglycan. IL-6 plays role in B cells differentiation, T cell proliferation, and acute phase proteins expression. In addition, IL-6 in synergism with TNF-α is able to induce the differentiation of osteoclast progenitors directly or stimulate the stromal cells to produce RANKL.

This cytokine exerts an important effect in the pathogenesis of periodontitis, mainly in bone metabolism. During the development of CP, multiple biological actions could be mediated by the IL-6, including hematopoiesis, angiogenesis induction, immunocyte activation, and osteoclast differentiation. The presence of IL-6 in serum, gingival crevicular fluid, and saliva suggested an altered production of IL-6 in patients with CP [46, 47].

2.3.4. Interleukin-17 (IL-17)

The IL-17 family contains six members: IL-17A, IL-17B, IL-17C, IL-17D, IL-17E (or IL-25) and IL-17F, and five receptors, IL-17RA-RD and SEF. Interleukin-17A is most homologous to IL-17F and the genes encoding them are proximally located on chromosome 6p12 (https://www.ncbi.nlm.nih.gov/gene/3605). The IL-17F activity is similar to IL-17A, but significantly weaker, and is related to induce the expression of various cytokines, chemokines, matrix metalloproteinases, antimicrobial peptides, and adhesion molecules by human fibroblasts, and airway epithelial cells and vein endothelial cells. IL-17A, IL-17B, IL-17C, IL-17D, and IL-17F are considered proinflammatory cytokines, and IL-17E is believed to have antiinflammatory properties. IL-17A, IL-17F and IL-22 are involved in neutrophilia, tissue remodeling, tissue repair, and production of antimicrobial products [48].

Many studies have demonstrated the presence of IL-17 in periodontal tissues, crevicular gingival fluid, saliva, and plasma of patients with periodontal disease. IL-17 contributes to inflammatory bone pathology and bone resorption by different ways: (i) stimulating the production and expression of TNF-α and IL-1β by human macrophages and IL-1β by OB; (ii) stimulating secretion of IL-6, CXCL8/IL-8, and PGE2 by fibroblasts, epithelial, and endothelial cells; (iii) increasing the expression of RANKL on OB; and (iv) stimulates the differentiation and activation of OC. In periodontal environment, IL-17 potentiates the innate immunity, mobilizing macrophages and neutrophils, and increasing TLR responsiveness in gingival epithelial cells. IL-17, when combined with IFN-γ, may modulate GF in periodontal disease by triggering the release of other proinflammatory, metalloproteinase and neutrophil-mobilizing cytokines [49].

2.3.5. Interleukin-18 (IL-18)

IL-18 is a member of IL-1 cytokine family and is codified by *IL18* gene located on chromosome 11q22 (https://www.ncbi.nlm.nih.gov/gene/3606) [50]. This proinflammatory cytokine is released at sites of chronic inflammation by APCs, such macrophages and DC, and non-immune cells, such epithelial and osteoblastic stromal cells. Its receptor IL-18RC is complex with two chains, the IL-18Rα and the IL-18Rβ chains; and the β protein contains the motif for sign-transducing. IL-18 has the property of stimulating both Th1/Th2 responses, depending on the immunological context. When the IL-12 is present, IL-18 drives to Th1 response, and in its absence, the Th2 cells' response is stimulated. IL-12 is able to increase the expression of IL-18Rβ. One of the major actions of IL-18 in Th1 response is to enhance the release of IFN-γ by TCD4⁺ cells and natural killer (NK). INF-γ acts as a positive regulator of Th1 differentiation through increased transcription of T-bet. In addition, proinflammatory properties of IL-18 are due to promotion of the increase of cell adhesion molecules, nitric oxide synthesis, and chemokines production. IL-18 induces the production of Th2 cytokines such as IL-4, IL-5, IL-10, and IL-13, stimulating allergic inflammation, and inducing PGE_2 production [36, 51].

There are low evidences according IL-18 participation in periodontitis. Some studies show that IL-18 is an inhibitor of OC formation by indirect effects mediated by T cells and granulocyte macrophage colony-stimulating factor (GM-CSF). GM-CSF binds to preosteoclast and inhibits its proliferation and differentiation. The IL-18RC was found on T cells and OC. The concentration of IL-18 was found increased in the gingival crevicular fluid and serum of gingivitis, aggressive, and chronic periodontitis [52].

2.3.6. Interleukin-10 (IL-10)

IL-10 is considered an antiinflammatory cytokine playing a key role in the regulation of immune mechanisms. The *IL10* gene (https://www.ncbi.nlm.nih.gov/gene/3586) is mapped on chromosome 1q31-q32, in a cluster with closely related interleukin genes, including IL-19, IL-20, and IL-24, and has several regulatory promoter sequences within the 1.3 kb region upstream of the transcription start site [53].

IL-10 is produced by monocytes, macrophages, and T cells and plays a role in the regulation of proinflammatory cytokines such as IL-1 and TNF-α. During bone loss, IL-10 was correlated to inhibition of OC formation direct and indirectly. Directly, IL-10 inhibits osteoclast progenitors by an effect associated with decreased RANK-induced activation of nuclear factor-kappaB and expression of NFATc1, c-Fos, and c-Jun. Indirectly, by decreasing RANKL and increasing osteoprotegerin in dental folic cells. IL-10 also had protective role toward periodontal tissue destruction, inhibiting MMPs. However, it has stimulatory effect on B lymphocyte and may also stimulate the production of autoantibodies. Autoantibodies may play a role in periodontitis. The high production of IL-10 by Treg was found in gingival tissue [54].

2.4. Immunopathogenesis of bone resorption

Skeletal homeostasis depend on a dynamic balance between the activities of the bone forming osteoblasts (OB) and bone-resorbing osteoclast (OC). The RANK/RANKL/OPG regulating system controls the bone resorption and deposition activity that occur during this bone remodeling. The receptor-activator of nuclear factor-kappaB (NF-κB) ligand (RANKL) binds to RANK on osteoclast precursors (monocyte/macrophage) causing them to differentiate into active cells (OC) that secrete enzymes that degrade bone. OPG (osteoprotegerin) is a soluble decoy receptor of RANKL that prevents the RANK-RANKL interaction. OPG inhibits the osteoclastogenesis and induces osteopetrosis when overexpressed [55]. In periodontitis, high levels of RANKL and low levels of OPG have been detected in gingival crevicular fluid. In response to LPS from periodontopathogens, for instances *P. gingivalis* and *A. actinomycetem-comitans*, RANKL expression has been increased in periodontal ligament fibroblasts; however, its major source is the activated immune cells, mainly Th1, Th17, and B cells [15, 56].

Several cytokines can synergize with RANKL in promoting osteoclastogenesis and increasing RANKL/OPG ratio. Cytokines, such as IL-1, TNF-α, IL-6, and IL-17, have the ability to stimulate bone resorption, whereas others, such as IL-4, IL-10, and TGF-β, act as inhibitors. TNF-α and also IL-1 have been shown to play an important role in periodontal bone loss in a dependent and independent RANKL pathway: TNF-α could promote the proliferation and differentiation of osteoclast precursors via NFATc1 activation. TNF-α also could lead to inhibition of OB differentiation. The TNF-related apoptosis inducing ligand (TRAIL) is expressed on OB after infection and induce the apoptosis of these cells. IL-17, when in high concentration, promotes osteoclastogenesis by enhanced RANKL expression on osteoblasts and CD4 T cells [57, 58].

The immune cells and cytokines produced by them involved in the protective and aggressive roles during CP are summarized in **Table 2**.

Immune response	Cells	Characteristic produced cytokines*	Protective actions	Deleterious actions
Innate immunity	Neutrophils	TNF-α IL-1 IL-6	No evidence	Proinflammatory RANKL inducers
	PDLFs	TNF-α IL-1 IL-6	No evidence	Proinflammatory RANKL inducers RANKL+
	Monocyte/macrophage		No evidence	Proinflammatory RANKL inducers OC differentiation
Adaptive immunity	T_H1	INF-γ	Antiosteoclastogenic	Proinflammatory RANKL+
	T_H2	IL-4	Antiosteoclastogenic	B cells lesions and autoimmunity B RANKL+
	T_H17	IL-17	No evidence	Proinflammatory RANKL inducers RANKL+
	Tregs	IL-10 TGF-β	Antiosteoclastogenic	No evidence

PDLFs: periodontal ligament fibroblasts; OC: osteoclasts.

Table 2. Immune cells and their characteristic cytokines involved in tissue damage and bone resorption in chronic periodontitis.

3. Immunomodulation and therapeutic approaches

Therapeutic approaches in periodontitis attempt to eliminate the periodontal plaque, manage the inflammation and minimize the tissue damage. The conventional treatment of CP is the mechanical removal of infectious agents in gingival tissues, which resulted in bacteria resistance and disease recurrence. Considering the complexity of periodontitis, immunopathogenesis and clinical manifestations of disease, many different approaches could be considered in order to interfere during immunity response. Amongst them, blocking the cytokines activity may be a promissory intervention. The effect of TNF-α and IL-1 antagonists on periodontitis showed a significant reduction of inflammation and bone resorption when administered either systemically or locally in the gingiva. The administration of antiTNF-α or TNF-α/Fc fusion protein had demonstrated significant reduction of the clinical and radiographic signals in rheumatoid arthritis and periodontal diseases [59]. IL-11 has antiinflammatory effects by induction of inhibition of TNF-α and other proinflammatory cytokines, thus the use of recombinant human IL-11 in the animal models showed significant reduction in the rate of clinical attachment and radiographic bone loss [60]. Similarly, the use of RANKL inhibitors in periodontitis, although limited in animal models [61] or *in vitro* assays [62], demonstrates a protective effect on bone resorption. The inhibition of PGE2 formation by nonsteroidal antiinflammatory drugs decreases osteoclasts formation and alveolar bone loss in humans and in animal experiments [63]. The United State Food Drug Administration approved the host modulator drug denominated subantimicrobial dose doxycycline (SDD), which inhibits matrix metalloproteinases and results in reduced progression of disease [64].

4. Genetic variants and the periodontitis risk

The development of periodontitis relies on multiple factors, and it is estimated that 50% of the expression of periodontitis could be attributed to genetic factors. The multifactorial etiology of the periodontitis and the development of sequencing technology enabled us to discuss whether the variations of host's immunity affect the occurrence and development of the disease. Several immune response genes have been related to the protection or predisposition to CP, such as those responsible for bacterial antigens presentation to lymphocytes, as well as soluble mediators or membrane receptors that initiate or amplify the inflammatory process and bone loss.

4.1. Human leukocyte antigen (HLA)

HLA comprises of high polymorphic cell-surface molecules that have a key role in antigen presentation and activation of T cells. Because of the capability to bind periodontopathogens peptides, HLA represents an important factor of risk or resistance to CP development. A metaanalysis focusing on Caucasian case-control studies demonstrated no associations between HLA and CP, although for aggressive periodontitis, HLA-A*09 and B*15 appeared to represent susceptibility factors, and HLA-A*02 and B*05 were potential protective factors

[65]. However, other studies provide evidence that class I and II HLA polymorphisms are associated with chronic periodontitis [66].

4.2. Pattern recognition receptors (PRRs)

PRRs play an important role in the recognition of periodontopathogens and genetic variations within the genes encoding them. They may have an important influence on immune response and in the pathogenesis of periodontal diseases [67].

TLR polymorphism may alter host susceptibility to periodontitis. The main studied polymorphism was related to *TLR4* gene because TLR-4 is responsible for LPS recognition. *TLR4* was associated with susceptibility of the periodontitis, although conflicting results are related [68]. *TLR2* and *TLR9* (except some TLR9 haplotypes) were not associated to CP development [69].

The *CD14* −159C>T and −260 C>T promoter polymorphisms are located upstream from the major transcriptional site, affecting the transcriptional activity and CD14 density. Individuals homozygous for the mutation have increased serum levels of soluble sCD14 and an increased density of CD14 in monocytes. Thus, patients without mutation lead to a reduced expression of the CD14 receptor and may be more susceptible to CP. No association of CD14 polymorphism and CP was found in a metaanalysis study [70].

Mannose-binding lectin (MBL) polymorphisms were also associated to the severity of CP. Therefore, it is possible to affirm that periodontitis susceptibility was partly controlled by PRR polymorphisms involved in the innate immunity [71].

4.3. Cytokines

4.3.1. IL1

The *IL1* genotypes appear to be the most studied genetic polymorphisms in CP. Associations between *IL1* family polymorphisms and CP were initially assessed by Kornman et al. [72]. The authors observed that the simultaneous occurrence of *IL1A* −889 and *IL1B* +3953 polymorphisms was associated with severe periodontitis in nonsmokers. To date, the following *IL1* genetic polymorphisms have been studied in association with CP: *IL1A* −889 (in linkage disequilibrium, LD, with +4845), *IL1B* −511 (in LD with −31), *IL1B* +3954 (also mentioned as +3953), and *IL1RN* VNTR (in LD with +2018). Different from others *IL1* SNPs, *IL1RN* VNTR variant-alleles seem to decrease gene transcription or the protein production levels. Taken altogether, the *IL1* gene cluster polymorphisms cannot be considered as risk factors for CP in the worldwide population. However, in Caucasians, an association between CP and *IL1A* −889 and *IL1B* +3953 mutate-allele may be genetic risk factors. The *IL1* promoter SNPs and periodontitis might reflect subpopulation effects and have to be interpreted with care [72–74].

4.3.2. TNF

Several case-control studies in both Caucasians and nonCaucasians have investigated genetic polymorphisms in the *TNF* gene as putative risk factors for periodontitis. SNPs in the gene encoding *TNF* are mainly studied in the promoter region at positions 1031, 863, 857, 376, 308, and 238 and also in the first intron at position +489. *TNF* −308 G/A and A/A genotypes were associated with increased CP risk in Asians, Caucasians, and nonsmoking Asians [75].

4.3.3. IL6

The *IL6* −174G>C was found to influence IL-6 expression and production, and the individuals with carrier mutation present low *IL6* gene transcriptional activity and low plasma levels of IL-6. Thus, the polymorphism may hamper individual's defense against periodontal pathogens. Many studies had been found that *IL6* −174 polymorphism may be associated with CP susceptibility and *A. actinomycetemcomitans* infection. However, a metaanalysis that included this polymorphism did not show any association for this polymorphism with CP [76, 77].

4.3.4. IL17

Two *IL17* polymorphisms had been found associated to diseases: *IL17A* G197A (rs2275913) and *IL17F* T7488C (His161Arg, rs763780). The *IL17A* 197A allele correlates to more efficient IL-17 secretion and higher affinity for the nuclear factor activated T cells (NAFT), which is a critical regulator of the *IL17* promoter gene. IL-17F activity is similar to IL-17A, but weaker, and the variant form of IL-17 protein suppresses the expression and the activity of wild type. *IL17A* AA genotype and A allele were associated with worse clinical and inflammatory periodontal parameters. *IL17F* polymorphisms were not associated to CP [78].

4.3.5. IL10

Several promoter polymorphisms have been described in the *IL10* gene: −1087 (−1082), −819 (−824), −627, −592 (−597), and −590. There is strong linkage disequilibrium between *IL10* 1082G>A, 819C>T, and 592C>A, and they form two common haplotypes on the basis of *IL10* −592 polymorphism. The allele A of the −592 has been associated with decreased synthesis of IL-10 *in vitro* and *in vivo*, and when present could modify the synthesis of IL-10 in response to inflammation. IL-10 has a protective role toward periodontal tissue destruction; therefore, the *IL10* −592 polymorphism may be less protected against bacterial challenge and contribute to a relative increase in the risk for CP [79].

5. Conclusion

Chronic periodontitis is an inflammatory disease of the teeth-supporting tissues. The imbalance between periodontopathogens and host factors is responsible for the transition of gingivitis into periodontitis and is estimated that 50% of the expression of periodontitis could be attributed to genetic factors. The genetic polymorphisms may in some situations cause a change in the protein or its expression possibly resulting in alterations in innate and adaptive immunity and may thus be deterministic in disease outcome. Thus, development and regulation of the immune response influence disease progression or resolution, and each person may have an individual response to the bacterial challenge. Most individuals are resistant to the disease and will not develop CP. The disease progression depends on the increased production of proinflammatory cytokines (IL-1α, IL-1β, IL-6, IL-8, and TNFα), metalloproteinases, and prostaglandins or decreased production of antiinflammatory cytokines (IL-10, TGFβ) and inhibitors of metalloproteinases. The knowledge of the immunopathogenesis mechanisms in the chronic periodontitis could contribute to new therapeutic approaches.

Acknowledgements

The authors wish to thank Coordenação de Aperfeiçoamento de Pessoal de Nível Superior (CAPES), Conselho Nacional de Desenvolvimento Científico e Tecnológico (CNPq), Fundação Araucária de Apoio ao Desenvolvimento Científico e Tecnológico do Estado do Paraná and the financial support by Laboratory of Immunogenetics-LIG-UEM (00639/99-DEG-UEM).

Author details

Ana Maria Sell[1]*, Josiane Bazzo de Alencar[1], Jeane Eliete Laguila Visentainer[1] and Cleverson de Oliveira e Silva[2]

*Address all correspondence to: anamsell@gmail.com

1 Department of Analysis Clinical and Biomedicine, Maringa State University, Parana, Brazil

2 Department of Dentistry, Ingá University Center (Uningá), Parana, Brazil

References

[1] Page RC, Offenbacher S, Schroeder HE, Seymour GJ, Kornman KS. Advances in the pathogenesis of periodontitis: Summary of developments, clinical implications and future directions. Periodontology 2000. 1997;**14**:216-248

[2] Socransky SS, Haffajee AD, Cugini MA, Smith C, Kent Jr RL. Microbial complexes in subgingival plaque. Journal of Clinical Periodontology. 1998;**25**(2):134-144

[3] Sun Y, Shu R, Li CL, Zhang MZ. Gram-negative periodontal bacteria induce the activation of Toll-like receptors 2 and 4, and cytokine production in human periodontal ligament cells. The Journal of Periodontology. 2010;**81**(10):1488-1496

[4] Marchesan JT, Morelli T, Lundy SK, Jiao Y, Lim S, Inohara N, et al. Divergence of the systemic immune response following oral infection with distinct strains of *Porphyromonas gingivalis*. Molecular Oral Microbiology. 2012;**27**(6):483-495

[5] Oppermann RV, Weidlich P, Musskopf ML. Periodontal disease and systemic complications. Brazilian Oral Research. 2012;**26**(Suppl 1):39-47

[6] Uriarte SM, Edmisson JS, Jimenez-Flores E. Human neutrophils and oral microbiota: A constant tug-of-war between a harmonious and a discordant coexistence. Immunological Reviews. 2016;**273**(1):282-298

[7] Fredriksson M, Gustafsson A, Asman B, Bergstrom K. Hyper-reactive peripheral neutrophils in adult periodontitis: generation of chemiluminescence and intracellular hydrogen peroxide after in vitro priming and FcgammaR-stimulation. Journal of Clinical Periodontology. 1998;**25**(5):394-398

[8] Ling MR, Chapple IL, Matthews JB. Peripheral blood neutrophil cytokine hyper-reactivity in chronic periodontitis. Innate Immunity. 2015;**21**(7):714-725

[9] Vitkov L, Klappacher M, Hannig M, Krautgartner WD. Extracellular neutrophil traps in periodontitis. Journal of Periodontal Research. 2009;**44**(5):664-672

[10] Scott DA, Krauss J. Neutrophils in periodontal inflammation. Frontiers of Oral Biology. 2012;**15**:56-83

[11] Sippert EA, de Oliveira e Silva C, Visentainer JE, Sell AM. Association of duffy blood group gene polymorphisms with IL8 gene in chronic periodontitis. PLoS One. 2013;**8**(12):e83286

[12] Zhu XQ, Lu W, Chen Y, Cheng XF, Qiu JY, Xu Y, et al. Effects of *Porphyromonas gingivalis* lipopolysaccharide tolerized monocytes on inflammatory responses in neutrophils. PLoS One. 2016;**11**(8):e0161482

[13] Baek KJ, Choi Y, Ji S. Gingival fibroblasts from periodontitis patients exhibit inflammatory characteristics in vitro. Archives of Oral Biology. 2013;**58**(10):1282-1292

[14] Bloemen V, Schoenmaker T, de Vries TJ, Everts V. Direct cell-cell contact between periodontal ligament fibroblasts and osteoclast precursors synergistically increases the expression of genes related to osteoclastogenesis. Journal of Cellular Physiology. 2010;**222**(3):565-573

[15] Di Benedetto A, Gigante I, Colucci S, Grano M. Periodontal disease: Linking the primary inflammation to bone loss. Clinical & Developmental Immunology. 2013;**2013**:503754

[16] Takeda K, Akira S. Toll-like receptors in innate immunity. International Immunology. 2005;**17**(1):1-14

[17] Drexler SK, Foxwell BM. The role of toll-like receptors in chronic inflammation. The International Journal of Biochemistry & Cell Biology. 2010;**42**(4):506-518

[18] Chrzeszczyk D, Konopka T, Zietek M. Polymorphisms of Toll-like receptor 4 as a risk factor for periodontitis: Meta-analysis. Advances in Clinical and Experimental Medicine. 2015;**24**(6):1059-1070

[19] Beklen A, Hukkanen M, Richardson R, Konttinen YT. Immunohistochemical localization of Toll-like receptors 1-10 in periodontitis. Oral Microbiology and Immunology. 2008;**23**(5):425-431

[20] Hayashi J, Masaka T, Ishikawa I. Increased levels of soluble CD14 in sera of periodontitis patients. In: McGhee JR, editor. Infection and Immunity. 1999;**67**:417-420

[21] Hedgpeth DC, Zhang X, Jin J, Leite RS, Krayer JW, Huang Y. Periodontal CD14 mRNA expression is downregulated in patients with chronic periodontitis and type 2 diabetes. BMC Oral Health. 2015;**15**:145

[22] Kinane DF. Regulators of tissue destruction and homeostasis as diagnostic aids in periodontology. Periodontology 2000. 2000;**24**:215-225

[23] Vokurka J, Klapusova L, Pantuckova P, Kukletova M, Kukla L, Holla LI. The association of MMP-9 and IL-18 gene promoter polymorphisms with gingivitis in adolescents. Archives of Oral Biology. 2009;**54**(2):172-178

[24] Li W, Zhu Y, Singh P, Ajmera DH, Song J, Ji P. Association of common variants in MMPs with periodontitis risk. Disease Markers. 2016;**2016**:1545974

[25] Pillai S, Abbas AK, Lichtman AHH. Imunologia Celular e Molecular. Brasil: Elsevier; 2015

[26] Silva N, Abusleme L, Bravo D, Dutzan N, Garcia-Sesnich J, Vernal R, et al. Host response mechanisms in periodontal diseases. Journal of Applied Oral Science. 2015;**23**(3):329-355

[27] Campbell L, Millhouse E, Malcolm J, Culshaw S. T cells, teeth and tissue destruction—What do T cells do in periodontal disease? Molecular Oral Microbiology. 2016;**31**(6):445-456

[28] Baker PJ, Boutaugh NR, Tiffany M, Roopenian DC. B cell IgD deletion prevents alveolar bone loss following murine oral infection. Interdisciplinary Perspectives on Infectious Diseases. 2009;**2009**:864359

[29] Weaver CT, Harrington LE, Mangan PR, Gavrieli M, Murphy KM. Th17: An effector CD4 T cell lineage with regulatory T cell ties. Immunity. 2006;**24**(6):677-688

[30] Hizawa N, Kawaguchi M, Huang SK, Nishimura M. Role of interleukin-17F in chronic inflammatory and allergic lung disease. Clinical and Experimental Allergy. 2006;**36**(9):1109-1114

[31] Ernst CW, Lee JE, Nakanishi T, Karimbux NY, Rezende TM, Stashenko P, et al. Diminished forkhead box P3/CD25 double-positive T regulatory cells are associated with the increased nuclear factor-kappaB ligand (RANKL+) T cells in bone resorption lesion of periodontal disease. Clinical and Experimental Immunology. 2007;**148**(2):271-280

[32] Buchwald ZS, Kiesel JR, DiPaolo R, Pagadala MS, Aurora R. Osteoclast activated FoxP3+ CD8+ T-cells suppress bone resorption in vitro. PLoS One. 2012;**7**(6):e38199

[33] Baker PJ, Howe L, Garneau J, Roopenian DC. T cell knockout mice have diminished alveolar bone loss after oral infection with *Porphyromonas gingivalis*. Immunology and Medical Microbiology. 2002;**34**(1):45-50

[34] Graves D. Cytokines that promote periodontal tissue destruction. The Journal of Periodontology. 2008;**79**(8 Suppl):1585-1591

[35] IL1B Interleukin 1 Beta [*Homo sapiens* (Human)] IL18 Interleukin 18 [Homo Sapiens (Human)] [Internet]. 2017. Available from: https://www.ncbi.nlm.nih.gov/gene/36062017. [Accessed: 06 February 2017]

[36] Dinarello CA. The IL-1 family and inflammatory diseases. Clinical and Experimental Rheumatology. 2002;**20**(5 Suppl 27):S1-13

[37] O'Neill LA. The interleukin-1 receptor/Toll-like receptor superfamily: 10 years of progress. Immunological Reviews. 2008;**226**:10-18

[38] Liu YC, Lerner UH, Teng YT. Cytokine responses against periodontal infection: protective and destructive roles. Periodontology 2000. 2010;**52**(1):163-206

[39] Gupta G. Gingival crevicular fluid as a periodontal diagnostic indicator—II: Inflammatory mediators, host-response modifiers and chair side diagnostic aids. Journal of Medicine and Life. 2013;**6**(1):7-13

[40] Al-Shammari KF, Giannobile WV, Aldredge WA, Iacono VJ, Eber RM, Wang HL, et al. Effect of non-surgical periodontal therapy on C-telopeptide pyridinoline cross-links (ICTP) and interleukin-1 levels. The Journal of Periodontology. 2001;**72**(8):1045-1051

[41] TNF Tumor Necrosis Factor [*Homo sapiens* (Human)] IL18 Interleukin 18 [Homo sapiens (Human)] [Internet]. 2017. Available from: https://www.ncbi.nlm.nih.gov/gene/36062017. [Accessed: 06 February 2017]

[42] Idriss HT, Naismith JH. TNF alpha and the TNF receptor superfamily: Structure-function relationship(s). Microscopy Research and Technique. 2000;**50**(3):184-195

[43] Pietschmann P. Principles of Osteoimmunology. Switzerland: Springer; 2011

[44] Singh P, Gupta ND, Bey A, Khan S. Salivary TNF-alpha: A potential marker of periodontal destruction. Journal of Indian Society of Periodontology. 2014;**18**(3):306-310

[45] IL6 Interleukin 6 [*Homo sapiens* (Human)] IL10 Interleukin 10 [Homo Sapiens (Human)] [Internet]. 2017. Available from: https://www.ncbi.nlm.nih.gov/gene/3586 [Accessed: 06 February 2017]

[46] Nibali L, Fedele S, D'Aiuto F, Donos N. Interleukin-6 in oral diseases: A review. Oral Diseases. 2012;**18**(3):236-243

[47] Costa PP, Trevisan GL, Macedo GO, Palioto DB, Souza SL, Grisi MF, et al. Salivary interleukin-6, matrix metalloproteinase-8, and osteoprotegerin in patients with periodontitis and diabetes. The Journal of Periodontology. 2010;**81**(3):384-391

[48] Dong C. TH17 cells in development: An updated view of their molecular identity and genetic programming. Nature Reviews Immunology. 2008;**8**(5):337-348

[49] Jovanovic DV, Di Battista JA, Martel-Pelletier J, Jolicoeur FC, He Y, Zhang M, et al. IL-17 stimulates the production and expression of proinflammatory cytokines, IL-beta and TNF-alpha, by human macrophages. Journal of Immunology. 1998;**160**(7):3513-3521

[50] IL18 Interleukin 18 [Homo sapiens (Human)] [Internet]. 2017. Available from: https://www.ncbi.nlm.nih.gov/gene/36062017. [Accessed: 06 February 2017]

[51] Cornish J, Gillespie MT, Callon KE, Horwood NJ, Moseley JM, Reid IR. Interleukin-18 is a novel mitogen of osteogenic and chondrogenic cells. Endocrinology. 2003;144(4):1194-1201

[52] Nair V, Bandyopadhyay P, Kundu D, Das S. Estimation of interleukin-18 in the gingival crevicular fluid and serum of Bengali population with periodontal health and disease. Journal of Indian Society of Periodontology. 2016;20(3):260-264

[53] IL10 interleukin 10 [Homo sapiens (Human)] [Internet]. 2017. Available from: https://www.ncbi.nlm.nih.gov/gene/3586. [Accessed: 06 February 2017]

[54] Laine ML, Loos BG, Crielaard W. Gene polymorphisms in chronic periodontitis. International Journal of Dentistry. 2010;2010:324719

[55] Theoleyre S, Wittrant Y, Tat SK, Fortun Y, Redini F, Heymann D. The molecular triad OPG/RANK/RANKL: Involvement in the orchestration of pathophysiological bone remodeling. Cytokine & Growth Factor Reviews. 2004;15(6):457-475

[56] Liu D, Xu JK, Figliomeni L, Huang L, Pavlos NJ, Rogers M, et al. Expression of RANKL and OPG mRNA in periodontal disease: Possible involvement in bone destruction. International Journal of Molecular Medicine. 2003;11(1):17-21

[57] Yarilina A, Xu K, Chen J, Ivashkiv LB. TNF activates calcium-nuclear factor of activated T cells (NFAT)c1 signaling pathways in human macrophages. Proceedings of the National Academy of Sciences of the United States of America. 2011;108(4):1573-1578

[58] Mori G, Brunetti G, Colucci S, Ciccolella F, Coricciati M, Pignataro P, et al. Alteration of activity and survival of osteoblasts obtained from human periodontitis patients: Role of TRAIL. Journal of Biological Regulators and Homeostatic Agents. 2007;21(3-4):105-114

[59] Kirkwood KL, Cirelli JA, Rogers JE, Giannobile WV. Novel host response therapeutic approaches to treat periodontal diseases. Periodontology 2000. 2007;43:294-315

[60] Leng SX, Elias JA. Interleukin-11 inhibits macrophage interleukin-12 production. Journal of Immunology. 1997;159(5):2161-2168

[61] Bartold PM, Cantley MD, Haynes DR. Mechanisms and control of pathologic bone loss in periodontitis. Periodontology 2000. 2010;53:55-69

[62] Deepak V, Kasonga A, Kruger MC, Coetzee M. Carvacrol inhibits osteoclastogenesis and negatively regulates the survival of mature osteoclasts. Biological & Pharmaceutical Bulletin. 2016;39(7):1150-1158

[63] Elavarasu S, Sekar S, Murugan T. Host modulation by therapeutic agents. Journal of Pharmacy & Bioallied Sciences. 2012;4(Suppl 2):S256-259

[64] Payne JB, Golub LM. Using tetracyclines to treat osteoporotic/osteopenic bone loss: From the basic science laboratory to the clinic. Pharmacological Research. 2011;63(2):121-129

[65] Stein J, Reichert S, Gautsch A, Machulla HK. Are there HLA combinations typical supporting for or making resistant against aggressive and/or chronic periodontitis? Journal of Periodontal Research. 2003;**38**(5):508-517

[66] Sippert EA, de Oliveira e Silva C, Ayo CM, Marques SB, Visentainer JE, Sell AM. HLA haplotypes and genotypes frequencies in Brazilian Chronic periodontitis patients. Mediators of Inflammation. 2015;**2015**:481656

[67] Han MX, Ding C, Kyung HM. Genetic polymorphisms in pattern recognition receptors and risk of periodontitis: Evidence based on 12,793 subjects. Human Immunology. 2015;**76**(7):496-504

[68] Jin SH, Guan XY, Liang WH, Bai GH, Liu JG. TLR4 polymorphism and periodontitis susceptibility: A meta-analysis. Medicine (Baltimore). 2016;**95**(36):e4845

[69] Holla LI, Vokurka J, Hrdlickova B, Augustin P, Fassmann A. Association of Toll-like receptor 9 haplotypes with chronic periodontitis in Czech population. Journal of Clinical Periodontology. 2010;**37**(2):152-159

[70] Zheng J, Hou T, Gao L, Wu C, Wang P, Wen Y, et al. Association between CD14 gene polymorphism and periodontitis: A meta-analysis. Critical Reviews in Eukaryotic Gene Expression. 2013;**23**(2):115-123

[71] Liukkonen A, He Q, Gursoy UK, Pussinen PJ, Grondahl-Yli-Hannuksela K, Liukkonen J, et al. Mannose-binding lectin gene polymorphism in relation to periodontal infection. Journal of Periodontal Research. 2017;**52**(3):540-545

[72] Kornman KS, Crane A, Wang HY, di Giovine FS, Newman MG, Pirk FW, et al. The interleukin-1 genotype as a severity factor in adult periodontal disease. Journal of Clinical Periodontology. 1997;**24**(1):72-77

[73] Zuccarello D, Bazzato MF, Ferlin A, Pengo M, Frigo AC, Favero G, et al. Role of familiarity versus interleukin-1 genes cluster polymorphisms in chronic periodontitis. Gene. 2014;**535**(2):286-289

[74] Fiebig A, Jepsen S, Loos BG, Scholz C, Schafer C, Ruhling A, et al. Polymorphisms in the interleukin-1 (IL1) gene cluster are not associated with aggressive periodontitis in a large Caucasian population. Genomics. 2008;**92**(5):309-315

[75] Ding C, Ji X, Chen X, Xu Y, Zhong L. TNF-alpha gene promoter polymorphisms contribute to periodontitis susceptibility: Evidence from 46 studies. Journal of Clinical Periodontology. 2014;**41**(8):748-759

[76] Nibali L, Donos N, Farrell S, Ready D, Pratten J, Tu YK, et al. Association between interleukin-6 −174 polymorphism and *Aggregatibacter actinomycetemcomitans* in chronic periodontitis. The Journal of Periodontology. 2010;**81**(12):1814-1819

[77] Nikolopoulos GK, Dimou NL, Hamodrakas SJ, Bagos PG. Cytokine gene polymorphisms in periodontal disease: A meta-analysis of 53 studies including 4178 cases and 4590 controls. Journal of Clinical Periodontology. 2008;**35**(9):754-767

[78] Zacarias JM, Sippert EA, Tsuneto PY, Visentainer JE, de Oliveira e Silva C, Sell AM. The influence of interleukin 17A and IL17F polymorphisms on chronic periodontitis disease in Brazilian patients. Mediators of Inflammation. 2015;**2015**:147056

[79] Albuquerque CM, Cortinhas AJ, Morinha FJ, Leitao JC, Viegas CA, Bastos EM. Association of the IL-10 polymorphisms and periodontitis: A meta-analysis. Molecular Biology Reports. 2012;**39**(10):9319-9329

5

Impact of Dental Plaque Biofilms in Periodontal Disease: Management and Future Therapy

Veronica Lazar, Lia-Mara Ditu, Carmen Curutiu,
Irina Gheorghe, Alina Holban, Marcela Popa and
Carmen Chifiriuc

Abstract

Oral cavity represents an ideal environment for the microbial cell growth, persistence, and dental plaque establishment. The presence of different microniches leads to the occurrence of different biofilm communities, formed on teeth surface, above gingival crevice or at subgingival level, on tongue, mucosa and dental prosthetics too. The healthy state is regulated by host immune system and interactions between microbial community members, maintaining the predominance of "good" microorganisms. When the complexity and volume of biofilms from the gingival crevice increase, chronic pathological conditions such as gingivitis and periodontitis can occur, predisposing to a wide range of complications. Bacteria growing in biofilms exhibit a different behavior compared with their counterpart, respectively planktonic or free cells. There have been described numerous mechanisms of differences in antibiotic susceptibility of biofilm embedded cells. Resistance to antibiotics, mediated by genetic factors or, phenotypical, due to biofilm formation, called also tolerance, is the most important cause of therapy failure of biofilm-associated infections, including periodontitis; the mechanisms of tolerance are different, the metabolic low rate and cell's dormancy being the major ones. The recent progress in science and technology has made possible a wide range of novel approaches and advanced therapies, aiming the efficient management of periodontal disease.

Keywords: dental plaque biofilm, periodontitis, host defense mechanisms, resistance mechanisms, therapeutic approaches

1. Introduction

Oral cavity represents an ideal environment (e.g., appropriate temperature and nutrients) for the microbial cell growth, survival and persistence, and subsequent dental plaque biofilm establishment. The exact number of species from the oral plaque is not known, because some of them are not cultivable, but it is estimated to be between 700 and 1000 species, reaching densities of 10^8 bacterial cells/mg, much of them being uncultivable [1]. However, bacteria are the most numerous group in the oral microbiota, accompanied by a diverse collection of archaea, fungi, protozoa, and viruses. The oral microorganisms are generally commensal species, maintaining relationships with the host based on mutual benefits. They do not produce disease, but instead impede pathogenic species to adhere to mucosal surfaces [2, 3].

Dental plaque biofilm represents a polymicrobial community that remains relatively stable in health, consisting in species belonging to *Streptococcus, Actinomyces, Veillonella, Fusobacterium, Porphyromonas, Prevotella, Treponema, Neisseria, Haemophilus, Eubacteria, Lactobacterium, Capnocytophaga, Eikenella, Leptotrichia, Peptostreptococcus, Staphylococcus*, and *Propionibacterium* genera.

The dental plaque biofilm formation follows many stages and begins at 1 h after washing, when the tooth surfaces are covered by an organic "pellicle" composed from salivary glyco-proteins, carbohydrates and immunoglobulins, which are adsorbed on the hydroxyapatite surface through electrostatic interactions between calcium ions and phosphate groups with the oppositely charged groups of the macromolecules from the saliva. In a second stage, bacteria adhere to the pellicle and between them through the interaction between specialized structures or adhesins (glycocalyx, capsule, and fimbriae) with complementary receptors. The first colonizers are gram-positive cocci (*Str. mutans, Str. mitis, Str. sanguis* or *Str. oralis, Rothia dentocariosa*, or *Staphylococcus epidermidis*), gram-positive rods, actinobacteria (*Actinomyces israelis* and *A. viscosus*) and few gram-negative cocci [4]. The attached species secrete exopoly-mers such as glucans that contribute to the development of biofilm matrix and allow associa-tion of other species. Although initially the oral cavity offers an aerobic condition, oxygen is rapidly consumed by the aerobic bacteria (e.g., *Neisseria* spp.) or facultative anaerobic (e.g., *Streptococcus* and *Actinomyces* spp.), which are first colonizers creating appropriate conditions for the survival of obligate anaerobe species. When biofilm reaches maturity, the oral cavity becomes colonized predominantly by anaerobic bacteria [5].

In the oral cavity, the presence of different microenvironments leads to the occurrence of different biofilm communities, like those formed on the surface of teeth above the gingival crevice (the supragingival plaque) or at the subgingival level (the subgingival plaque), on the tongue, on the mucosal surfaces, or biofilms developed on dental prosthetics and fill-ings. Some microbial species are better adapted to some location. For example, based on their oxygen requirements, species could be classified as obligate aerobes, obligate anaer-obes (as *Veillonella* and *Fusobacterium*), facultative anaerobes (as most streptococci and *Actinomyces*), and microaerophilic species that prefer low concentrations of O_2 (from 2 to 10%) and capnophilic (species that grow best at high CO_2 concentrations, from 5 to 10%, as *Neisseria*) [3].

When the complexity and volume of biofilms located in the gingival crevice increase, path-ological conditions such as periodontitis or chronic gingivitis can occur. Literature of the last decades has shown that almost all forms of the periodontal disease are consequences of the chronic, nonspecific or specific bacterial infections. If in the healthy individuals, the oral biofilms are comprised mainly of gram-positive facultative anaerobes (*Streptococcus anginosus* and *A. naeslundii*), in the above mentioned pathologic conditions, the percentage of gram-negative anaerobic bacteria increases and may include *Aggregatibacter* (previously *Actinobacillus*) *actinomycetemcomitans, Porphyromonas gingivalis, P. intermedia, Bacteroides forsythus, Campylobacter rectus, Eikenella sp., Peptostreptococcus micros, Streptococcus intermedius, Prevotella sp., Fusobacterium sp., Capnocytophaga sp., Veillonella sp., Treponema* and other on-cultivable spirochetes, and the bacterial counts associated with the disease are up to 10(5) times larger than those of the same species found in healthy individuals [6, 7].

Perhaps, the three best-studied periodontal pathogens are *Porphyromonas gingivalis, Aggregatibacter actinomycetemcomitans,* and, more recently, *Bacteroides forsythus,* all three carrying pathogenicity islands and having the ability to secrete a number of virulence factors, including invasion of gingival epithelial cells and an abundant array of extracellular proteases. The last ones are responsible for the increase in vascular permeability and in the flow of gingival crevicular fluid (GCF), thus providing a rich source of nutrients for the subgingival plaque community.

Porphyromonas gingivalis is one of the most important periodontal pathogens, exhibiting the ability to adhere and invade epithelial tissue of the oral cavity *in vitro*. *Aggregatibacter (A.) actinomycetemcomitans* is associated with periodontal disease in preteen ages. *Fusobacterium nucleatum* is an important periodontal agent, especially in the rapid and progressive periodontal disease forms. *Prevotella intermedia* is black-pigmented, while *Bacteroides (B.) forsythus* an unpigmented gram-negative bacterium; *B. forsythus* has several virulence factors, including the production of trypsin-like proteases and polysaccharides, the ability to penetrate the host cell, or inducing of apoptosis. *Capnocytophaga* species are involved in the onset of the juvenile periodontal disease and in the periodontal disease of adults. These bacteria produce pro-inflammatory lipopolysaccharides and extracellular proteases that could destroy sIgA immunoglobulins. Prevalence *of Peptostreptococcus micros* in advanced periodontitis in adults has been reported as 58–63%. It was also positively associated with dental implant failure. Spirochetes were observed in a greater proportion in patients with periodontal disease than in healthy individuals [8]. Two important spirochetes species, i.e., *Troponema vincentii* and *T. denticola,* are also involved in periodontal disease. Both produce pro-inflammatory lipopolysaccharides and unusual metabolic products, such as indole, hydrogen sulfide and ammonia that are potentially toxic to the host cells.

Besides the microbial component, genetic, physiological, and behavioral factors are also involved in the pathogenesis of periodontal disease. Some people may be genetically susceptible to periodontal disease, but the genetic background involved is not clear. The hormonal changes associated with teen age and pregnancy could contribute to gingival enlargement. Smoking is among the factors that increase the probability to develop a periodontal disease. In smokers, reduced gingival blood flow, impaired wound healing, and increased production of inflammation-mediating cytokines were observed comparing with healthy persons. Smoking seems to increase the severity of periodontal disease, but also the response of the gingival tissues to periodontal therapy is reduced, fact that contributes to a greater incidence of refractory disease and to the risk to lose teeth. Regarding age, the researches indicate that older people have the highest rates of periodontal disease. Other factors which may contribute to evolution of periodontitis are diet, stress, obesity, and some other underlying diseases such as diabetes, cardiovascular disease, osteoporosis, and rheumatoid arthritis. Certain medications could also be inappropriate for the evolution of periodontal disease. Also, a bad oral hygiene, tooth decay and tooth positioned incorrectly may also increase the risk of periodontal disease [9].

The management and therapy of periodontal diseases may be diverse and is usually adjusted depending on particularities of each case/patient (**Figure 1**). Since periodontal disease occurs when a bacterial biofilm (dental plaque) adheres to the boundary between the teeth and gingiva, causing chronic inflammation and progressively destroying the periodontal tissue that supports the teeth, the periodontal treatment involves scaling and root planning, which mechanically removes the causative bacteria biofilm together with the necrotic cementum from the surface of the tooth root. Appropriate application of this therapy eliminates periodontal tissue inflammation and stops the process of destruction of the same tissue. However, removing the cause of the disease does not regenerate the lost periodontal tissue to its original state [10].

The main approaches considered in the current therapeutic procedures include the following:

(1) *Nonsurgical periodontal therapy* aims in motivating and instructing the patient in adequate self-care, followed by periodical re-evaluation of the oral hygiene status. The primary goal of nonsurgical periodontal therapy is to control microbial periodontal infection by removing bacterial biofilm, calculus and toxins from the involved periodontal root surfaces [11].

A new nonsurgical therapy is the ozone-therapy; the disinfection power of ozone over other antiseptics makes the use of ozone in dentistry a very good alternative and/or an additional disinfectant to standard antiseptics. Due to safety concerns, initially only dissolved ozone in water and ozonated oils were recommended, but a new device used for the gas application

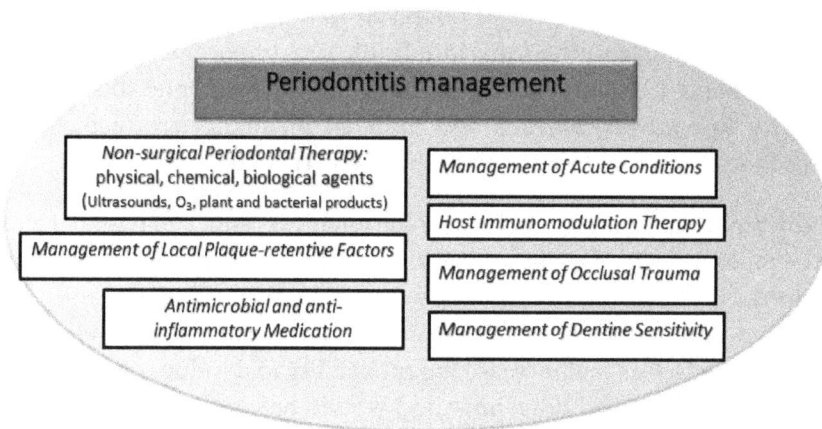

Figure 1. Periodontitis management—innovative strategies for reversing the chronic infectious and inflammatory condition.

with a suction feature allows now its safe intra-oral use, with better diffusion even in the dental hard tissues, for its healing and tissue regeneration properties, being indicated in all stages of gingival and periodontal diseases [12].

(2) *Management of local plaque-retentive factors* which refer to mal-positioned teeth, overhanging restorations, crown and bridgework, partial dentures and fixed and removable orthodontic appliances that can increase the risk of periodontal disease and can also prevent successful treatment and resolution of associated pockets. Local irritation and plaque retention caused by untreated carious lesions, subgingival and approximate overhanging crown margins can affect the attachment loss at patients with chronic periodontitis [13].

(3) *Antimicrobial medication* may refer to: full mouth disinfection (consisting in the instrumentation of all periodontal pockets in two steps within 24 h in combination with the adjunctive use of chlorhexidine mouthwash and gel to disinfect any bacterial reservoirs in the oral cavity), local antimicrobials (i.e., disinfectants such as chlorhexidine and locally delivered antibiotics or antiplaque mouthwashes) which have bacteriostatic and bactericidal activity and can inhibit the development of gingivitis, but despite this proved effect, they have a much reduced effect on established plaque and cannot prevent the progression of periodontitis [14], and systemic antibiotics (which are prescribed as an adjunct to root surface instrumentation) have been proposed to act by suppressing the bacterial species responsible for biofilm growth, leading to a less pathogenic oral environment [15].

(4) *Management of acute conditions* should be made as much as possible by local treatment, avoiding the use of systemic antibiotics if there is no significant sign of infection. The main acute conditions that may be associated with periodontal disease refer to periodontitis associated with endodontic lesions (which is a combined perio-endo lesion characterized by clinical attachment loss but also a tooth with a necrotic, or partially necrotic, pulp), periodontal abscess (occasionally occurring in patients with periodontitis, characterized by localized pain and swelling due to nondraining infection of a periodontal pocket), and necrotizing ulcerative gingivitis and periodontitis (characterized by marginal gingival ulceration with loss of the interdental papillae and a gray sloughing on the surface of the ulcers) [9].

(5) *Management of occlusal trauma* have been linked with periodontal disease for many years, but the role of occlusion in the etiology and pathogenesis of inflammatory periodontitis is still not completely understood [16].

(6) *Management of dentine sensitivity* is a condition some patients may experience following root surface instrumentation, especially those with sensitive teeth prior to treatment. Identification and treatment of the causative factors of dentine sensitivity help to prevent the condition from occurring or recurring. There are various treatment modalities available which can be used at home or may be professionally applied, such as toothpastes, mouthwashes, or chewing gums, and they act by either occluding the dentinal tubules or blocking the neural transmission [17].

(7) *Host modulation therapy* aims to modulate the destructive aspects of the host's immune-inflammatory response to the microbial biofilm by utilizing the anti-inflammatory drugs or oral products (i.e., sub-inhibitory doses of tetracycline). This approach has led to the emergence of a new field of "Perioceutics" which is based on the use of pharmaco-therapeutic

agents including antimicrobial drugs, as well as host modulatory therapy for the management of periodontitis. These host-modulating agents could be successfully used as adjunct components to the balance between periodontal health and disease progression in the direction of a healing response [18].

(8) *Dental prophylaxis* refers to various approaches including plaque elimination by regular tooth brushing, periodical professional removing of mineralized dental plaque or tartar, oral examination and evaluation of periodontal disease progression [19].

2. Oral microbiota: host interactions

In 2001, Joshua Lederberg introduced the term microbiome signifying "the ecological community of commensal, symbiotic, and pathogenic microorganisms that literally share our body space and have been all but ignored as determinants of health and disease" [20]. These complex communities of microbes and their genes play a fundamental role in controlling the host physiology (metabolism, nutrition, immune system development, regulation of gastrointestinal and cardiovascular systems, etc.) [21] and also support the innate and adaptive host defenses in excluding exogenous (and often pathogenic) microorganisms [22]. The healthy microbiome in any individual patient has relatively lower taxonomic diversity, remaining relatively constant over time, this natural balance being termed "microbial homeostasis," but its exact composition differs significantly across individuals [23].

The healthy state is highly regulated by the host immune system, and interactions between the microbial community members and with the host maintain a community dominated by "good" microbes, usually gram-positive *Actinobacteria* or streptococci (**Figure 2**) [24].

2.1. Host defense mechanisms

Host defenses play an important role in maintaining the homeostasis of the oral cavity. The alliance between the immune system and oral microbiota is responsible for the maintenance of tolerance to microbial antigens, the host monitoring and responding permanently to the colonizing microorganisms. Any changes in this symbiotic relationship induced by antibiotics, diet, and elimination of normal microbiota constitutive species increase the risk for autoimmune and inflammatory disorders [21].

Regarding the prenatal development of cellular components associated with the oral mucosa associated immune system, it was observed that the initial organization of Peyer's patches can be immunohistologically detected at 11 weeks of gestation [25]. Epithelial cells positive for the secretory component of the sIgA and immunocytes positive for IgM can be detected in salivary gland tissue by 19–20 weeks and continue to predominate during gestation. After birth, immunocytes secreting IgA begin to dominate, but no IgA can be detected in saliva at birth. sIgA was detected in the neonates' saliva as early as 3 days after birth, and its concentration increased more rapidly during the first 6 months after birth in infants exclusively breast fed [26]. Salivary IgA in young infants has the molecular characteristics of secretory IgA and predominates in saliva. Both IgA subclasses are present in the proportions characteristic of

HOMEOSTASIS/DISEASE STATE OF THE ORAL CAVITY

LOCAL IMMUNE SYSTEM

balanced/disbalanced relationship

ORAL MICROBIOTA

- **Antimicrobial salivary components of innate immunity** (mucin, lysozyme, lactoferrin, salivary peroxidase, histidine rich proteins);
- **Gingival crevicular fluid** with molecular and cellular components: complement components and antibodies, K^+, Na^+ – electrolytes, enzymes (MMPs - matrix metalloproteinase), enzymes inhibitors, neutrophils and plasma cells;
- **Mucosal epithelial cells** that play an integral role in innate immune defense by: physical barrier against pathogens, antimicrobial peptides, interleukin synthesis.
- **Neutrophils and macrophages** that play key role in both nonspecific and specific mucosal immunity, but in chronic inflammation too;
- **Complement system** as major component of the innate immune response involved in recognizing and destroying microorganisms.

PHYLUM:
- FIRMICUTES (~ 52%)
- BACTEROIDETES (~ 40%)
- PROTEOBACTERIA (~ 8%)

GENERA ans species:
- Streptococcus,
- Actinomyces,
- Veillonella,
- Fusobacterium,
- Porphyromonas,
- Prevotella,
- Aggregatibacter,
- Treponema,
- Neisseria,
- Haemophilus,
- Eubacteria,
- Lactobacterium,
- Capnocytophaga,
- Eikenella,
- Leptotrichia,
- Peptostreptococcus,
- Staphylococcus,
- Propionibacterium.

DENTAL PLAQUE/ BIOFILM

involved in the stimulation of the local defense mechanisms, but in vesicles formation too, chronic inflammation, gingivitis and periodontal disease.

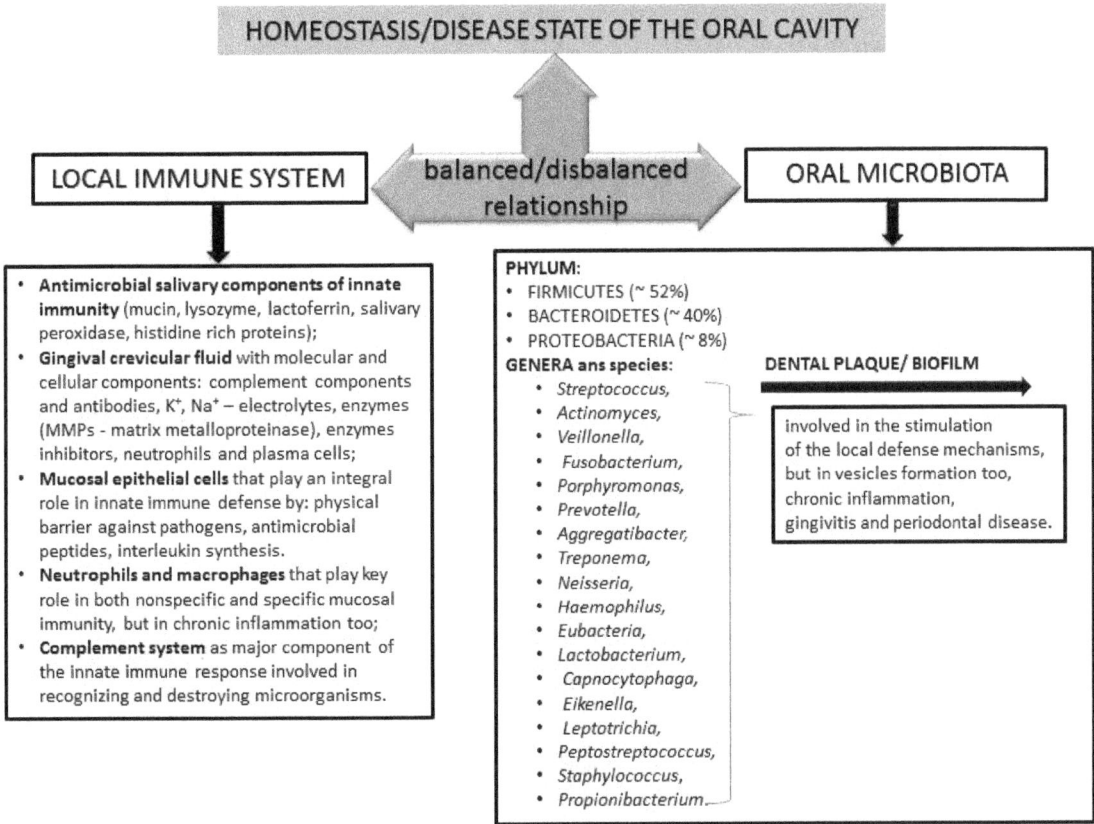

Figure 2. The microbiota plays a fundamental role on the induction, training and function of the host immune system, the interactions between mucosal surfaces and microbiota accomplishing a key role in host defense, health and disease.

adult in 1- to 2-month-old infants, although the appearance of IgA2 is delayed in some subjects [27]. The infant apparently can activate mucosal immune responses quite early in life. For example, salivary antibody specific to organisms that originally colonize the oral cavity (e.g., *S. mitis, S. salivarius)* can be detected by 1–2 months of age. Most of these antibodies are sIgA, although some IgM antibodies can also be initially detected. Salivary sIgA1 and sIgA2 specific to *S. mitis* and *S. salivarius* components increase qualitatively and quantitatively during the first few years of life [28]. Salivary IgA specific to components of streptococci that require hard surfaces for colonization (e.g., *S. sanguis* and *mutans* streptococci) generally appear after tooth eruption [29]. The maternal placental–derived IgG with specificity toward oral microbiota is replaced by the *de novo* synthesis stimulated by the teething process. The collective contributions in the oral cavity of innate and antibody-based immune elements from the saliva, gingival crevicular fluid (and milk if breast feeding) may be considered together with diet, infectious dose, salivary receptors, and tooth integuments, as factors that can determine the outcome of initial colonization events on erupting tooth surfaces [25].

Saliva plays an important role in maintaining the oral homeostasis, through the flushing effects and its antimicrobial constituents like mucin, lysozyme, lactoferrin, salivary peroxidase, and histidine-rich proteins, which are all components of innate immunity [25]. Moreover, local concentrations of these proteins near the mucosal surfaces, periodontal sulcus (gingival crevicular fluid), and oral wounds reinforced by immune and/or inflammatory reactions of the oral mucosa are primarily responsible for innate immunity [30]. *Lysozyme* is a hydrolytic enzyme that cleaves the carbohydrate components of the cell wall peptidoglycan, resulting in cell lysis. This enzyme is active against both gram-negative and gram-positive microorganisms; its targets include *Veilonella* species and *Actinobacillus actinomycetencomitans* [30]. *Lactoferrin* is an iron-binding glyco-protein that links to free iron in the saliva, causing bactericidal or bacteriostatic effects on various microorganisms requiring iron for their survival. Lactoferrin also provides fungicidal, antiviral, anti-inflammatory, and immunomodulatory functions [31–33]. The *lactoperoxidase-thiocyanate sys-tem* in saliva has been shown to be bactericidal on some strains of *Lactobacillus* and *Streptococcus* by preventing the accumulation of lysine and glutamic acid, both of which being essential for bacterial growth [34, 35]. The *histatins*, a family of *histidine-rich peptides,* have antimicrobial activ-ity against some strains of *Streptococcus mutans* and inhibit hemagglutination activity of the peri-odontopathogenic *P. gingivallis.* Also, they neutralize the lipopolysaccharides of gram-negative bacteria and exhibit fungicidal activity against several *Candida* species, *Aspergillus fumigatus,* some strains of *Saccharomyces cerevisiae,* and *Cryptococcus neoformans* [36, 37]. Some defense proteins, like chaperones HSP70/HSPAs (70 kDa heat shock proteins), are also involved in both innate and acquired immunity [30]. In addition, saliva contains abundant CD14 amounts from salivary glands in a soluble form, although LPS-binding protein was below detectable levels, suggesting that saliva CD14 is important for the maintenance of oral health [38].

Gingival crevicular fluid (GCF) is a fluid coming from the junctional epithelium of the gingiva that carries all key molecular (complement components and antibodies, K, Na–electrolytes, enzymes and enzymes inhibitors) and cellular (neutrophils and plasma cells) components of the immune response that are necessary to prevent tissue invasion by subgingival plaque bacteria [39, 40]. Composition of the GCF is the result of the interaction between bacterial biofilm adherent to the tooth surfaces and the cells of the periodontal tissues [41]. The GCF induces permanently changes in microbiota composition, playing an important role in the introduction of immune cells, and being a source of nutrients for resident microorganisms. A number of enzymes can be detected in GCF, including collagenases and elastases which are derived from phagocytic cells and are responsible for the destruction of gingival tissues [42]. Therefore, GCF components might serve as potential diagnostic or prognostic markers for the progression of periodontitis [23, 39]. Although the presence of cytokines was highlighted in GCF, there is no clear evidence of their involvement in the disease. However, interleukin-1 (IL-1) alpha and IL-1 beta are known to increase the binding of PMNs and monocytes to endo-thelial cells, stimulate the production of prostaglandin E2, release of lysosomal enzymes and bone resorption. On the other hand, interferon (IFN) alpha present in GCF has a protective role in periodontal disease because of its ability to inhibit bone resorption activity of IL-1 beta [43].

Mucosal epithelial cells play an integral role in innate immune defense by sensing signals from the external environment, generating various molecules to affect growth, development, function of other cells and maintaining the balance between health and disease [44]. Mucosal epithelial cells produce antimicrobial peptides that include the β-defensin family, cathelicidin (LL-37), calprotectin, and adrenomedullin. These epithelial antimicrobial peptides are impor-tant for wound healing and cell proliferation or exert chemotactic effect to immune cells [45]. It is now recognized that the antimicrobial peptide hBD-2 found in the supra-basal layer of epithe-lium, stimulates antigen-presenting dendritic cells that signal the adaptive immune system, in addition to its antimicrobial activity [44, 46]. Also, it has been proposed that LL-37, the only anti-microbial peptide from the cathelicidin family, detected in gingival epithelium may be the product of neutrophils migrated through gingival epithelium rather than epithelial cells themselves [47]. LL37 is active against both gram-negative and gram-positive bacteria including established periodontopathogens, like *P. gingivalis* and *A. actinomycetemcomitans* [48].

Calprotectin is constitutively produced by neutrophils, monocytes, macrophages, and epithelial cells, its levels being positively correlated with the severity of periodontitis in GCF [49]. The antimicrobial activity of calprotectin is provided by its ability to bind calcium, zinc, copper, and manganese ions. These ions are essential for usual microbial functioning; thus, calprotectin is a growth inhibitory type of host defense [50].

Oral mucosal cells such as epithelial cells are thought to act as a physical barrier against the invasion of pathogenic organisms, but they have also the ability to produce inflammatory cytokines and express adhesion molecules. Gingival tissue of clinically healthy human also expresses low levels of a wide range of toll-like receptors (TLRs), including TLR1-TLR9 that mediate the response to a broad range of microorganisms [51, 52]. However, oral epithelial cells are refractory to many bacterial components, although they express toll-like receptors/MyD88 and acquire responsiveness after priming with IFN-gamma. When the cells are stimulated with lipopolysaccharides and neutrophil protease (PR3) after IFN-gamma priming, the cells produce interleukin 8 (IL-8), which is critical to Th1 and Th2 responses. PR3 itself is able to activate the cells through G protein-coupled protease-activated receptor-2 on the cell surface.

Also, gingival fibroblasts are well equipped to respond to bacterial components and may contribute to the IL-8 levels observed in clinically healthy tissue [53]. Studies in germ-free mice show that there are low levels of innate immunity mediators present in the periodontal tissue [54, 55], indicating that a basic level of cytokine expression is genetically programmed, without bacterial challenge. Any changes of dental plaque composition modify cytokine expression [54, 56]. As an example, an *in vitro* study is showing that the TLR response can be manipulated by *P. gingivalis* toward two types of lipopolysaccharides: PgLPS1690 (type I) and PgLPS1435/1449 (type II). Type I is a TLR4 agonist, thus activating the immune system, while type II is a TLR4 antagonist inhibiting the immune response to *P. gingivalis* [57]. The expression of these two types of LPS is regulated by the concentration of iron from the hemin found in the GCF [58]. During inflammatory process, *P. gingivalis* type II LPS expression increases which reduces the TLR4 response. It was proposed that this could facilitate survival and multiplication of the entire microbial community [59]. *P. gingivalis* can block gingival epithelial cells IL-8 production *in vitro*, by secreting a serine phosphatase that inhibits the synthesis of IL-8 [60]. This process can delay the recruitment of neutrophils preventing the proper formation of the neutrophil wall, facilitating initial microbial colonization of the periodontium [61]. Other bacteria such as *T. denticola* are also able to manipulate the interleukin response of the host by yet not understood mechanism(s) [62].

2.1.1. Neutrophils

The primary function of both nonspecific and specific mucosal immunity is to protect the teeth, jaws, gingiva, and oral mucosa against infection. In healthy individuals, periodontal tissue contains a wall of neutrophils, between the plaque and the epithelial surface, and cellular infil-trate located in juxtaposition to the colonized tooth surface, closest to the dental plaque bio-film [63]. Expression of mediators such as interleukin 8 (IL-8), intercellular adhesion molecule (ICAM), E-selectin and β defensin molecules 1, 2 and 3 are required to form this neutrophil defense wall [64–66]. E-selectin is required for neutrophil migration from the highly vascular-ized gingival tissue, IL-8 is a key neutrophil chemo-attractant produced by epithelial cells, and ICAM facilitates adhesion of neutrophils to the tissue allowing formation of this wall [67, 68].

2.1.2. Complement system

The complement system is a major component of the innate immune response involved in recognizing and destroying microorganisms, with complex roles in homeostasis and disease. Activated complement fragments are abundantly found in the GCF of periodontitis patients, whereas they are absent or present in lower concentrations in healthy individuals [69, 70]. To be a successful pathogen in humans (and any other mammal), a microorganism needs to be able to avoid complement-mediated detection and killing. *In vitro* studies have shown that periodontal bacteria, such as *P. gingivalis*, *T. denticola* and *Prevotella intermedia* could interact with the complement system in complex ways that either inhibit or activate specific comple-ment components [71]. One of the best-studied species from the oral cavity is *P. gingivalis* that produces membrane bound and soluble arginine-specific cysteine proteinases called "gingipains" that can destroy complement factors (C3 and C5) and thus render the bacteria resistant to the bacteriolytical activity of complement system [72, 73].

2.2. Oral microbiome dysbiosis and periodontitis

Recent discussions on the definition of general health have led to the proposal that human health is the ability of the individual to adapt to physiological changes, a condition known as *allostasis* [74]. The *allostasis* in the oral cavity is a complex phenomenon, since the relation-ship between the oral microbiome and its host is dynamic and any physiological or hormonal changes of the host can affect the balance of the species within these communities [75]. The idea that the accumulation of dental plaque is responsible for oral disease, but without dis-criminating between the different virulence levels of bacteria, has led to the "Non-Specific Plaque Hypothesis" [76]. The two most common oral diseases, caries and periodontal disease, are highly abundant among the population of industrialized countries, having a major impact on the populations' well-being and healthcare providers [77].

The factors responsible for the transition from periodontal health to either gingivitis or peri-odontitis are the acquisition of certain species/combinations of species (**Table 1**) and less than optimal host response, which in extreme cases removes the local environment by causing loss of dentition to protect the host from life-threatening bacterial infections [78]. Although the peri-odontal disease microbiomes are more diverse in terms of community structure, that structure is quite similar across different patients [79]. Gingivitis is associated with an increased microbial load (10^4 to 10^6 organisms) and a corresponding increase in the percentage of gram-negative organisms (15–50%) [80]. An interesting finding is that the microbiota of older subjects, with no prior history of gingivitis, had up to 45% gram-negative species including *Fusobacterium*

Normal	Gingivitis	Periodontitis
Streptococcus oralis	*Streptococcus oralis*	*Porphyromonas gingivalis*
Streptococcus sanguis	*Streptococcus sanguis*	*Aggregatibacter actinomycetemcomitans*
Streptococcus mutans	*Capnocytophaga ochracea*	*Treponema denticola other spirochetes*
Streptococcus anginous	*Capnocytophaga gingivalis*	*Bacteroides intermedius* *B. pneumosintes*
Actinomyces odontolyticus subsp. nucleatum	*Actinomyces iraelii, Act. naeslundii*	*Fusobacterium nucleatum*
Eubacterium nodatum	*Actinomyces odontolyticus*	*Selenomonas sputigena*
Campylobacter gracilis	*Eubacterium brachy*	*Lactobacillus sp.*

Table 1. The specific composition of subgingival bacterial plaque in gingivitis and periodontitis.

nucleatum, P. gingivalis, P. intermedia, Campylobacter rectus, Eikenella corrodens, Leptotrichia, and *Selenomonas* species, demonstrating that an individual is more likely to carry gram-negative bacteria and periodontal pathogens in healthy sites with increasing age [59, 81]. It is likely that the presence of these periodontal pathogens in healthy sites alters the host response, rendering these sites more susceptible to active disease in the future.

The microbiota associated with periodontal disease seems to display a significant enrichment in specific metabolic pathways, compatible with an oxygen poor environment, and the availability of amino acids and lipids as major carbon and nitrogen sources [82]. The unbalanced microbiota is rich in lipid-degradation pathways, as well as other known virulence-related activities, such as lipopolysaccharide (LPS) biosynthesis with local inflammatory effect [83].

The presence of pathogens within this community can lead to the clinical manifestations of periodontal disease, which in turn can lead to additional changes in the community due to the increased availability of nutrients released by the damaged tissue.

Although the bacteria rarely invade the tissues and cause acute infections (e.g., *Prevotella intermedia* invades both epithelial cells and macrophages), they could release substances that penetrate the gum and directly causes the tissue destruction by the enzymes and endotoxins action or indirectly through the induction and maintenance of the chronic inflammatory process, leading to the progressive destruction of collagen in the connective tissue that hold teeth in the gum [84, 85]. The presence of *P. gingivalis* and high colonization by *A. actinomycetemcomitans, T. denticola* and *P. intermedia* plays an important role in severe periodontitis.

The presence of *P. gingivalis* in the dental plaque biofilm results in the inhibition of components of the innate host defense system. This is caused by the lack of IL-8 that normally guides leukocytes to the site of bacterial colonization. In addition, E-selectin that facilitates leukocyte exit from the vasculature into surrounding tissue is absent. The local inhibition of these inflammatory mediators results in the lack of sufficient leukocytes to properly control dental plaque growth, proposed to be one of the major factors in the development of periodontitis. Also, it has been demonstrated that individuals co-infected with *T. denticola* and *P. intermedia* were more likely to have periodontitis than were those infected with a single pathogen [86].

Gram-negative bacteria in particular are known to release large amounts of cell wall material as outer membrane vesicles containing lipopolysaccharide, lipid and protein that are believed to represent a normal mechanism of membrane turnover. In addition, the release of membrane vesicles and cell wall fragments serves to protect bacteria in the biofilm by acting as decoys that bind and activate innate host defense components (i.e., alternative pathways of activation of complement system) and that would otherwise bind to the surface of viable bacteria and kill them; in the same time, the total amount of LPS and the consecutive inflammatory effect are increasing [59].

Lipopolysaccharide has been reported to pass through an intact epithelial cell barrier and concentrate around blood vessels in the *lamina propria*, interacting with nearly all cell types present in the periodontium, inducing a large increase in the numbers of leukocytes, especially neutrophils, in the sulcus or pocket, causing ulcerations [87]. At an early stage, the infiltrate is dominated by B and T (Th1 and Th2) lymphocytes. Subsequently, the lesion becomes dominated by B cells, and less T cells, macrophages and neutrophils, all of which becoming activated. As the disease worsens, periodontal pockets deepen, the components of the extracellular matrix of the gingiva and periodontal ligament are destroyed, and alveolar bone is desorbed [88]. On the other hand, bacterial LPS can subsequently interact with macrophage or dendritic cell receptors, including CD14 and TLRs, to stimulate the production of inflammatory cytokines, especially IL1, and other proinflammatory mediators [89].

The collagen and other components of the perivascular extracellular matrix are destroyed, by the release of lysosomal enzymes by phagocytes and the production of cytokines that stimulate the release of metalloproteinases (including collagenase) by connective tissue cells or cytokines that activate bone resorption [90]. Four distinct pathways may be involved with this destruction: plasminogen dependent, phagocytic, osteoclastic and matrix metalloproteinase (MMP) pathway which is the most prevalent, as revealed by the larger amounts of collagenase and gelatinase (MMP1, MMP2, MMP9, and MMP13) found in the crevicular gingival fluid of patients with periodontitis [91–93]. Cleavage of collagen I by MMP13 seems to be the initial step of the entire bone resorption process [94, 95], and subsequently, denatured collagen fragments are also degraded by gelatinases, MMP2 and MMP9 [96].

Several species, in the subgingival plaque constitution, produce volatile fatty acids (butyrate, propionate, and isobutirat) and peptide N-formyl-methionyl-leucyl-phenylalanine, as sulfide ions, hydrogen sulfide, and methyl mercaptan with cytotoxic effect on endothelial cells and gingival fibroblasts [97, 98].

The bacterial products and epithelial response activate perivascular mast cells to release histamine that activates vascular endothelial cells to release IL-8 within the vessels to assist in localizing neutrophils. B and T lymphocytes are activated by antigens or unspecific mitogens to proliferate and give rise to clones of effector cells; B cells are driven to differentiate into clones of antibody producing plasma cells [99, 100]. Bacterial material released in the periodontium provides thus a major form of communication between dental plaque and the host [78].

Bacteria could activate myeloid cells (e.g., monocytes or neutrophils) to elicit IL-1, and this cytokine then activates a nonmyeloid cell (e.g., fibroblasts, endothelial, or epithelial cells) to secrete additional inflammatory mediators, interleukins 6, 10 and 12, tumor necrosis factor alpha, prostaglandin E2, interferon gamma, and a series of chemotactic substances: monocyte chemoattractant protein, macrophage inflammatory protein, and RANTES (regulated on activation, normal T-cell expressed, and secreted) [88, 101].

After the trend of 1950s and early 1960s, when periodontal treatment was based on the nonspecific plaque hypothesis, criteria for defining periodontal pathogens have been developed.

In periodontal disease, the precise identification of certain organisms (e.g., a particular clone (JP2) of *Aggregatibacter actinomycetemcomitans*) is required to identify the risk factors for localized aggressive periodontitis in young adults. Taking into account the difficulties of periodonto-pathogen cultivation, new techniques have been developed in order to detect bacterial species associated with periodontal disease: PCR-based methods in single or multiplexed approaches, sequencing 16S rRNA gene fragments or a housekeeping gene, next-generation sequencing [102]. Now, the Human Oral Microbiome Database project is undergoing, which aims to catalog all bacterial species found in the oral cavity. However, the molecular techniques are limited to the detection of a selected number of pathogens, so other important disease factors arising from the deregulation of the local host response could be missed [103].

3. Mechanisms of dental plaque resistance to antimicrobials and strategies to fight them

Dental plaque displays properties that are typical for biofilms, being structurally and functionally organized polyspecific communities embedded in an extracellular matrix of exopolymers on mucosal and dental surfaces [104], functionally organized and benefiting of increased metabolic efficiency, pathogenic synergism and enhanced virulence, greater resistance to host stress factors and tolerance to all kind of antimicrobials [105].

Resistance to antibiotics (genetic or phenotypical, due to biofilm formation) is the most important cause of nonefficient therapy of biofilm-associated infections from the oral cavity, and it is multifactorial.

One of the main reasons for the antibiotics ineffectiveness against the periodontal pathogen bacteria is that they grow in biofilms, becoming increasingly powerful, aggressive, and difficult to destroy. The antibiotics effective doses and the minimum concentration to eradicate biofilms are very difficult to achieve *in vivo*, especially in the local treatments. Biofilm penetration by biocides or antibiotics is typically strongly hindered. To increase the efficiency of new treatment strategies against bacterial and fungal infections, factors that lead to biofilm growth inhibition, biofilm disruption, or biofilm eradication are being sought. These factors could include antibiotics, e.g., chlorhexidine, triclosan, povidone-iodine active against *P. gingivalis* and *F. nucleatum* biofilms [106]—azithromycin and other macrolides could block quorum sensing mechanism and the alginate polymer formation [107].

The widespread use of antibiotics has evolutionary and ecological consequences, leading to the recruitment of more genes into the *resistome* and *mobilome*, with adverse consequences for human welfare [108], so new approaches are urgently needed to help regain control over infectious diseases, including periodontal disease.

There are theories which support that horizontal gene transfer of resistance determinants can occur in the oral biofilm [109–112]. This strongly suggests that exchange of mobile genetic elements between commensals and pathogenic bacteria can contribute to the emergence of drug resistance in the oral cavity. Oral microbiota exhibits different resistance mechanisms, presumably due to the complex microbial interactions and the genetic fluidity in oral biofilms. The possibility of conjugation among oral bacteria using an erythromycin-resistant (Erm) shuttle plasmid, from *T. denticola* to *S. gordonii*, was revealed [112].

Amoxicillin and penicillin resistance have been described in *Veillonella* sp., *Fusobacterium*, and *Prevotella denticola* isolated from root canals [113, 114]. High levels of penicillin resistance have been demonstrated in the α-hemolytic streptococci (*Streptococcus mutans, S. salivarius, S.oralis,* and *S. mitis*) and represent a cause for concern.

Generally, the α-hemolytic streptococci are very highly resistant to cephalosporins; *Enterococcus* sp. isolated from root canal exudates patients with periodontal lesions revealed high-level of cephalosporins resistance [115]. In contrast, Kuriyama et al. found that the genera *Porphyromonas* and *Fusobacterium* showed susceptibility to all cephalosporins, while *Prevotella* species were highly resistant [114].

Mechanisms of metronidazole resistance include mutations in the enzymes responsible for reduction of the antibiotic to its active form, mutations resulting in decreased entry of the antibiotic into the cell and mutations in transporters causing the efflux of the antibiotic. These mechanisms have been demonstrated in different species, e.g., *Lactobacillus* sp., *Gemella morbillorum, Actinomyces israelii, Clostridium butyricum, Eikenella corrodens,* and *A. actinomycetemcomitans* [116]. Four genes, *nimA, nimB, nimC,* and *nimD,* chromosomal or plasmid located, able to confer moderate to high-level metronidazole resistance have been revealed in *Bacteroides* sp. [117].

Mechanisms of tetracycline resistance include efflux proteins, production of ribosome protection proteins, and enzymatic modification of the antibiotic. Tetracycline resistance is encoded by *tet* genes. Antibiotic profiling of α-hemolytic streptococci isolated from the oropharynx of healthy Greek children showed a high percent of tetracycline resistant isolates [118], the majority of isolates being represented by *S. mitis*. Okamoto et al. [119] studied the prevalence of *tetQ* gene in genus *Porphyromonas* and *Prevotella* sp. They have been demonstrated that *tet*(M) represented the most common gene, which encodes a ribosomal protection protein, carried on Tn916/Tn1545-like conjugative transposons in *Streptococcus sp., Granulicatella sp., Veillonella sp.* and *Neisseria* sp., from the oral cavity [120].

Resistance to erythromycin is commonly conferred by the acquisition of *erm* gene, antibiotic inactivation by an enzyme encoded by *mph*, and efflux of macrolides by an ATP-binding transporter encoded by *msrA* expressed by *S. aureus* isolates [116]. Low-level macrolide resistance in the oral microbiota may also be associated with the expression of genes from the *mef* family, encoding another efflux pump, and recently have been found on a conjugative transposon Tn*1207.3* in *Streptococcus pyogenes* [121]. There have been described [122] erythromycin-resistant α-hemolytic streptococci, such as *S. oralis*, *S. salivarius* and *S. sanguis* in healthy Greek children. *P. intermedia* isolates carried erm(F) alone or tetQ alone, but in other oral anaerobes, macrolide resistance often occurred in conjunction with tetracycline resistance. In *Gemella* sp. and commensal viridans streptococci isolates from oral cavity, macrolide resistance was associated with the *aphA-3* gene [123].

There are studies which support that the resistance to chlorhexidine resistance in *Streptococcus mutans* and S. *sobrinus* isolates from dental plague is plasmid-mediated [124, 125].

Bacteria growing in biofilms often exhibit differing phenotypes compared with their counterpart, respectively planktonic or free cells. There have been described numerous mechanisms for the differences in antibiotic susceptibilities in biofilms relative to planktonic state growth cells. Among these, there have been demonstrated by several studies that oxygen limitation [126], antibiotic penetration into the biofilm [127], the presence of persister cells [128], biofilm-associated cells that grow significantly more slowly than planktonic cells and, as a result, take up antimicrobial agents more slowly [83], and also the maturity of the biofilm might also be important contributors to increased resistance. Results of previous studies have demonstrated also other important mechanisms responsible for resistance to antibiotics [129]: biofilm growth is associated with an increased number of mutations, leading to generation of antibiotic-resistant phenotypes of bacteria, and genes involved in antibiotic resistance are correlated with biofilm phenotype [130]; the production of the exopolysaccharide matrix contributes to an increased cell survival by slowing down antimicrobial diffusion speed; and the differences in metabolic activity among bacteria. It has been revealed that slow-growing and nongrowing bacteria contribute to increased biofilm resistance to antibiotics [131]. The up-regulation of efflux pump proteins and activation of quorum sensing systems reduces and neutralizes incoming antibiotics.

Altered gene expression represents another difference between bacteria grown in biofilms compared with planktonic cells. There are numerous genes that are either positively or negatively regulated by the complex regulatory networks, efflux pumps when the bacteria are growing as a biofilm compared with planktonic cultures [132, 133].

Numerous plants are used in traditional medicine against various diseases. Furthermore, plant extracts have pronounced antimicrobial activities when used at sub-inhibitory concentrations, which are usually very low concentrations with minimal or no effect against host cells. Using sub-inhibitory concentrations of an antimicrobial compound, namely concentrations which do not interfere with bacteria growth, but only with their behavior, leads to reduced risk of developing resistance to that compound. The most recent strategies propose the targeting of communication control, as QS signaling, since quorum sensing is not an essential process, and QS mutants in general have not displayed growth defects, but this signaling controls virulence and biofilms. The quorum sensing mechanism involves the production, release and detection of chemical signaling molecules, which permits communication between microbial cells and gene expression regulation in a cell-density-dependent manner. Granted, interfering with the regulation of virulence factor production developing resistance mechanisms against quorum-inhibiting therapies, may be a difficult proposition for bacteria, which could help promote long-term efficacy of anti-QS therapies [134].

Recent studies revealed that numerous plant-derived compounds and essential oils (EOs) exhibit increased antimicrobial properties, by interfering with QS controlled phenotypes such as adherence, biofilm, formation, motility and pigment production, affecting also antibiotic susceptibility, or revealing microbiostatic properties [135–137]. Not only plant extracts, but also propolis extracts have proved to possess a broad spectrum activity against various gram-positive and gram-negative bacteria: *Staphylococcus* spp., *Streptococcus* spp., *Listeria* spp., *Bacillus* spp., *Enterobacteria* (*Klebsiella pneumoniae*, *Escherichia coli*), *Pseudomonas aeruginosa*, and *Helicobacter pylori* [138, 139]. The antibacterial activity of propolis is mainly correlated with caffeic acids, flavonoids, phenolic esters, and aromatic compounds [140].

Relatively few research works on propolis ability to inhibit biofilm formation have been published. Duarte et al. have shown that propolis inhibits the growth of oral microorganisms and the activity of bacteria-derived glucosyltransferases (GTFs), responsible for glucan synthesis which favors bacterial adhesion and plays an essential role in the development of pathogenic dental plaque [141]. Bulman et al. showed that propolis contains compounds that inhibit signaling mediated by N-acyl-homoserin-lactone in *Pseudomonas aeruginosa PAO1* [142]. Our studies have shown that the 30% Romanian propolis tincture presented antibacterial activity toward *S. aureus, E. coli, K. pneumoniae* and *P. aeruginosa*, and antibiofilm activity against *S. aureus*) [139]. Associated with the use of some antibiotics, the efficacy and duration of propolis extract action is more pronounced, and these organisms do not develop antibiotics resistance, as demonstrated for dexpanthenol associated with propolis against *P. aeruginosa* and *S. aureus* strains isolated from infected wounds.

These data confirm that natural extracts have anti-QS, antiseptic, and antivirulence properties and can easily inhibit biofilm formation as well as disrupt the mature biofilm structure. Thus, plant and/or bee extracts in combination with other antimicrobial strategies could provide an effective microbicidal tool for the treatment of various bacterial and yeast infections. However, due to difficulties in cultivating anaerobic periodontal pathogens, there are only few studies concerning the efficiency of vegetal extracts against periodontal pathogenic strains. Chifiriuc et al. (2009) demonstrated that usnic acid selectively inhibited the biofilm development by Gram-positive bacteria and the expression of hemolytic properties of strains isolated from the dental plaque [143].

It has been shown that mouthwash with essential oils (EO) might be a reliable alternative to chlorhexidine (CHX) for controlling gingival inflammation, dental plaque development, bacteremia with anaerobic bacteria in patients with mild-to-moderate gingivitis and oral malodor [144, 145]. Moreover, the diluted EO displayed no detectable detrimental effects on human gingival and periodontal ligament fibroblasts, while diluted CHX reduced both cell migration and long-term survival [146]. The regular long-term use of the EO-based mouth rinse improved the efficacy of a 0.05% cetylpyridinium chloride- and fluoride-containing mouth rinse [144]. Linalool and α-terpineol exhibited strong antimicrobial activity against periodontopathic and cariogenic bacteria [147]. *Salvadora persica* root stick extracts and its active component benzyl isothiocyanate are very efficient against oral pathogens involved in periodontal disease as well as against other gram-negative bacteria [148]. The adjunctive use of EO has been shown to promote significant clinical attachment level gain and probing pocket depth reduction in deep residual pockets [149]. A gel containing 10% *Lippiasidoides* (LS) was evaluated and has been shown to reduce plaque, bleeding, and gingival index within the experimental period of 21 days [150].

These scientific data suggest that the antibiofilm compounds should be used in various combinations, in order to develop innovative early combinatory strategies [151] which may potentially strongly support classical treatments and cause an increase of their effectiveness in case of chronic infections, such the periodontal ones.

Other strategies in the improvement of the biological activity used in the management of periodontal diseases are based on the encapsulation of therapeutic drugs in appropriate shuttles. Drug delivery by liposomes with different encapsulated bioactive molecules (such as bacteriocins, enzymes, antiseptics, antibiotics, and vegetal compounds) can assure a controlled delivery of some antimicrobial substances at infection's situs, with a great efficiency in dental caries and every other biofilm-associated infection [152]. Encapsulation technologies, which may shield substances such as nisin from degradation by digestive enzymes and effectively deliver the encapsulated contents at the same time, represent new direction in the field of preventive medicine [153].

4. Future perspectives for the therapeutic management of periodontitis

Despite numerous current approaches, periodontitis still remains one of the most common disease, causing moderate-to-very-severe health damage and complications in a high number of individuals. Perspectives for future and advanced therapies aiming for efficient management of periodontal conditions flourished in the last decade, and the recent progress in science and technology made possible a wide range of novel approaches to be successfully applied.

4.1. Periodontal tissue regenerative therapy

This approach was formulated in 1993 by Langer, who proposed tissue engineering as a possible technique for regenerating lost periodontal tissues. This rapidly emerging research field represents the interface between materials science and biocompatibility and integrates cells, natural, or synthetic scaffolds, and specific signals to obtain new tissues [154].

Tissue engineering applied for bone and periodontal regeneration combines three key elements to enhance regeneration: use of progenitor cells, design of scaffolds or supporting matrixes, and selection of suitable signaling molecules. Cell sources of progenitor cells may be represented by periodontal ligament-derived cells, periodontal ligament-derived mesenchymal stromal cells, periosteal cells, gingival epithelium and fibroblast cells but also bone marrow–derived mesenchymal stem cells [154].

Scaffolds and supporting matrices are required to offer a three-dimensional (3D) support and assist periodontal tissue regeneration. These structures have important roles, such as: (1) suitable framework, which maintains the shape of the defect; (2) physical support for the healing area, so that there is no collapse of the surrounding tissue into the wound site; (3) 3D substratum for cellular adhesion, migration, proliferation and production of extracellular matrix; (4) selective barrier to restrict cellular migration; and (5) delivery vehicle for growth factors and differentiation molecules [154]. Biomaterials utilized for efficient scaffolds are very diverse, and they may be included in various categories, such as: ceramics (i.e., hydroxy-apatite, beta tricalcium phosphate), polymers (i.e., synthetic: polyglycolic acid, polylactic acid and polycaprolactone; natural: collagen fibrin, albumin, hyaluronic acid, cellulose, chitosan, polyhydroxyalkanoates, alginate, agarose, polyamino acids, etc.), and synthetic polyesters (i.e., polyglycolic acid, polylactic acid and polylactic-co-glycolic acid) [155].

In order to increase efficiency, regenerative therapy relies on the incorporation of various bioactive molecules into scaffolding materials, to improve cellular development and tissue healing. The incorporation of specific bioactive molecules within the scaffold is aiming to ensure a sustained and controlled release of bioactive molecules for longer periods of time. These bioactive molecules can be incorporated directly into the scaffolding material or with along with a delivery vector, which ensures its stability and controlled release.

The most utilized bioactive molecules to be integrated in scaffolds designed for periodontal tissue regenerative therapy are as follows: platelet-derived growth factor (potent mediator of periodontal tissue regeneration, currently approved for the treatment of periodontal defects—commercially available as Gem-21 (Osteohealth, Shirley, NY)); fibroblast growth factor (which has a profound effect on periodontal soft tissue and bone healing and also stimulates angiogenesis) [156]; bone morphogenetic proteins (disulfide-linked homodimer that promotes periodontal healing) [157]; insulin-like growth factor (which has mitogenic effects on periodontal ligament fibroblastic cells and can stimulate the synthesis of DNA in periodontal ligament fibroblasts) [158]; transforming growth factor beta (act as bone coupling factor linking bone resorption to bone formation) [159]; and periodontal ligament-derived growth factor (it is a highly specific autocrine chemotactic agent for human periodontal ligament cells, which is 1000-fold more potent than many known growth factors, and has no chemotactic effect on gingival fibroblast or epithelial cells, thereby promising its utility for biological therapeutic regime needed for cell-specific periodontal regeneration) [159].

Recent progress in tissue engineering has allowed the delivery of such molecular factors by various means. Gene therapy and nano-delivery represent the most investigated approaches for the delivery of bio-active molecules, useful for regenerative medicine applied for periodontal disease.

4.2. Gene therapy

Gene therapy presents certain advantages when compared to other therapies. Because both cell transplantation and laboratory cell culturing are not needed, gene therapy may be safer and more cost-effective than cell-based therapies [154, 160]. Platelet-derived growth factor and bone morphogenetic proteins are the most utilized for delivery in periodontal regenerative therapy. Plasmid and circular vector-based delivery of platelet-derived growth factor proved safety favorable characteristics for clinical use. Moreover, the expression of platelet-derived growth factor genes was prolonged for up to 10 days in gingival wounds, when administered through this approach. It seems that continuous exposure of cementoblasts to platelet-derived growth factor has inhibitory effect on cementum mineralization, possible via the upregulation of osteopontin and subsequent enhancement of multinucleated giant cells in cementum-engineered scaffolds [161].

The delivery of genes that encode the bone morphogenetic proteins stimulate the formation of periodontal tissue formation. Moreover, the expression of this gene promoted successful regeneration of alveolar bone defects around dental implants [161]. Ribonucleic acid mediated silencing, a novel approach, is based on the principle of RNA interference (RNAi), a novel mechanism of action whereby the expression of certain genes detrimental to the tissue regeneration process is silenced by RNAs. The first siRNA-based therapeutic tested in human clinical trials was the vascular endothelial growth factor (VEGF)–targeted RNA for the treatment of macular degeneration of the retina. Tumor necrosis factor-α-targeted siRNA can suppress osteolysis induced by metal particles in a murine calvaria model, opening the way to the application of RNAi in orthopedic and dental implant therapy [162]. The use of RNA-based therapeutics for tissue regeneration is still in its early stages. Nevertheless, RNAi promises to be an effective therapeutic tool and may be successful in periodontal regeneration [154].

5. Conclusions

Dental plaque is a model of polyspecific biofilm, very studied mainly due to its accessibility, but also to its implications in dental caries, periodontitis, and periodontal disease—this one being an irreversible affection once launched, very spread in the world. It is of great interest for the field of dentistry and for medicine too, due to its complications, more or less severe, local and at distance too, infectious and noninfectious. A lot of scientific knowledge is accumulated, and therapeutically progresses are done in this field, but the topic still needs improvements and remains a challenge.

Studies have shown that almost all forms of the periodontal disease are consequences of the dental plaque biofilms and of chronic, nonspecific or specific bacterial infections and chronic inflammation too. Along with dental plaque, the occurrence of periodontal diseases is influenced by numerous other factors, such as the virulence and resistance mechanisms of involved microbial species but also host-related factors. Understanding the complex organization of dental plaque biofilms, the interactions between commensal and pathogenic species in this community but also the relation with the host is vital for elucidating the mechanisms of periodontal diseases and drawing novel therapeutic perspectives.

Although traditional preventive and therapeutic approaches relying on adequate hygiene, mechanical removal of the dental plaque, surgery, and antibiotic treatment are still widely utilized, recent strategies propose the utilization of numerous modern techniques to specifically target particular aspects of periodontal disease. Their implementation depends on the extensive knowledge regarding intimate biological parameters of various periodontal conditions and could be more effective in both the prevention and therapy of such diseases.

Author details

Veronica Lazar[1,2], Lia-Mara Ditu[1,2]*, Carmen Curutiu[1,2], Irina Gheorghe[1,2], Alina Holban[1,2], Marcela Popa[2] and Carmen Chifiriuc[1,2]

*Address all correspondence to: lia_mara_d@yahoo.com

1 Department of Microbiology and Immunology, Faculty of Biology, University of Bucharest, Bucharest, Romania

2 Research Institute of the University of Bucharest, Bucharest, Romania

References

[1] Singh S, Sharma P, Shreehari AK. Dental plaque biofilm: An invisible terror in the oral cavity. In: Méndez-Vilas A, editor. The Battle Against Microbial Pathogens: Basic Science, Technological Advances and Educational Programs. 2015; pp. 422-428; Formatex Research Center, C/ Zurbaran 1, 2nd floor office 1, Badajoz 06002 Spain

[2] Lazar V., Bezirtzoglou E. Microbial biofilms. In Medical Sciences, Encyclopedia of life support systems (EOLSS) Publishing, France (2011); pp. 1-44. http://www.eolss.net/Sample-Chapters/C03/E6-59-89-00

[3] Avila M, Ojcius DM, Yilmaz O. The oral microbiota: Living with a permanent guest. DNA and Cell Biology. 2009;**28**(8):405-411

[4] Lazar V, Chifiriuc C, Bucur M, Burlibasa M, Sfeatcu R, Stanciu G, Savu B, Traistaru T, Cernat R, Suciu I, Suciu N. Investigation of dental-plaque formers biofilms by optic and confocal laser scanning microscopy and microbiological tools. Revista Medico-Chirurgicală a Societăţii de Medici şi Naturalişti din Iaşi. 2008;**112**(3):812-820

[5] Marsh PD, Moter A, Devine DA. Dental plaque biofilms: Communities, conflict and control. Periodontology 2000. 2011;**55**:16-35

[6] Noiri Y, Li L, Ebisu S. The localization of periodontal-disease-associated bacteria in human periodontal pockets. Journal of Dental Research. 2001;**80**(10):1930-1934

[7] Ismail FB, Ismail G, Dumitriu AS, Baston C, Berbecar V, Jurubita R, Andronesi A, Dumitriu HT, Sinescu I. Identification of subgingival periodontal pathogens and association with the severity of periodontitis in patients with chronic kidney diseases: A cross-sectional study. BioMed Research International. 2015;**2015**:370314

[8] Kesic L, Milasin J, Igic M, Obradovic R. Microbial etiology of periodontal disease. Medicine and Biology. 2008;**15**:1-6

[9] Scottish Dental. Prevention and Treatment of Periodontal Diseases in Primary Care Dental Clinical Guidance. 2014. ISBN: 978 1 905829 17 0. Available from: http://www.sdcep.org. uk/wp-content/uploads/2015/01/SDCEP+Periodontal+Disease+Full+Guidance.pdf

[10] Murakami S. Emerging regenerative approaches for periodontal regeneration: The future perspective of cytokine therapy and stem cell therapy. Interface Oral Health Science; Springer International Publishing AG. Part of Springer Nature, Romania 2016. pp. 135-14

[11] Aimetti M. Nonsurgical periodontal treatment. International Journal of Esthetic Dentistry. 2014;**9**(2):251-267

[12] Gupta G, Mansi B. Ozone therapy in periodontics. Journal of Medicine and Life. 2012;**5**(1):59-67

[13] Kovács V, Tihanyi D, Gera I. The incidence of local plaque retentive factors in chronic periodontitis. Fogorvosi Szemle. 2007;**100**(6):295-300

[14] Yousefimanesh H, Amin M, Robati M, Goodarzi H, Otoufi M. Comparison of the antibacterial properties of three mouthwashes containing chlorhexidine against oral microbial plaques: An in vitro study. Jundishapur Journal of Microbiology. 2015;**8**(2):e17341

[15] Zandbergen D, Slot DE, Niederman R, Van der Weijden FA. The concomitant administration of systemic amoxicillin and metronidazole compared to scaling and root planning alone in treating periodontitis: A systematic review. BMC Oral Health. 2016;**16**:27

[16] Davies SJ, Gray RJM, Lindenb GJ, James JA. Occlusal considerations in periodontics. British Dental Journal. 2001;**191**:597-604

[17] Miglani S, Aggarwal V, Ahuja B. Dentin hypersensitivity: Recent trends in management. Journal of Conservative Dentistry. 2010;**13**(4):218-224

[18] Gulati M, Anand V, Govila V, Jain N. Host modulation therapy: An indispensable part of perioceutics. Journal of Indian Society of Periodontology. 2014;**18**(3):282-288

[19] Chawla TN, Nanda RS, Kapoor KK. Dental prophylaxis procedures in control of periodontal disease in Lucknow (rural) India. Journal of Periodontology. 1975;**46**(8):498-503

[20] Lederberg J, Mccray AT. 'Ome sweet 'omics—A genealogical treasury of words. Scientist. 2001;**15**:8-10

[21] Marsh PD, Head DA, Devine DA. Prospects of oral disease control in the future—An opinion. Journal of Oral Microbiology. 2014;**6**:26176. DOI: 10.3402/jom.v6.26176

[22] Kilian M, Chapple ILC, Hannig M, Marsh PD, Meuric V, Pedersen AML, Tonetti MS, Wade WG, Zaura E. The oral microbiome—An update for oral healthcare professionals. British Dental Journal. 2016;**221**:657-666

[23]   Faran Ali SM, Tanwir F. Oral microbial habitat a dynamic entity. Journal of Oral Biology and Craniofacial Research. 2012;**2**(3):181-187

[24]   Belkaid Y, Hand T. Role of the microbiota in immunity and inflammation. Cell. 2014;**157**(1):121-141. DOI: 10.1016/j.cell.2014.03.011

[25]   Smith DJ, Taubman MA. Ontogeny of immunity to oral microbiota in humans. Critical Reviews in Oral Biology & Medicine. 1992;**3**(1-2):109-133

[26]   Fitzsimmons SP, Evans MK, Pearce CL, Sheridan MJ, Wientzen R, Cole MF. Immunoglobulin A subclasses in infants' saliva and in saliva and milk from their mothers. Journal of Pediatrics. 1994;**124**(4):566-573

[27]   Fagerås M, Tomičić S, Voor T, Björkstén B, Jenmalm MC. Slow salivary secretory IgA maturation may relate to low microbial pressure and allergic symptoms in sensitized children. Pediatric Research. 2011;**70**:572-577. DOI: 10.1203/PDR.0b013e318232169e

[28]   Smith DJ, Taubman MA. Emergence of immune competence in saliva. Critical Reviews in Oral Biology and Medicine. 1993;**4**(3/4):335-341

[29]   Nogueira RD, Talarico Sesso MC, Castro Loureiro Borges M, Mattos-Graner RO, Smith DJ, Paes Leme Ferriani V. Salivary IgA antibody responses to *Streptococcus mitis* and *Streptococcus mutans* in preterm and fullterm newborn children. Archives of Oral Biology. 2012;**57**(6):647-653

[30]   Fábián TK, Hermann P, Beck A, Fejérdy P, Fábián G. Salivary defense proteins: Their network and role in innate and acquired oral immunity. International Journal of Molecular Sciences. 2012;**13**(4):4295-4320

[31]   Actor JK, Hwang SA, Kruzel ML. Lactoferrin as a natural immune modulator. Current Pharmaceutical Design. 2009;**15**(17):1956-1973

[32]   Siqueiros-Cendón T, Arévalo-Gallegos S, Iglesias-Figueroa BF, García-Montoya IA. Immunomodulatory effects of lactoferrin. Acta Pharmacologica Sinica. 2014;**35**(5): 557-566

[33]   García-Montoya IA, Cendón TS, Arévalo-Gallegos S, Rascón-Cruz Q. Lactoferrin a multiple bioactive protein: An overview. Acta Pharmacologica Sinica. 2014;**35**(5):557-566

[34]   Bafort F, Parisi O, Perraudin JP, Jijakli MH. Mode of action of lactoperoxidase as related to its antimicrobial activity: A review. Enzyme Research. 2014;**2014**:517164. DOI: 10.1155/2014/517164

[35]   Welk A, Meller C, Schubert R, Schwahn C, Kramer A, Below H. Effect of lactoperoxidase on the antimicrobial effectiveness of the thiocyanate hydrogen peroxide combination in a quantitative suspension test. BMC Microbiology. 2009. Available from: http://bmcmicrobiol.biomedcentral.com/articles/10.1186/1471-2180-9-134 [open access]

[36]   Jang WS, Edgerton M. Salivary histatins: Structure, function, and mechanisms of antifungal activity. In Calderone R, Clancy C (ed), Candida and Candidiasis, Second Edition. ASM Press, Washington, DC. DOI: 10.1128/9781555817176.ch13

[37] Melino S, Santone C, Di Nardo P, Sarkar B. Histatins: Salivary peptides with copper(II)- and zinc(II)-binding motifs: Perspectives for biomedical applications. FEBS Journal. 2014;**281**(3):657-672

[38] Sugawara S, Uehara A, Tamai R, Takada H. Innate immune responses in oral mucosa. Journal of Endotoxin Research. 2002;**8**(6):465-468

[39] Gupta G. Gingival crevicular fluid as a periodontal diagnostic indicator-I: Host derived enzymes and tissue breakdown products. Journal of Medicine and Life. 2012;**5**(4):390-397

[40] Taylor JJ, Preshaw PM. Gingival crevicular fluid and saliva. Periodontology 2000. 2016;**70**(1):7-10

[41] Champagne CME, Buchanan W. Potential for gingival crevice fluid measures as predictors of risk for periodontal diseases. Periodontology 2000. 2003;**31**:167-180

[42] Gupta G. Gingival crevicular fluid as a periodontal diagnostic indicator-II: Inflammatory mediators, host-response modifiers and chair side diagnostic aids. Journal of Medicine and Life. 2013;**6**(1):7-13

[43] Rahnama M, Czupkałło L, Kozicka-Czupkałło M, Łobacz M. Gingival crevicular fluid—Composition and clinical importance in gingivitis and periodontitis. Polish Journal of Public Health. 2014;**124**(2):96-98. ISSN: 2083-4829 (online). DOI: 10.2478/pjph-2014-0022

[44] Linden SK, Sutton P, Karlsson NG, Korolik V, McGuckin MA. Mucins in the mucosal barrier to infection. Mucosal Immunology. 2008;**1**:183-197

[45] Hans M, Hans MV. Epithelial antimicrobial peptides: Guardian of the oral cavity. International Journal of Peptides. 2014;**2014**:370297

[46] Premratanachai P, Joly S, Johnson GK, McCray PB Jr, Jia HP, Guthmiller JM. Expression and regulation of novel human β-defensins in gingival keratinocytes. Oral Microbiology and Immunology. 2004;**19**(2):111-117

[47] Dale BA, Kimball JR, Krisanaprakornkit S, Roberts F, Robinovitch M, O'Neal R, Valore EV, Ganz T, Anderson GM, Weinberg A. Localized antimicrobial peptide expression in human gingiva. Journal of Periodontal Research. 2001;**36**(5):285-294

[48] Bachrach G, Chaushu G, Zigmond M, Yefenof E, Stabholz A, Shapira J, Merrick J, Chaushu S. Salivary LL-37 secretion in individuals with down syndrome is normal. Journal of Dental Research. 2006;**85**(10):933-936

[49] Dhas BBD, Vishnu Bhat B, Bahubali Gane D. Role of calprotectin in infection and inflammation. Current Pediatric Research. 2012;**16**(2):83-94

[50] Damo SM, Kehl-Fie TE, Sugitani N, Holta ME, Rathia S, Murphya WJ, Zhangb Y, Betzc C, Hencha L, Fritzc G, Skaarb EP, Chazina WJ. Molecular basis for manganese sequestration by calprotectin and roles in the innate immune response to invading bacterial pathogens. Proceedings of the National Academy of Sciences of the United States of America. 2013;**110**(10):3841-3846

[51] Sugawara Y, Uehara A, Fujimoto Y, Kusumoto S, Fukase K, Shibata K, Sugawara S, Sasano T, Takada H. Toll-like receptors, NOD1, and NOD2 in oral epithelial cells. Journal of Dental Research. 2006;**85**(6):524-529

[52] Ren L, Leung WK, Darveau RP, Jin L. The expression profile of lipopolysaccharide-binding protein, membrane-bound CD14, and toll-like receptors 2 and 4 in chronic periodontitis. Journal of Periodontology. 2005;**76**(11):1950-1959

[53] Mahanonda R, Sa-Ard-Iam N, Montreekachon P, Pimkhaokham A, Yongvanichit K, Fukuda MM, Pichyangkul S. IL-8 and IDO expression by human gingival fibroblasts via TLRs. Journal of Immunology. 2007;**178**(2):1151-1157

[54] Dixon DR, Reife RA, Cebra JJ, Darveau RP. Commensal bacteria influence innate status within gingival tissues: A pilot study. Journal of Periodontology. 2004;**75**:1486-1492

[55] Orozco A, Gemmell E, Bickel M, Seymour GJ. Interleukin-1beta, interleukin-12 and interleukin-18 levels in gingival fluid and serum of patients with gingivitis and periodontitis. Oral Microbiology and Immunology. 2006;**21**(4):256-260

[56] Kumar A, Begum N, Prasad S, Lamba AK, Verma M, Agarwal S, Sharma S. Role of cytokines in development of pre-eclampsia associated with periodontal disease—Cohort study. Journal of Clinical Periodontology. 2014;**41**:357-365. DOI: 10.1111/jcpe.12226

[57] Coats SR, Pham TT, Bainbridge BW, Reife RA, Darveau RP. MD-2 mediates the ability of tetra-acylated and penta-acylated lipopolysaccharides to antagonize *Escherichia coli* lipopolysaccharide at the TLR4 signaling complex. Journal of Immunology. 2005;**175**:4490-4498

[58] Coats SR, Do CT, Karimi-Naser LM, Braham PH, Darveau RP. Antagonistic lipopolysaccharides block *E. coli* lipopolysaccharide function at human TLR4 via interaction with the human MD-2 lipopolysaccharide binding site. Cellular Microbiology. 2007;**9**:1191-1202. DOI: 10.1111/j.1462-5822.2006.00859

[59] Darveau RP. Periodontitis: A polymicrobial disruption of host homeostasis. Nature Reviews Microbiology. 2010;**8**:481-490. DOI: 10.1038/nrmicro2337

[60] Hasegawa Y, Tribble GD, Baker HV, Mans JJ, Handfield M, Lamont RJ. Role of *Porphyromonas gingivalis* SerB in gingival epithelial cell cytoskeletal remodeling and cytokine production. Infection and Immunity. 2008;**76**:2420-2427. DOI: 10.1128/IAI.00156-08

[61] Dixon DR, Bainbridge BW, Darveau RP. Modulation of the innate immune response within the periodontium. Periodontology 2000. 2004;**35**:53-74

[62] Ji Y, Ferracci G, Warley A, Ward M, Leung KY, Samsuddin S, Leveque C, Queen L, Reebye V, Pal P, Gkaliagkousi E, Seager M, Ferro A. β-Actin regulates platelet nitric oxide synthase 3 activity through interaction with heat shock protein 90. Proceedings of the National Academy of Sciences of the United States of America. 2007;**104**(21):8839-44

[63] Kornman KS, Page RC, Tonetti MS. The host response to the microbial challenge in periodontitis: Assembling the players. Periodontology 2000. 1997;**14**:33-53

[64] Moughal NA, Adonogianaki E, Thornhill MH, Kinane DF. Endothelial cell leukocyte adhesion molecule-1 (ELAM-1) and intercellular adhesion molecule-1 (ICAM-1) expression in gingival tissue during health and experimentally-induced gingivitis. Journal of Periodontal Research. 1992;**27**(6):623-630

[65] Tonetti MS. Molecular factors associated with compartmentalization of gingival immune responses and transepithelial neutrophil migration. Journal of Periodontal Research. 1997;**32**(1 Pt 2):104-109

[66] Lu Q, Samaranayake LP, Darveau RP, Jin L. Expression of human beta-defensin-3 in gingival epithelia. Journal of Periodontal Research. 2005;**40**(6):474-481

[67] Darveau RP. The oral microbial consortium's interaction with the periodontal innate defense system. DNA and Cell Biology. 2009;**28**(8):389-395

[68] Tonetti MS, Imboden MA, Lang NP. Neutrophil migration into the gingival sulcus is associated with transepithelial gradients of interleukin-8 and ICAM-1. Journal of Periodontology. 1998;**69**(10):1139-1147

[69] Challacombe, S J; Shirlaw, P J; Mestecky, J (Editor); Lamm, M E (Editor); Strober, W (Editor); Bienenstock, J (Editor); McGhee, J R (Editor); Mayer, L (Editor) / Immunology of diseases of the oral cavity. Chapter 89. Local immune responses in tuberculosis. Academic Press UK, 2005. p. 1517-1546

[70] Hajishengallis G. Complement and periodontitis. Biochemical Pharmacology. 2010;**80**(12): 1992-2001

[71] Wang M, Krauss JL, Domon H, Hosur KB, Liang S, Magotti P, Triantafilou M, Triantafilou K, Lambris JD, Hajishengallis G. Microbial hijacking of complement-toll-like receptor crosstalk. Science Signaling. 2010;**3**(109):ra11

[72] Imamura R, Wang Y, Kinoshita T, Suzuki M, Noda T, Sagara J, Taniguchi S, Okamoto H, Suda T. Anti-inflammatory activity of PYNOD and its mechanism in humans and mice. Journal of Immunology. 2010;**184**:5874-5884

[73] Popadiak K, Potempa J, Riesbeck K, Blom AM. Biphasic effect of gingipains from *Porphyromonas gingivalis* on the human complement system. Journal of Immunology. 2007;**178**(11):7242-7250

[74] Zaura E, ten Cate JM. Towards understanding oral health. Caries Research. 2015;**49**(Suppl 1):55-61

[75] Marsh PD, Head DA, Devine DA. Ecological approaches to oral biofilms: Control without killing. Caries Research. 2015;**49**(Suppl 1):46-54

[76] Loesche WJ. Chemotherapy of dental plaque infections. Oral Science Reviews. 1976;**9**:65-107

[77] Petersen PE, Lennon MA. Effective use of fluorides for the prevention of dental caries in the 21st century: The WHO approach. Community Dentistry and Oral Epidemiology. 2004;**32**(5):319-321

[78] Darveau RP, Tanner A, Page RC. The microbial challenge in periodontitis. Periodontology 2000. 1997;**14**:12-32

[79] Hajishengallis G. Immunomicrobial pathogenesis of periodontitis: Keystones, pathobionts, and host response. Trends in Immunology. 2014;**35**(1):3-11

[80] Marsh PD, Martin MV. Oral Microbiology. 5th ed. Edinburgh: Churchill Livingstone; 2009

[81] Carrouel F, Viennot S, Santamaria J, Veber P, Bourgeois D. Quantitative molecular detection of 19 major pathogens in the interdental biofilm of periodontally healthy young adults. Frontiers in Microbiology. 2016;**7**:840. DOI: 10.3389/fmicb.2016.00840

[82] Mason MR, Preshaw PM, Nagaraja HN, Dabdoub SM, Rahman A, Kumar PS. The subgingival microbiome of clinically healthy current and never smokers. ISME Journal. 2015;**9**(1):268-272

[83] Donlan RM, Costerton JW. Biofilms: Survival mechanisms of clinically relevant microorganisms. Clinical Microbiology Reviews. 2002;**15**:167

[84] Page RC. Host response tests for diagnosing periodontal diseases. Journal of Periodontology. 1992;**63**:356-366

[85] Page RC. The role of inflammatory mediators in the pathogenesis of periodontal disease. Journal of Periodontal Research. 1991;**26**:230-242

[86] Torrungruang K, Jitpakdeebordin S, Charatkulangkun O, Gleebbua Y. *Porphyromonas gingivalis, Aggregatibacter actinomycetemcomitans*, and *Treponema denticola/Prevotella intermedia* co-infection are associated with severe periodontitis in a Thai population. PLoS One. 2015;**10**(8):e0136646. DOI: 10.1371/journal. pone.0136646

[87] Silva N, Abuslem L, Bravo D, Dutzan N, Garcia-Sesnich J, Hernández M, Gamonal J. Host response mechanisms in periodontal diseases. Journal of Applied Oral Science. 2015;**23**(3):329-55. DOI: 10.1590/1678-775720140259

[88] Kornman K, Roy S, Page C, Tonetti M. The host response to the microbial challenge in periodontitis: Assembling the players. Periodontology 2000. 1997;**14**:12-32

[89] Bascones-Martínez A, Muñoz-Corcuera M, Noronha S, Mota P, Bascones-Ilundain C, Campo-Trapero J. Host defence mechanisms against bacterial aggression in periodontal disease: Basic mechanisms. Medicina Oral Patologia Oral y Cirugia Bucal. 2009;**14**:680-685

[90] Nalini HE, Mathew S, Padmanaban J, Sundaram E, Devi Ramamoorthy R. Perioceutics: Matrix metalloproteinase inhibitors as an adjunctive therapy for inflammatory periodontal disease. Journal of Pharmacy and Bioallied Sciences. 2012;**4**(Suppl 2):S417-S421

[91] Birkedal-Hansen H. Role of matrix metalloproteinase in human periodontal diseases. Journal of Periodontology. 1993;**64**(5 Suppl):474-484

[92] Ejeil AL, Igondjo-Tchen S, Ghomrasseni S, Pellat B, Godeau G, Gogly B. Expression of matrix metalloproteinases (MMPs) and tissue inhibitors of metalloproteinases (TIMPs) in healthy and disease human gingiva. Journal of Periodontology. 2003;**74**:188-195

[93] Kim S, Ahn SH, Lee JS, Song JE, Cho SH, Jung S, Kim SK, Kim SH, Lee KP, Kwon KS, Lee TH. Differential matrix metalloprotease (MMP) expression profiles found in aged gingiva. PLoS One. 2016;**11**(7):e0158777 [Epub: July 8, 2016]

[94] Inui T, Ishibashi O, Origane Y, Fujimori K, Kokubo T, Nakajima M. Matrix metalloproteinases and lysosomal cysteine proteases in osteoclasts contribute to bone resorption through distinct modes of action. Biochemical and Biophysical Research Communications. 1999;**29**:173-178

[95] Séguier S, Gogly B, Bodineau A, Godeau G, Brousse N. Is collagen breakdown during periodontitis linked to inflammatory cells and expression of matrix metalloproteinases and tissue inhibitors of metalloproteinases in human gingival tissue. Journal of Periodontology. 2001;**72**:1398-1406

[96] Talic NF. The mechanisms of mineralized tissue resorption by clast cells in relation to orthodontic tooth movement and root resorption. Journal of Dentistry and Oral Biology. 2016;**1**(3):1014

[97] Ready D, D'Aiuto F, Spratt DA, Suvan J, Tonetti MS, Wilson M. Disease severity associated with presence in subgingival plaque of *Porphyromonas gingivalis*, *Aggregatibacter actinomycetemcomitans*, and *Tannerella forsythia*, singly or in combination, as detected by nested multiplex PCR. Journal of Clinical Microbiology. 2008;**46**(10):3380-3383

[98] Dashper SG, Seers CA, Tan KH, Reynolds EC. Virulence factors of the oral Spirochete *Treponema denticola*. Journal of Dental Research. 2011;**90**(6):691-703

[99] Ebersole JL, Dawson DR, Morford LA, Peyyala R, Miller CS, González OA. Periodontal disease immunology: 'Double indemnity' in protecting the host. Periodontology 2000. 2013;**62**(1):163-202

[100] Bickel M. The role of interleukin-8 in inflammation and mechanisms of regulation. Journal of Periodontology. 1993;**64**(5 Suppl):456-460

[101] Dosseva-Panova VT, Popova CL, Panov VE. Subgingival microbial profile and production of proinflammatory cytokines in chronic periodontitis. Folia Medica (Plovdiv). 2014;**56**(3):152-160

[102] Maheaswari R, Kshirsagar JT, Lavanya N. Polymerase chain reaction: A molecular diagnostic tool in periodontology. Journal of Indian Society of Periodontology. 2016;**20**(2):128-135

[103] Chen T, Yu WH, Izard J, Baranova OV, Lakshmanan A, Dewhirst FE. The human oral microbiome database: A web accessible resource for investigating oral microbe taxonomic and genomic information. Database. 2010;**2010**:baq013. DOI: 10.1093/database/baq013

[104] Do T, Devine D, Marsh PD. Oral biofilms: Molecular analysis, challenges, and future prospects in dental diagnostics. Clinical, Cosmetic and Investigational Dentistry. 2013;**5**:11-19

[105] Marsh PD. Dental plaque: Biological significance of a biofilm and community life-style. Journal of Clinical Periodontology. 2005;**32**(Suppl 6):7-15

[106] Hosaka Y, Saito A, Maeda R, Fukaya C, Morikawa S, Makino A, Ishihara K, Nakagawa T. Antibacterial activity of povidone-iodine against an artificial biofilm of *Porphyromonas gingivalis* and *Fusobacterium nucleatum*. Archives of Oral Biology. 2012;**57**(4):364-368

[107] Hoffmann N, Lee B, Hentzer M, Rasmussen TB, Song Z, Johansen HK, Givskov M, Høiby N. Azithromycin blocks quorum sensing and alginate polymer formation and increases the sensitivity to serum and stationary-growth-phase killing of *Pseudomonas aeruginosa* and attenuates chronic *P. aeruginosa* lung infection in Cftr(−/−) mice. Antimicrobial Agents and Chemotherapy. 2007;**51**(10):3677-3687

[108] Gillings MR. Evolutionary consequences of antibiotic use for the resistome, mobilome and microbial pangenome. Frontiers in Microbiology. 2013;**4**:4. DOI: 10.3389/fmicb.2013.00004 [published online: January 22, 2013]

[109] Roberts MC. Antibiotic resistance in oral/respiratory bacteria. Critical Reviews in Oral Biology and Medicine. 1998;**9**:522-540

[110] Roberts AP, Cheah G, Ready D, Pratten J, Wilson M, Mullany P. Transfer of TN916-like elements in microcosm dental plaques. Antimicrobial Agents and Chemotherapy. 2001;**45**:2943-2946

[111] Mercer DK, Scott KP, Melville CM, Glover LA, Flint HJ. Transformation of an oral bacterium via chromosomal integration of free DNA in the presence of human saliva. FEMS Microbiology Letters. 2001;**200**:163-167

[112] Wang BY, Chi B, Kuramitsu HK. Genetic exchange between *Treponema denticola* and *Streptococcus gordonii* in biofilms. Oral Microbiology and Immunology. 2002;**17**:108-112

[113] Teng LJ, Hsueh PR, Chen YC, Ho SW, Luh KT. Antimicrobial susceptibility of viridans group streptococci in Taiwan with an emphasis on the high rates of resistance to penicillin and macrolides in *Streptococcus oralis*. Journal of Antimicrobial Chemotherapy. 1998;**41**:621-627

[114] Kuriyama T, Karasawa T, Nakagawa K, Nakamura S, Yamamoto E. Antimicrobial susceptibility of major pathogens of orofacial odontogenic infections to 11 β-lactam antibiotics. Oral Microbiology and Immunology. 2002;**17**:285-289

[115] Noda M, Komatsu H, Inoue S, Sano H. Antibiotic susceptibility of bacteria detected from the root canal exudate of persistent apical periodontitis. Journal of Endodontics. 2000;**26**(4):221-224

[116] Roberts MC. Antibiotic toxicity, interactions and resistance development. Periodontology 2000. 2000;**28**:280-297

[117] Trinh S, Reysset G. Identification and DNA sequence of the mobilization region of the 5-nitroimidazole resistance plasmid pIP421 from *Bacteroides fragilis*. Journal of Bacteriology. 1997;**179**:4071-4074

[118] Ioannidou S, Tassios PT, Kotsovili-Tseleni A, Foustoukou M, Legakis NJ, Vatopoulos A. Antibiotic resistance rates and macrolide resistance phenotypes of viridans group streptococci from the oropharynx of healthy Greek children. International Journal of Antimicrobial Agents. 2001;**17**:195-201

[119] Okamoto M, Takano K, Maeda N. Distribution of the tetracycline resistance determinant tet Q gene in oral isolates of black pigmented anaerobes in Japan. Oral Microbiology and Immunology. 2001;**16**:224-228

[120] Lancaster H, Bedi R, Wilson M, Mullany P. The maintenance in the oral cavity of children of tetracycline-resistant bacteria and the genes encoding such resistance. Journal of Antimicrobial Chemotherapy. 2005;**56**:524-531

[121] King A, Bathgate T, Phillips I. Erythromycin susceptibility of viridans streptococci from the normal throat flora of patients treated with azithromycin or clarithromycin. Clinical Microbiology and Infection. 2002;**8**:85-92

[122] Santagati M, Iannelli F, Cascone C, Campanile F, Oggioni MR, Stefani S, Pozzi G. The novel conjugative transposon Tn*1207.3* carries the macrolide efflux gene *mef*(A) in *Streptococcus pyogenes*. Microbial Drug Resistance. 2003;**9**:243-247

[123] Cerdá Zolezzi P, Laplana LM, Calvo CR, Cepero PG, Erazo MC, Gómez-Lus R. Molecular basis of resistance to macrolides and other antibiotics in commensal viridans group streptococci and *Gemella* spp. and transfer of resistance genes to *Streptococcus pneumoniae*. Antimicrobial Agents and Chemotherapy. 2004;**48**:3462-3467

[124] Emilson CG, Westergren G. Effect of chlorhexidine on the relative proportions of *Streptococcus mutans* and *Streptococcus sanguis* in hamster plaque. Scandinavian Journal of Dental Research. 1979;**87**:288-295

[125] Yamamoto T, Tamura Y, Yokota T. Antiseptic and antibiotic resistance plasmid in *Staphylococcus aureus* that possesses ability to confer chlorhexidine and acrinol resistance. Antimicrobial Agents and Chemotherapy. 1988;**32**:932-935

[126] Borriello G, Werner E, Roe F, Kim AM, Ehrlich GD, Stewart PS. Oxygen limitation contributes to antibiotic tolerance of *Pseudomonas aeruginosa* in biofilms. Antimicrobial Agents and Chemotherapy. 2004;**48**(7):2659-2664

[127] Anderl JN, Franklin MJ, Stewart PS. Role of antibiotic penetration limitation in *Klebsiella pneumoniae* biofilm resistance to ampicillin and ciprofloxacin. Antimicrobial Agents and Chemotherapy. 2000;**44**(7):1818-1824

[128] Lewis K. Persister cells and the riddle of biofilm survival. Biochemistry (Moscow). 2005;**70**(2):267-274

[129] Drenkard E. Antimicrobial resistance of *Pseudomonas aeruginosa* biofilms. Microbes and Infection. 2003;**5**:1213-1219

[130] Mah TF, O'Toole GA. Mechanisms of biofilm resistance to antimicrobial agents. Trends in Microbiology. 2001;**9**:34-39

[131] Steward PS. Mechanisms of antibiotic resistance in bacterial biofilms. International Journal of Medical Microbiology. 2002;**292**:107-113

[132] Yamanaka T, Furukawa T, Matsumoto-Mashimo C, Yamane K, Sugimori C, Nambu T, Mori N, Nishikawa H, Walker CB, Leung KP, Fukushima H. Gene expression profile and pathogenicity of biofilm-forming *Prevotella intermedia* strain 17. BMC Microbiology. 2009;**16**:11

[133] Chang YM, Jeng WY, Ko TP, Yeh YJ, Chen CK, Wang AH. Structural study of TcaR and its complexes with multiple antibiotics from *Staphylococcus epidermidis*. Proceedings of the National Academy of Sciences of the United States of America. 2010;**107**:8617-8622

[134] LaSarre B, Federle MJ. Exploiting quorum sensing to confuse bacterial pathogens. Microbiology and Molecular Biology Reviews. 2013;**77**(1):73

[135] Ravichandiran V, Shanmugam K, Anupama K, Thomas S, Princy A. Structure-based virtual screening for plant-derived SdiA-selective ligands as potential antivirulent agents against uropathogenic *Escherichia coli*. European Journal of Medicinal Chemistry. 2012;**48**:200-205

[136] Issac Abraham SV, Palani A, Ramaswamy BR, Shunmugiah KP, Arumugam VR. Antiquorum sensing and antibiofilm potential of *Capparis spinosa*. Archives of Medical Research. 2011;**42**(8):658-668

[137] Jakobsen TH, van Gennip M, Phipps RK, Shanmugham MS, Christensen LD, Alhede M, Skindersoe ME, Rasmussen TB, Friedrich K, Uthe F, Jensen PØ, Moser C, Nielsen KF, Eberl L, Larsen TO, Tanner D, Høiby N, Bjarnsholt T, Givskov M. Ajoene, a sulfur-rich molecule from garlic, inhibits genes controlled by quorum sensing. Antimicrobial Agents and Chemotherapy. 2012;**56**(5):2314-2325

[138] Sforcin JM, Bankova V. Propolis: Is there a potential for the development of new drugs? Journal of Ethnopharmacology. 2011;**133**:253-260

[139] Stan T, Marutescu L, Chifiriuc MC, Mateescu C, Lazar V. Antimicrobial and antibiofilm activity of Romanian propolis. Biointerface Research in Applied Chemistry. 2013;**3**(2): 541-550

[140] Katircioglu H, Mercan N. Antimicrobial activity and chemical compositions of Turkish propolis from different regions. African Journal of Biotechnology. 2006;**5**:1151-1153

[141] Duarte S, Koo H, Bowen WH, Hayacibara MF, Cury JA, Ikegaki M, Rosalen PL. Effect of a novel type of propolis and its chemical fractions on glucosyltransferases and on growth and adherence of mutans streptococci. Biological & Pharmaceutical Bulletin. 2003;**26**(4):527-531

[142] Bulman Z, Le P, Hudson AO, Savka MA. A novel property of propolis (bee glue): Anti-pathogenic activity by inhibition of N-acyl-homoserine lactone mediated signaling in bacteria. Journal of Ethnopharmacology. 2011;**138**:788-797

[143] Chifiriuc MC, Diţu LM, Oprea E, Liţescu S, Bucur M, Mǎruţescu L, Enache G, Saviuc C, Burlibaşa M, Trǎistaru T, Tǎnǎse G, Lazǎr V. In vitro study of the inhibitory activity of usnic acid on dental plaque biofilm. Roumanian Archives of Microbiology and Immunology. 2009;**68**(4):215-222

[144] Cortelli JR, Cogo K, Aquino DR, Cortelli SC, Ricci-Nittel D, Zhang P, Araujo MW. Validation of the anti-bacteremic efficacy of an essential oil rinse in a Brazilian population: A cross-over study. Brazilian Oral Research. 2012;**26**(5):478-484

[145] Cortelli SC, Cortelli JR, Wu MM, Simmons K, Charles CA. Comparative antiplaque and antigingivitis efficacy of a multipurpose essential oil-containing mouthrinse and a cetylpyridinium chloride-containing mouthrinse: A 6-month randomized clinical trial. Quintessence International. 2012;**43**(7):e82-e94

[146] Tsourounakis I, Palaiologou A, Stoute D, Maney P, Lallier TE. Effect of essential oil and chlorhexidine mouthwashes on gingival fibroblast survival and migration. Journal of Periodontology. 2012;**47**(5):563-571

[147] Lakhdar L, Hmamouchi M, Rida S, Ennibi O. Antibacterial activity of essential oils against periodontal pathogens: A qualitative systematic review. Odonto-Stomatologie Tropicale. 2012;**35**(140):38-46

[148] Sofrata A, Santangelo EM, Azeem M, Borg-Karlson AK, Gustafsson A, Pütsep K. Benzyl isothiocyanate: A major component from the roots of *Salvadora persica* is highly active against gram-negative bacteria. PLoS One. 2011;**6**(8):e23045

[149] Feng HS, Bernardo CC, Sonoda LL, Hayashi F, Romito GA, De Lima LA, Lotufo RF, Pannuti CM. Subgingival ultrasonic instrumentation of residual pockets irrigated with essential oils: A randomized controlled trial. Journal of Clinical Periodontology. 2011;**38**(7):637-643

[150] Rodrigues IS, Tavares VN, Pereira SL, Costa FN. Antiplaque and antigingivitis effect of *Lippia sidoides*: A double-blind clinical study in humans. Journal of Applied Oral Science. 2009;**17**(5):404-407

[151] Christensen LD, van Gennip M, Jakobsen TH, Alhede M, Hougen HP, Høiby N, Bjarnsholt T, Givskov M. Synergistic antibacterial efficacy of early combination treatment with tobramycin and quorum-sensing inhibitors against *Pseudomonas aeruginosa* in an intraperitoneal foreign-body infection mouse model. Journal of Antimicrobial Chemotherapy. 2012;**67**(5):1198-1206

[152] Zora R, Željka V. Current trends in development of liposomes for targeting bacterial biofilms. Pharmaceutics. 2016;**8**:18. DOI: 10.3390/pharmaceutics8020018

[153] Tsumori H., Shimizu Y., Nagatoshi K., Sakurai Y., Yamakami K. (2015) Prospects for Liposome-Encapsulated Nisin in the Prevention of Dental Caries. In: Sasaki K., Suzuki O., Takahashi N. (eds) Interface Oral Health Science; Springer, Tokyo: 2014.pp 305-316

[154] Dabra S, Chhina K, Soni N, Bhatnagar R. Tissue engineering in periodontal regeneration: A brief review. Dental Research Journal (Isfahan). 2012;**9**(6):671-680

[155] Available from:https://www.fda.gov/ohrms/dockets/dockets/05m0474/05m-0474-aav00 01-04-Labeling-vol1.pdf

[156] Terranova VP, Odziemiec C, Tweden KS, Spadone DP. Repopulation of dentin surfaces by periodontal ligament cells and endothelial cells. Effect of basic fibroblast growth factor. Journal of Periodontology. 1989;**60**:293-301

[157] Schliephake H, Aref A, Scharnweber D, Bierbaum S, Roessler S, Sewing A. Effect of immobilized bone morphogenic protein 2 coating of titanium implants on periimplant bone formation. Clinical Oral Implants Research. 2005;**16**:563-569

[158] Blom S, Holmstrup P, Dabelsteen E. The effect of insulin like growth factor 1 and human growth hormone on periodontal ligament fibroblast morphology, growth pattern, DNA synthesis and receptor binding. Journal of Periodontology. 1992;**63**:960-968

[159] Position Paper. The potential role of growth and differentiation factors in periodontal regeneration. Journal of Periodontology. 1996;**67**:545-553

[160] Franceschi RT. Biological approaches to bone regeneration by gene therapy. Journal of Dental Research. 2005;**84**:1093-1103

[161] Ramseier CA, Abramson ZR, Jin Q, Giannobile WV. Gene therapeutics for periodontal regenerative medicine. Dental Clinics of North America. 2006;**50**:245-263

[162] Intini G. Future approaches in periodontal regeneration: Gene therapy, stem cells and RNA interference. Dental Clinics of North America. 2010;**54**:141-155

6

Biomarkers of Periodontal Tissue Remodeling during Orthodontic Tooth Movement in Mice and Men: Overview and Clinical Relevance

Fabrizia d'Apuzzo, Ludovica Nucci,
Abdolreza Jamilian and Letizia Perillo

Abstract

Tooth movement by orthodontic force application is dependent on remodeling in periodontal ligament and alveolar bone, involving the activation of complex cellular and molecular mechanisms correlated with several macro- and microscopic biological changes. The orthodontic process involves the activation of many complex cellular and molecular mechanisms mediated by the release of chemical substance cascades by many cells of the periodontium. Mainly during the early stage of application of orthodontic forces, an inflammatory process can occur in the periodontium as a physiological response to the tissue stress. Several potential biomarkers of the biological alterations after an orthodontic force application expressing bone resorption and formation, periodontal ligament changes, and vascular and neural responses, may be detected. The appropriate choice of the mechanical force to achieve the highest rate of tooth movement in the shortest time of treatment avoiding adverse consequences is a primary objective of a specialist. Thus, an insight into the biological phenomena occurring during the orthodontic therapies by evaluating these biomarkers may be quite relevant for the clinicians. In this chapter, two models of study, i.e., mice and men, were used to describe the clinical usefulness of some biomarkers in orthodontics.

Keywords: orthodontics, periodontal ligament, tooth movement, gingival crevicular fluid, biomarkers

1. Introduction

Tooth movement by orthodontic force application is dependent on remodeling in periodontal ligament (PDL) and alveolar bone, correlated with several macro- and microscopic biological changes.

After more than 100 years, since the first article on the theory of tooth movement was published by Carl Sandstedt (1904–1905), the specialists have reasonably good understanding of the sequence of events involved in the orthodontic tooth movement at tissue and cellular levels [1]. Orthodontic movements represent a continual and balanced process characterized by bone deposition in tension sites and bone resorption in the pressure ones. The mechanical stress from the application of orthodontic forces induces the activation of many cellular and molecular mechanisms mediated by the release of chemical substance cascade allowing the transmission of signals from extracellular matrix. These alterations lead to a gradual remodeling of the mineralized (alveolar bone) and nonmineralized (periodontium) tooth supporting tissues during the orthodontic movement [2].

Mainly during the early stage of application of orthodontic forces, an inflammatory process can occur in the periodontium as a physiological response to the tissue stress. Several potential biomarkers of the biological alterations after an orthodontic force application may be detected, specifically expressing bone resorption and formation, periodontal ligament changes, and vascular and neural responses.

The appropriate choice of the mechanical force to induce the highest rate of tooth movement in the shortest period of treatment avoiding adverse consequences is a primary objective of a specialist. To identify the degree of remodeling occurring in the periodontal tissues during an orthodontic treatment by monitoring the levels of certain biochemical mediators may be a clinically useful procedure.

In this chapter, the importance of evaluating the levels of substances as valid biomarkers of periodontal effects of an orthodontic treatment is emphasized through a description of the specific role of each of them. Only studies on mice and rats have been considered as animal models, whereas in order to monitor the expression of these biomarkers noninvasively in humans, changes in the composition of gingival crevicular fluid (GCF) during orthodontic and orthopedic tooth movement have been selected as first choice. Substances involved in bone remodeling are produced by periodontal ligament cells in sufficient quantities to diffuse into the gingival crevicular fluid. Thus, by means of two different study models "mice and men," the clinical usefulness of some biomarkers in orthodontics is properly analyzed.

2. Anatomy and function of periodontal ligament and alveolar bone

"Periodontium" comes from the Greek "what is around the tooth." It includes all structures that anchor the tooth to the alveolar bone surrounding forming a strong support structure [3]. Its components are gingiva, periodontal ligament, cement, and alveolar bone (**Figure 1**).

The periodontal ligament is the structure interposed between the tooth root and the alveolar bone, with an area of 0.25–0.5 mm. It is a connective tissue whose main component is represented by a set of elastic collagen fibers, parallel to each other, inserted on one side in the cementum and on the other in the lamina dura of the alveolar bone (Sharpey's fibers). The oblique direction of these supporting fibers on the tooth surface provides the tooth with enough elasticity to distribute the masticatory forces over a large surface of the alveolar process, allowing the

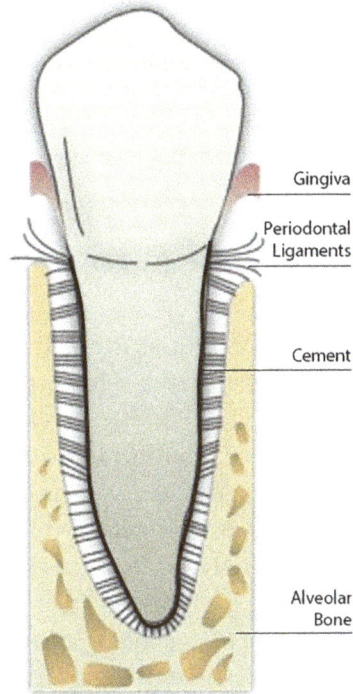

Figure 1. The tooth and its supporting tissues: gingiva, periodontal ligament, cement, and alveolar bone.

tooth to oppose a greater resistance to forces exerted during masticatory function. The other component of the periodontal ligament is the cellular element consisting of undifferentiated mesenchymal cells and their lines of differentiation in fibroblasts and osteoblasts, together with the neural elements, and vascular tissue fluid from the circulatory system.

The alveolar bone or cortex alveolaris is the portion of the jaws functionally dependent on the teeth. The alveolar bone forms the socket where the tooth is located. Under physiological conditions, the alveolar bone is located approximately 2 mm apical to the cement-enamel junction (CEJ). In general, the bone is a mineralized connective tissue, which consists of organic material. Bone is a very dynamic tissue remodeling continuously throughout life. Histologically, it is a particular type of connective tissue of support, consisting of cells dispersed in an abundant extracellular matrix, formed by fibers, and amorphous substance of glycoproteic origin. The bone tissue is composed of two associated phases: organic and mineral inorganic. The organic phase is constituted for 90% of collagen type I. The mineral phase is constituted by calcium and phosphorus combined in a little crystallized hydroxyapatite, and other ions which usually are found in the surface layers.

Osteoblasts and osteoclasts constitute the bone cellular components. The former synthesize and secrete the organic matrix. Osteoblastic cells, after the deposition of the matrix that is subsequently mineralized, remain embedded in it turning into osteocytes, which remain in mutual connection via cytoplasmic extensions, and also in vasal connection through a series of small channels. The osteoclasts, instead, are multinucleated cells formed by fusion of precursor cells consisting of hematopoietic stem cells from the family of mononuclear phagocytes. They are the mediators of the continuous resorption of bone. Osteoclasts occupy small depressions on the bone's surface, called Howship's lacunae, caused by erosion of the bone by specific enzymes.

The characteristic trabecular structure is constituted by external component of the compact bone and the inner cancellous bone, providing a great resistance to mechanical stress [4].

3. Periodontal and bone responses to physiologic masticatory activity

Orthodontic therapy applies light and continuous forces to the teeth and to the related facial structures. The term biomechanics in orthodontics refers to the complex reactions in response to a specific orthodontic force application [5]. Each tooth is attached to the surrounding alveolar bone by the periodontal ligament (PDL), a robust structure collagen support around the tooth root with cellular components and tissue fluids. These last two elements play a key role in normal physiological masticatory system. The collagen of the ligament, the alveolar process and cementum are constantly subjected to remodeling and renovation during normal masticatory activities [6]. The fibroblasts in the periodontal ligament have similar features to osteoblasts and, standing out from the focal cell population, produce new tissue bone. Osteoclasts and cementoclasts remove alveolar bone and cementum, respectively. During the physiological process of mastication, dental and periodontal structures are subjected to both heavy and intermittent forces. In particular, the teeth are subjected to loads that vary from 1 to 2 kg when chewing soft food up to 50 kg for tough food. During heavy masticatory loads lasting maximum 1 second, the displacement of a single tooth in the periodontal space is prevented by the naturally incompressible fluid, and the loading force is transmitted to the alveolar process walls, which are consequently flexed. They generate currents stimulating bone regeneration and repair, thus allowing the adaptation of the bone architecture to the changed function.

4. Periodontal and bone responses to the application of orthodontic forces

Bone and periodontal responses to orthodontic treatment mainly depend on the force duration and its intensity applied to the teeth. The orthodontic biological mechanisms can be evaluated considering two different theories: bioelectrical theory and pressure-tension theory. According to the first theory, the bone subjected to bending generates piezoelectric currents that determine changes in bone metabolism. These currents are constituted by electrons ($e-$) moving from side to side of the network of a crystalline material; thus, the orthodontic forces routinely produce an alveolar bone deflection, and these strains lead to changes in the periodontal ligament. For the theory of the pressure tension, the cell differentiation and the subsequent tooth movement are controlled by chemical signals. A continuous force induces a compression of the ligament in some areas, with reduction of oxygen tension and then of blood flow, whereas in other areas, a traction of the ligament with increased oxygen tension and equal or increased blood flow (**Figure 2**) [5].

Modifications of the irroration are accompanied by rapid chemical changes, which can stimulate the differentiation and activation of specialized cells for bone and periodontal remodeling. Cellular destruction and injury of capillaries lead to an inflammatory reaction followed by formation of new capillaries and connective cells. In particular, the compression of the periodontal fibers causes the "hyalinization" [7] characterized by the disappearance and/or pycnosis of cell nuclei and the convergence of the collagen fibers in a gelatinous-like substance. Reitan in his papers on the histological changes following orthodontic force application [8] reported that the hyalinization refers to cell-free areas within the PDL, in which the normal tissue architecture and staining characteristics of collagen in the processed histological material have been lost. He observed that the hyalinization occurred within the PDL following the application of even minimal force. After the elimination of the hyalinized tissue, a direct resorption occurs thanks to the activation of the osteoclasts from the PDL, and then, an indirect resorption with cellular elements from the blood flow occurred. The pressure exerted on the periodontal ligament is directly proportional to the reduction of the blood flow inside the PDL until a complete collapse of the blood vessels and to a consequent ischemia. If the pressure applied to the tooth is light and lasting for 1–2 seconds, the PDL is partially compressed to the displacement of the fluids outside of the periodontal space following the displacement of the tooth in its alveolus; after 3–5 seconds, the blood vessels are passively compressed by the pressure side and dilated from the tension side; fibers and cells of the PDL appear mechanically distorted. A slight pressure maintained for a few minutes causes changes in the blood flow and variations of oxygen tension, with a simultaneous release of prostaglandins and inflammatory cytokines. After at least 4 hours, metabolic changes occur by induction of several chemical modulators, increased cyclic Adenosine Monophosphate (cAMP), and cell differentiation within the periodontal ligament. After 48 hours, the orthodontic tooth movement starts after the alveolar

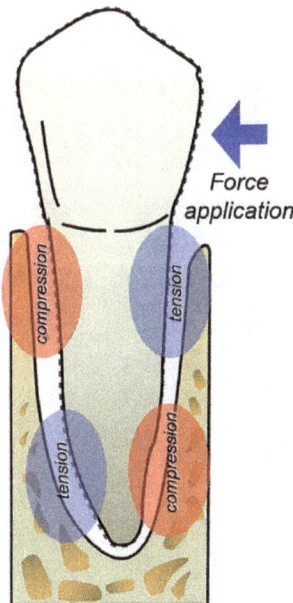

Figure 2. Compression and tension areas after force application.

bone remodeling that occurs through the combined activity of osteoclasts and osteoblasts. If pressure on dental structure is high, after 3–5 seconds, the blood vessels in the PDL collapse on the compression side, and after a few minutes, the interruption of blood circulation occurs in that area of PDL, with sterile necrosis and disappearance of the cellular component (areas of hyalinization). In this case, the remodeling takes place thanks to cells from contiguous areas, which begin to invade the necrosis causing an indirect resorption, since the action of osteoclasts starts from the outer part of the lamina dura. Consequently, the mechanisms of hyalinization and resorption indirectly involve an inevitable delay in the displacement of the tooth, in addition to the pain caused to the patient, due to the presence of ischemic and inflamed areas in the PDL. The ideal intensity for orthodontic forces is when it promotes tooth movement producing cell differentiation without the complete occlusion of the blood vessels in the periodontal ligament, and, therefore, the biological effect of an orthodontic force depends on its intensity and area of PDL involved, or by the pressure on the tooth.

Therefore, orthodontic tooth movement could be divided in three phases: the initial phase, the lag phase, and the postlag phase. The initial phase is characterized by immediate and rapid tooth movement and occurs from 24 to 48 hours after the first application of force. This rate is largely attributed to the displacement of the tooth in the PDL space. The lag phase lasts from 20 to 30 days and shows relatively little tooth displacement. This phase is marked by PDL hyalinization in the region of compression. No subsequent tooth movement occurs until the cells complete the removal of the main part of the necrotic tissues. The lag phase is followed by the postlag phase, during which the rate of movement increases [9].

The sequence of events following orthodontic tooth movement can be characterized using suitable biomarkers (**Figure 3**).

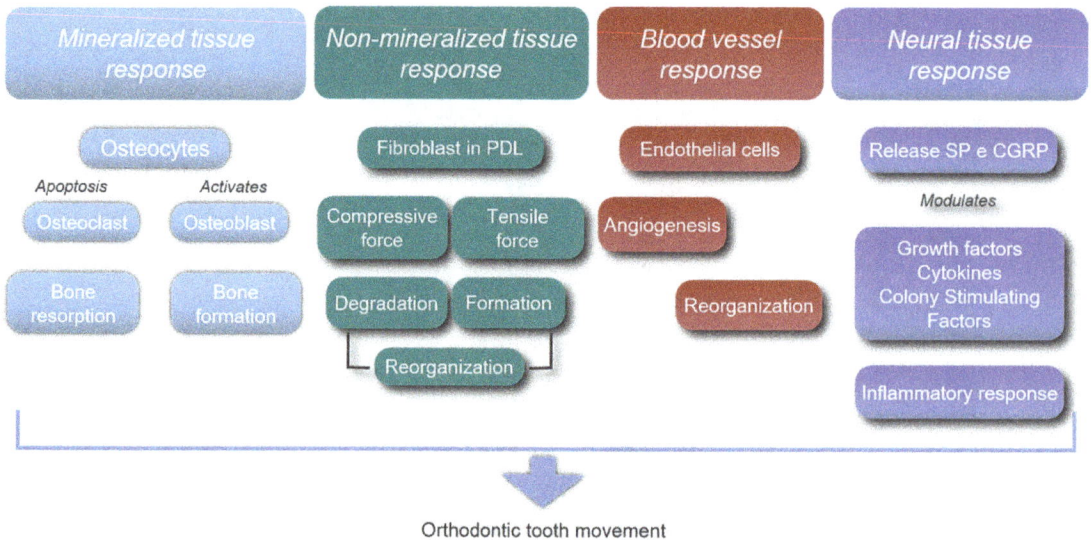

Figure 3. Effects of orthodontic force application on periodontal tissues.

5. Two different models "mice and men" to analyze the orthodontic tooth movement

5.1. Mice as models of study of periodontal and bone tissue remodeling after orthodontic tooth movement

Up to now, a large number of studies in various species of animals have been carried out to evaluate the biological response on the periodontal ligament after a force application. Mice are the most widely used animals to study tooth movement (**Figure 4**), even if there are advantages or disadvantages [10].

To note among the disadvantages, the alveolar bone of mice is denser than in humans, and there are no osteons. Indeed, the animal osteoid tissue along the alveolar bone surface is less, a few mucopolysaccharides are contained in the extracellular matrix, and the calcium concentration is more controlled by intestinal absorption than by the bony tissue. Some disparities have also been reported in the arrangement of the peritoneal fibers, in the supporting structures, as well as in root formations that are faster. However, mice are considered a good model to study the orthodontic tooth movement consequences. They are relatively inexpensive facilitating the use of a large sample and the housing for a long period of time; the histological preparation of their material is easier than in other animals; most antibodies required for cellular and molecular biological techniques are only available for mice and rats; moreover, transgenic strains are almost exclusively developed in small rodents. The difference between mice and rats poses greater difficulty in placing an effective orthodontic appliance in the smaller mouth of a mouse. A systematic review on the literature for experimental tooth movement in rodents showed several shortcomings in part related to the physiology of the animals and on the other hand to the design of the orthodontic appliance [11]. In consideration of this critical evaluation, the animal model was useful to achieve the current knowledge on experimental orthodontic tooth movement.

5.2. Evaluation of bone and periodontal tissue responses to orthodontic movement in men with the gingival crevicular fluid

The gingival crevicular fluid (GCF) is an exudate derived from epithelium lining of the gingival sulcus has been recognized for over a century. However, the exact nature of the fluid, its origins, and its composition have been the subject of controversy for decades [12, 13]. Investigations into the protein content of the GCF reported that in healthy gingival crevices, the GCF has a similar protein concentration to interstitial fluid, which was notably lower than in serum [14–16]. On the contrary, an inflamed gingiva has GCF with raised protein concentrations that are thus similar to those of serum [17]. Subsequently, upon local inflammation or injury, the GCF would become an inflammatory exudate. The increased GCF flow contributes to host defense by flushing bacterial colonies and their metabolites away from the sulcus, thus restricting their penetration into the tissue [18].

The range of the GCF constituents is very large, as it can contain both human and bacterial cells and many different molecules. Among the most representative cellular components of the GCF, there are the leukocytes, especially neutrophils, which have important roles in the

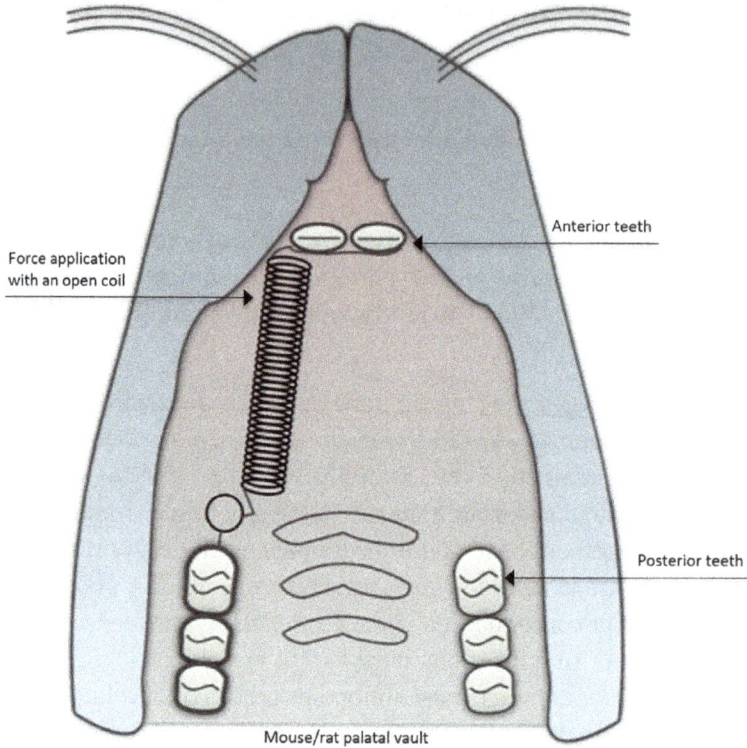

Figure 4. A schematic drawing of the animal model with the application of a force by an open coil between anterior and posterior teeth to induce a tooth movement.

antimicrobial defense of the periodontium [19]. However, while the bacterial and cellular components of the GCF are of primary concern for clinicians and researchers, its molecular contents represent a promising source of biomarkers in dentistry and in orthodontics for the monitoring of site-specific tissue remodeling leading to the tooth movement [20] and, as revealed more recently, for the evaluation of skeletal maturation on an individual basis [21].

The host molecular content of the GCF includes a large variety of molecules that have the potential to be classified as biomarkers of cell death, tissue damage, inflammation, bone resorption, bone deposition, and others, according to their specific biological functions. For several of these biomarkers, associations between their levels and specific clinical conditions have been shown along with the predictive value for the biomarkers; for instance, in terms of tissue destruction due to periodontitis. Several recent studies on orthodontic tooth movement have used biochemical assay analysis of GCF as a simple and noninvasive procedure for repetitive sampling from the same site [22].

5.2.1. Methods of collection of gingival crevicular fluid

The GCF can be collected by different methods. The most used methods in the literature are (1) the gingival washing technique; (2) the capillary tubing or micropipettes; and (3) the use of absorbent filter paper strips.

5.2.1.1. The gingival washing technique

This technique was described a long time ago [23]. The gingival crevice is perfused with a determined volume of an isotonic solution ejected from a microsyringe and then re-aspirated from the gingival crevice at the interdental papilla. The fluid collected represents a dilution of the GCF, and it will contain both cells and soluble constituents, such as plasma proteins. As a major disadvantage, this procedure can fail to recover all the instilled fluid or the GCF contents during the re-aspiration. Thus, an accurate quantification of the GCF volume or composition is not guaranteed as the precise dilution factor cannot be determined. This technique is particularly valuable for harvesting cells from the gingival crevice region.

5.2.1.2. Capillary tubing or micropipettes

This collection method was described more than 40 years ago [24]. It consists on the use of capillary tubes of specific internal diameter inserted into the gingival crevice after the isolation and drying of the area. Due to the known internal diameter of the capillary tubes, it is possible to determine the exact GCF volume collected, through the measure of the GCF migration along the capillary tubing. However, it is difficult to collect an adequate volume of GCF in a short period, unless the sites are inflamed and contain large volumes of fluid. In fact, collection times from an individual site may exceed 30 minutes, thus making the capillary holding difficult and possibly traumatic for periodontal tissues. Moreover, this can cause the release of a serum-derived fluid that may alter volume and composition of the GCF [25]. A further disadvantage of this method is the challenging removal of the full GCF sample from the capillary tubes.

5.2.1.3. Absorbent filter paper strips

The use of adsorbent paper strips represents the procedure most used for GCF collection today [25, 26]. In this procedure, the standardized absorbent paper strips are inserted into the gingival crevice and left *in situ* for 5–60 seconds. The advantages of the technique are that it is quick and easy to use and can be applied to individual sites, and it is the least traumatic when correctly used. The main variations are the reduced timing of sampling and the volume estimation of the collected sample. Because of this methodological variability, the data from different studies need to be interpreted with caution, considering how exactly the collection of the GCF was performed with the paper strips. The methods of collection may be broadly divided into the intracrevicular and extracrevicular techniques. The former depends on the strip inserted at least 3 mm into the gingival crevice or into a periodontal pocket [27], whereas in the latter, the strips are inserted until the "minimum resistance" is felt [28] in an attempt to minimize trauma. A problem with GCF collection and data interpretation may be the sample contamination by blood, saliva, or bacterial plaque. A careful isolation should be performed to minimize the potential GCF contamination. Before performing any biochemical analysis, the volume of the GCF sample must be determined. To achieve the recovery of strips, it is necessary to separate the GCF from the filter paper strips, and protein recovery is close to 100% using a centrifugal elution technique [29].

6. Biomarkers of periodontal and bone responses to orthodontic force application

Orthodontic tooth movement induces a series of orchestrated cellular and molecular events responsible for connective tissue remodeling and osteoclast activation [30].

Thus, the sequence of cascades following the mechanical stress from orthodontic appliances can be characterized using suitable biomarkers.

6.1. Pro-inflammatory cytokines: interleukin-1 (IL-1β), interleukin-6 (IL-6), interleukin-8 (IL-8), tumor necrosis factor-(TNF-α), and prostaglandins E (PGE1-PGE2)

IL-1β is one of the most abundant cytokines in the periodontium during the initial stage of orthodontic tooth movement [3]. In the early stages of tooth movement (at 12 and 24 hours), the following cells stained positively for IL-1β: fibroblasts, macrophages, cementoblasts, cementoclasts, osteoblasts, and osteoclasts [31, 32]. IL-1β seems to be primarily secreted by macrophages, whereas macrophage accumulation in compressed periodontal areas has been detected at later stages of the treatment. Thus, during the initial stage of tooth movement, IL-1β derives from other periodontal cell types, like the osteoclasts, as immediate response to mechanical stress.

The experimental tooth movement leads to significantly increased recruitment of cells belonging to the mononuclear phagocytic system. It was suggested that the neuroimmune interactions may be of primary importance in the initial inflammatory response, as well as the regenerative processes of the periodontal ligaments are incident to orthodontic tooth movement [33]. IL-1β is involved in the survival, fusion, and activation of osteoclasts. This role is significant since the rate of tooth movement correlates with the quantity of bone remodeling in the alveolar process [34]. Higher levels of expression of inflammatory cytokines and their related receptors have been shown after an inflammatory process induced by perforating the buccal cortical plate of orthodontically treated rats. The concentration of the IL-1β mRNA in the rats' periodontal ligament is increased within 3 hours after orthodontic force loading, mainly on the pressure side [35, 36].

The particular function as pro-inflammatory cytokine of IL-1β has been demonstrated by the administration of exogenous IL-1 receptor antagonist (IL-1RA) [37]. IL-1RA treated mice showed a 66% decrease in the levels of IL-1β when compared to the experimental tooth movement of vehicle treated mice, and this was associated with a reduction of the number of osteoclasts in the pressure side of periodontal tissues after histological characterization. Therefore, IL-1RA down-regulates orthodontic tooth movement because of the lower rate of tooth displacement in mice treated with IL-RA therapy. IL-1β is also considered a potent inducer of IL-6 production: it overlaps with IL-6 and TNF-α in their actions [38]. IL-6 regulates immune responses in inflammation sites [39], and it has an autocrine/paracrine activity stimulating osteoclast formation and the bone-resorbing activity of preformed osteoclasts [40]. IL-6 production increases after 24 hours [41].

Tumor necrosis factor-α (TNF-α) is another pro-inflammatory cytokine shown to elicit acute or chronic inflammation and stimulate bone resorption [32]. TNF-α directly stimulates the differentiation of osteoclast progenitors to osteoclasts in concert with the macrophage-colony stimulating factor (M-CSF). Tuncer et al. [42] reported the increased levels of IL-8 at PDL tension sites and proposed it as triggering factor for bone remodeling.

Many studies of the gingival crevicular fluid have confirmed the increased levels of these pro-inflammatory cytokines during periodontal tissue remodeling after orthodontic tooth movement [41, 43, 44].

Other clinical and animal investigations have also identified a primary role of prostaglandins E (PGE1 and PGE2) in stimulating bone resorption [45, 46]. Prostaglandins are produced from the arachidonic acid, which in turn derives from phospholipids. The liberation of prostaglandins constitutes the first response to the pressure stimulus; it occurs when cells are mechanically deformed, and the consequent mobilization of membrane phospholipids leads to the formation of inositol phosphate (IP), an important chemical messenger. PGE2, in particular, is able to mediate inflammatory responses and induce bone resorption by osteoclastic cell activation [9]. The literature reports that prostaglandins directly stimulate osteoclast production and their capacity to form ruffled border and effect bone resorption. In addition, the PGE2 level in GCF reflects the biologic activity in the periodontium during orthodontic tooth movement, and it is significantly increased in both tension and compression sides [47].

6.2. RANK/RANKL/osteoprotegerin (OPG) system

During orthodontic movement, a variety of proliferation markers are expressed: KI-67 and receptor activator of nuclear factor-Kappa β ligand (RANKL) [48, 49] indicate the recruitment of osteoclasts in compression areas, whereas Runx2 [50], Col1-GFP, and BSP-GFP expression cells express the increase of differentiated osteoblasts in tension areas [51]. To note, the TNF-related ligand, the receptor activator of nuclear factor-Kappa β ligand (RANKL), and its decoy receptor RANK, as well as the osteoprotegerin (OPG), were found to play important roles in the regulation of bone metabolism. RANKL is a downstream regulator of osteoclast formation and activation, through which many hormones and cytokines produce their bone resorption effect. In the bone tissue, RANKL is expressed on osteoblast cell lineage and exerts its effect by binding the RANK receptor on osteoclast lineage cells. This binding leads to rapid differentiation of hematopoietic osteoclast precursors to mature osteoclasts. OPG is a decoy receptor produced by osteoblastic cells in competition with RANK for RANKL binding. The biological effects of OPG on bone cells include inhibition of terminal stages of osteoclast differentiation, suppression of activation of matrix osteoclasts, and induction of apoptosis. Thus, bone remodeling is controlled by a balance between RANK-RANKL binding and OPG production. Kanzaki et al. [52] reported that OPG gene inhibited RANKL-mediated osteoclastogenesis and experimental tooth movement in rats. Thus, the inhibition of the activity of RANKL in its promoting osteoclast differentiation could be very helpful in preventing, for instance, tooth anchorage during orthodontic treatment and relapse during the posttreatment period.

6.3. Macrophages-colony-stimulating factors (M-CSFs)

Colony-stimulating factors (CSFs) comprise those related to granulocytes (G-CSFs), macrophages (M-CSFs), or to both cell types (GM-CSFs). They have a great implication in bone remodeling through osteoclast formation and thereby during tooth movement [9]. These molecules are specific glycoproteins interacting to regulate production, maturation, and function of granulocytes and monocyte macrophages. Therefore, M-CSF plays an important role during the early osteoclast differentiation, which increases the rate of osteoclastic recruitment and differentiation during initial phases of orthodontic tooth movement [50]. In particular, optimal dosages of M-CSF are correlated with measurable changes in tooth movement and gene expression, providing potential for clinical studies in accelerating tooth movement.

6.4. Vascular endothelial growth factor (VEGF) as a key factor of neovascularization

Vascular endothelial growth factor (VEGF) is the primary mediator of angiogenesis and increases vascular permeability during tissue neoformation, always associated to the presence of blood vessels [53]. During orthodontic tooth movement, compressive forces induce angiogenesis of periodontal ligaments and the activation of the vascular endothelial growth factor [54]. A study performed the localization of VEGF *in vivo* in the periodontal tissues of 15 male Wistar rat during an experimental tooth movement. A compressive force at 150 mN was applied by a standardized compressive spring placed between the right and left upper first molars in each rat's mouth. The maxillary bone was analyzed with immunohistochemical staining. VEGF immunoreactivity was in vascular endothelial cells, osteoblasts, osteoclasts in resorption lacunae, in fibroblasts adjacent to hyalinized tissue, a local necrotic area in compressed zone, and in mononuclear cells in periodontal tissues from animals. VEGF mRNA was also found in fibroblasts and osteoblasts in tension area of mice periodontal ligament during experimental tooth orthodontic movement [55]. The protocol included 10 mice, divided between experimental and control animals, and provided the assessment of premaxillary bone frontal sections [56].

Therefore, VEGF has a relevant role in remodeling periodontal ligament as well as in bone resorption and formation.

6.5. Neuropeptides during neural tissue response to orthodontic tooth movement

During orthodontic tooth movement, a neurogenic inflammation occurs in the periodontium with an increased concentration of specific proteins. Somatosensory neurons disseminate signals from periodontal peripheral nerve fibers to the central nervous system. With application of physiologic orthodontic force, periodontal peripheral nerve fibers release calcitonin gene-related peptide (CGRP) and substance P, acting as neurotransmitters. Moreover, CGRP and substance P are vasodilators, inducers of increased vascular flow and permeability (diapedesis), and stimulators of plasma extravasation and leukocyte migration into tissues (transmigration).

CGRP activates the bone formation through osteoblast proliferation and osteoclast inhibition. Receptors for CGRP are revealed on osteoblasts, monocytes, lymphocytes, and mast cells. Receptor activation results in amplified intercellular communication, promoting cytokine (inflammatory mediator molecules) synthesis and release.

Healthy periodontal and alveolar bone innervation promotes maximum blood flow during orthodontic tooth movement, whereas denervation reduces blood flow and bone formation [57]. Substance P (SP) is another sensory neuropeptide released from the peripheral endings of sensory nerves. It can modify the secretion of pro-inflammatory cytokines from immunocompetent cells during periodontal tissue remodeling. Worthy of note, SP stimulated the production of PGE2 [58].

6.6. Enzymes reflecting biological activity in periodontium: caspase-1, β-glucuronidase (β-G), aspartate aminotransferase (AST), and lactate dehydrogenase (LDH)

In conjunction with the inflammatory process, there is an apoptotic process occurring to eliminate the hyalinized periodontal tissue formed during the early stages of orthodontic movement. Caspase-1 is the most important mediator of inflammation and apoptotic responses, activated by inflammatory signals as alterations in the intracellular ionic milieu. It has the role to process and activate pro-IL-1β and other pro-inflammatory cytokines. In a rat model under orthodontic treatment, caspase-1 mRNA expression is increased, and the level of caspase-1 changes with different temporal phases of orthodontic tooth movement [59]. An irreversible root resorption and deformation of periodontal tissues might emerge: an excessive local orthodontic force application or in some diseases like rheumatoid arthritis related to the hyperexpression of caspase-1. In these cases, a method to preserve the structure of periodontal ligaments may be the administration of the inhibitors of caspase-1 activity such as VX-765 [60] and Pralnacasan [61]. A biomarker of primary granule release from polymorphonuclear leukocytes is the lysosomal enzyme β-glucuronidase (βG). Increased levels of this enzyme have been found in the GCF of adolescents treated with rapid maxillary expander, thus during orthodontic and orthopedic movement. Moreover, βG, similar to other biochemical mediators as IL-1β, correlates to both direct and indirect application of mechanical stimuli, with an increased level that is higher following stronger forces [62].

Aspartate aminotransferase (AST) and lactate dehydrogenase (LDH) are soluble enzymes usually confined to the cytoplasm of cells but released to the extracellular environment upon cell necrosis. The AST and LDH activities into the GCF have also been assessed during orthodontic treatment. The GCF AST activity is significantly increased in both the tension and compression sites at days 7 and 14. This amount is explained as a consequence of a controlled trauma that leads to an increased cell necrosis after the mechanical stress on the periodontal ligaments and alveolar bone. A low increase of GCF AST activity reflects the application of orthodontic force on teeth, particularly on compression side, while an occlusal trauma leads to a higher amount of enzymatic level [63]. The enzyme lactate dehydrogenase, likewise, is normally limited to cytoplasm, and it is only released extracellularly after cell death and tissue breakdown [64]. This enzymatic activity is greater in compression sites because of the typical process that occurs during periodontal remodeling resulting from orthodontic tooth movement: there is an early wave of resorption of 3–5 days followed by its reverse process of 5–7 days, and a late wave of formation that lasts for 7–14 days, on both the pressure and the tension sides of the alveolar wall.

6.7. Enzymes involved in bone cell activities: alkaline phosphatase (ALP) and acid phosphatase (ACP)

The biological alteration due to the orthodontic tooth movement involves alterations above all in the surrounding bone tissue [65]. Bone metabolism is associated with alkaline phosphatase (ALP) and acid phosphatase (ACP) expressed by osteoblasts and osteoclasts, respectively. ALP is a ubiquitous tetrameric enzyme associated with the plasma membrane of cells, also found in liver, intestine, and placenta, and it is observed during healing of bone fractures and physiologic bone growth. The bone isoenzyme predominates in childhood and particularly during puberty [66]. These are 507 amino acid proteins encoded by the same gene but differ in their degree of glycosylation. The enzymes catalyze the hydrolysis of monoesters of phosphoric acid and a transphosphorylation reaction with large concentrations of phosphate acceptors [67]. Alkaline and acid phosphatases are released by injured, damaged, or dead cells into extracellular tissue fluid, and, in general, high enzyme activity is an expression of greater cellular activity. ALP activity is found at much higher levels in the periodontal ligament than in other connective tissues [68]. After an orthodontic force application, these enzymes are produced in the periodontium and diffuse in the site-specific GCF. Thus, the monitoring of phosphatase activities in the GCF could be suggestive of the tissue changes occurring during orthodontic tooth movement. In fact, experimental studies in rats and clinical studies in humans correlate alveolar bone remodeling with changes in GCF phosphatase activities [26, 69–72]. To identify and understand the enzymatic changes occurring during the early stages of orthodontic tooth movement and to coincide with initial and lag phases of tooth movement, the studies consider an orthodontic cycle of duration 21 days. It was observed that the ALP activity peaked on the 14th day in most patients, followed by a sharp fall by the 21st day. The activity decrease is related to removal of the hyalinized zone. When the enzyme activity is high, the tooth movement rate is greater. This implies that the ALP activity follows the rate of tooth movement during the initial phases. In the hard bony tissues, the ALP has been implicated in the process of mineralization. Active osteoblasts and osteocytes give an intense staining reaction for alkaline phosphatase. No enzyme activity is found in bone matrix, except when it is in close association with matrix-synthesizing cells. The osteogenic cells in the periodontal ligament react to the tensional forces with an increase in the maturation level. The fibroblast proliferation and collagen have been shown to increase in the tension sites. The ALP activity is lower in the compressed hyalinized zones of the periodontal ligament, whereas ACP activity is higher. After 7–14 days of orthodontic force application, the bone deposition occurs in both tension and pressure sites of the alveolar wall. The main bone remodeling activity at the early times in a remodeling cycle is resorptive, but in the later phase, resorption and deposition become synchronous. This might be due to increased acid phosphatase activity that has been observed in the early phases of orthodontic tooth movement. High levels of alkaline phosphatase have been described after 7 days, when bone deposition begins, and a significant peak occurs on day 14. It is obvious that, as a forerunner to bone formation, the number of fibroblasts and osteoblasts increases in areas of tension. This occurs as a result of increase in cell number by mitotic cell division. The histologic studies showed that in marginal tensional areas, cell proliferation occurs between 36 and 50 hours and lasts for 10–21 days. The tension causes shape changes, and osteoblasts move slightly apart. On the compression side, bone resorption would occur, and osteoclastic activity would be high with little or no osteoblastic activity.

To note, ALP activity is influenced by clinically detectable dental displacements and also by mechanical stress and gingival inflammation.

In conclusion, the analysis of the ALP associated with bone metabolism, under healthy gingival conditions, is a suggestive indicator of the histological and biochemical changes in bone turnover and therefore of the rate/amount of tooth movement. Moreover, the properties of the GCF ALP activity distinguishing between clinically moving and nonmoving teeth show that this enzyme should be further studied as a diagnostic tool in orthodontics [22].

7. Conclusions and clinical relevance

When exposed to different degrees of magnitude, frequency, and duration of mechanical loading, alveolar bone and periodontal ligaments show extensive macroscopic and microscopic changes. Force application on the tooth also alters periodontal tissue vascularity and blood flow, resulting in the local synthesis and release of various molecules, such as cytokines, growth factors, colony-stimulating factors, enzymes, and neurotransmitters [73].

A biomarker is a substance that can be objectively measured revealing any process occurring during a therapeutic treatment. The several potential biomarkers of the biological alterations after an orthodontic force application described in this chapter may be significantly useful to perform an appropriate choice of the mechanical force to achieve the right rate of tooth movement and to accelerate the orthodontic time, avoiding adverse effects such as root resorption or bone loss [74–76].

Finally, a clinical use of these biomarkers for the specialists may be mandatory to improve orthodontic therapies.

The different experimental and clinical methods for the collection and assessment of these potential biological markers were described in both animal and human models. GCF analysis, especially, offered several advantages for its simple, quick, and noninvasive collection.

Overall, a detailed knowledge of the ongoing process occurring in periodontal tissues during orthodontic procedures can lead to proper choice of mechanical loading with the aim of shortening the period of treatment and avoiding adverse consequences associated with orthodontic treatment.

Author details

Fabrizia d'Apuzzo[1], Ludovica Nucci[1], Abdolreza Jamilian[2] and Letizia Perillo[1*]

*Address all correspondence to: letizia.perillo@unina2.it

1 Multidisciplinary Department of Medical-Surgical and Dental Specialties, University of Campania "Luigi Vanvitelli", Naples, Italy

2 Orthodontic Department, Craniomaxillofacial Research Center, Tehran Dental Branch, Islamic Azad University, Tehran, Iran

References

[1] Meikle MC. The tissue, cellular, and molecular regulation of orthodontic tooth movement: 100 years after Carl Sandstedt. European Journal of Orthodontics. 2006;**28**:221-240

[2] Camerlingo C, d'Apuzzo F, Grassia V, Perillo L, Lepore M. Micro-Raman spectroscopy for monitoring changes in periodontal ligaments and gingival crevicular fluid. Sensors. 2014;**14**(12):22552-22563

[3] Wolf HF, Rateitschak M, Rateitschak KH, Simion M. Parodontologia. Milano: Masson; 2005

[4] Lindhe J, Lang NP, Karring T. Parodontologia clinica e implantologia orale. Milano: Edi-Ermes; 2009

[5] Proffit WR, Fields HW, Sarver DM. Contemporary Orthodontics, 5th edition. Mosby Elsevier, US; 2013

[6] Bumann A, Carvalho RS, Scwarzer CL, Yen EH. Collagen synthesis from human PDL cells following orthodontic tooth movement. European Journal of Orthodontics. 1997;**19**(1):29-37

[7] Stuteville OH. Injuries to the teeth and supporting structures caused by various orthodontic appliances and methods of preventing these injuries. The Journal of the American Dental Association and the Dental Cosmos. 1937;**24**(9):1494-1507

[8] Reitan K, Righ P. Biomechanical principles and reactions. In: Graber TH, Vanarsdall TM, editors. Orthodontics, Current Principles and Techniques. 2nd ed. St Louis: CV Mosby; 1994. pp. 96-192

[9] Krishnan V, Davidovitch Z. Cellular, molecular, and tissue-level reactions to orthodontic force. American Journal of Orthodontics and Dentofacial Orthopedics. 2006;**129**(4):469.e1-e32

[10] Ren Y, Maltha JC, Kuijpers-Jagtman AM. The rat as a model of orthodontic tooth movement-a critical review and a proposed solution. European Journal of Orthodontics. 2004;**73**:86-92

[11] Ren Y, Maltha JC, Van 't Hof MA, Kuijpers-Jagtman AM. Age effect on orthodontic tooth movement in rats. Journal of Dental Research. 2003;**82**(1):38-42

[12] Brill N, Bjom H. Passage of fluid into human gingival pockets. Acta Odontologica Scandinavica. 1959;**17**:11-21

[13] Brill N. Influence of capillary permeability on flow of tissue fluid into gingival pockets. Acta Odontologica Scandinavica. 1959a;**17**:23-33

[14] Pashley DH. A mechanistic analysis of gingival fluid production. Journal of Periodontal Research. 1976;**11**:121-134

[15] Alfano MC, Brownstein CN, Chasens AI, Kaslick RS. Passively generated increase in gingival crevicular fluid flow from human gingiva. Journal of Dental Research. 1976;**55**:1132

[16] Bang JS, Cimasoni G. Total protein in human crevicular fluid. Journal of Dental Research. 1971;**50**:1683

[17] Curtis MA, Griffiths GS, Price SJ, Coulthurst SK, Johnson NW. The total protein concentration of gingival crevicular fluid. Variation with sampling time and gingival inflammation. Journal of Clinical Periodontology. 1988;**15**:628-632

[18] Pöllänen MT, Salonen JI, Uitto VJ. Structure and function of the tooth–epithelial interface in health and disease. Periodontology 2000. 2003;**31**:12-31

[19] Delima AJ, Van Dyke TE. Origin and function of the cellular components in gingival crevice fluid. Periodontology 2000. 2003;**31**:55-76

[20] Kavadia-Tsatala S, Kaklamanos EG, Tsalikis L. Effects of orthodontic treatment on gingival crevicular fluid flow rate and composition: Clinical implications and applications. The International Journal of Adult Orthodontics & Orthognathic Surgery. 2002;**17**:191-205

[21] Perinetti G, Di Leonardo B, Di Lenarda R, Contardo L. Repeatability of gingival crevicular fluid collection and quantification, as determined through its alkaline phosphatase activity: Implications for diagnostic use. Journal of Periodontal Research. 2013;**48**:98-104

[22] Perinetti G, D'Apuzzo F, Contardo L, Primozic J, Rupel K, Perillo L. Gingival crevicular fluid alkaline phosphate activity during the retention phase of maxillary expansion in prepubertal subjects: A split-mouth longitudinal study. American Journal of Orthodontics and Dentofacial Orthopedics. 2015;**148**:90-96

[23] Skapski H, Lehner T. A crevicular washing method for investigating immune components of crevicular fluid in man. Journal of Periodontal Research. 1976;**11**:19-24

[24] Sueda T, Bang J, Cimasoni G. Collection of gingival fluid for quantitative analysis. Journal for Dental Research. 1969;**48**:159

[25] Lamster IB, Mandella RD, Gordon JM. Lactate dehydrogenase activity in gingival crevicular fluid collected with filter paper strips: Analysis in subjects with non-inflamed and mildly inflamed gingiva. Journal of Clinical Periodontology. 1985;**12**:153-161

[26] Perinetti G, Paolantonio M, D'Attilio M, D'Archivio D, Tripodi D, Femminella B, et al. Alkaline phosphatase activity in gingival crevicular fluid during human orthodontic tooth movement. American Journal of Orthodontics and Dentofacial Orthopedics. 2002;**122**:548-556

[27] Loe H, Holm-Pedersen P. Absence and presence of fluid from normal and inflamed gingivae. Periodontics. 1965;**149**:171-177

[28] Brill N. The gingival pocket fluid. Studies of its occurrence, composition, and effects. Acta Odontologica Scandinavica. 1962;**20**:1-115

[29] Griffiths GS. Formation, collection and significance of gingival crevice fluid. Periodontol 2000. 2003;**31**:32-42

[30] Rody Jr WJ, Wijegunasinghe M, Wiltshire WA, Dufault B. Differences in the gingival crevicular fluid composition between adults and adolescents undergoing orthodontic treatment. The Angle Orthodontist. 2014;**84**:120-126

[31] Alhashimi N, Frithiof L, Brudvik P, Bakhiet M. Orthodontic tooth movement and de novo synthesis of proinflammatory cytokines. American Journal of Orthodontics and Dentofacial Orthopedics. 2011;**119**:307-312

[32] Davidovitch Z, Nicolay O, Ngan PW, Shanfeld JL. Neurotransmitters, cytokines and the control of alveolar bone remodeling in orthodontics. Dental Clinics of North America. 1988;**32**:411-435

[33] Vandevska-Radunovic V, Kvinnsland IH, Kvinnsland S, Jonsson R. Immunocompetent cells in rat periodontal ligament and their recruitment incident to experimental orthodontic tooth movement. European Journal of Oral Sciences. 1997;**105**:36-34

[34] Teixeira CC, Khoo E, Tran J, Chartres I, Liu Y, Thant LM, Khabensky I, Gart LP, Cisneros G, Alikhani M. Cytokine expression and accelerated tooth movement. Journal of Dental Research. 2010;**89**:1134-1141

[35] Baba S, Kuroda N, Arai C, Nakamura Y, Sato T. Immunocompetent cells and cytokine expression in the rat periodontal ligament at the initial stage of orthodontic tooth movement. Archives of Oral Biology. 2011;**56**:466-473

[36] Lee TY, Lee KJ, Bais HS. Expression of IL-1,MMP-9 and TIMP-1 on the Pressure Side of Gingiva under orthodontic loading. The Angle Orthodontist. 2009;**79**:733-739

[37] Salla JT, Taddei SRA, Queiroz-Junior CM, Andrade Junior I, Teixeira MM, Silva TA. The effect of IL-1 receptor antagonist on orthodontic tooth movement in mice. Archives of Oral Biology. 2012;**57**:519-524

[38] Linkhart TA, Linkhart SG, MacCharles DC, Long DL, Strong DD. Interleukin-6 messenger RNA expression and interleukin-6 protein secretion in cells isolated from normal human bone: Regulation by interleukin-1. Journal of Bone and Mineral Research. 1991;**6**:1285-1294

[39] Okada N, Kobayashi M, Mugikura K, Okamatsu Y, Hanazawa S, Kitano S, Hasegawa K. Interleukin-6 production in human fibroblasts derived from periodontal tissues is differentially regulated by cytokines and a glucocorticoid. Journal of Periodontal Research. 1997;**32**:559-569

[40] Kurihara N, Bertolini D, Suda T, Akiyama Y, Roodman GD. Interleukin-6 stimulates osteoclast-like multinucleated cell formation in long-term human marrow cultures by inducing IL-1 release. Journal of Immunology. 1990;**144**:426-430

[41] Uematsu S, Mogi M, Deguchi T. Interleukin (IL)-1β, IL-6, tumor necrosis factor-α, epidermal growth factor, and β2 microglobulin levels are elevated in gingival crevicular fluid during human orthodontic tooth movement. Journal for Dental Research. 1996;**75**:562-567

[42] Tuncer BB, Ozmeriç N, Tuncer C, Teoman I, Cakilci B, Yücel A, Alpar R, Balos K. Levels of interleukin-8 during tooth movement. The Angle Orthodontist. 2005;**75**:539-544

[43] Lowney JJ, Norton LA, Shafer DM, Rossomando EF. Orthodontic force increases tumor necrosis factor-α in the human gingival sulcus. American Journal of Orthodontics and Dentofacial Orthopedics. 1995;**108**:519-524

[44] Grieve WG III, Johanson J, Moore RN, Reinhardt RA, Dubois LM. PGE and IL-1β levels in gingival crevicular fluid during human orthodontic tooth movement. American Journal of Orthodontics and Dentofacial Orthopedics. 1994;**105**:369-374

[45] Lee W. Experimental study of the effect of prostaglandin administration on tooth movement with particular emphasis on the relationship to the method of PGE1 administration. American Journal of Orthodontics and Dentofacial Orthopedics. 1990;**98**:238-241

[46] Klein DC, Raisz LG. Prostaglandins: Stimulation of bone resorption in tissue culture. Endocrinology. 1970;**86**:1436-1440

[47] Dudic A, Kiliaridis S, Mombelli A, Giannopoulou C. Composition changes in gingival crevicular fluid during orthodontic tooth movement: Comparisons between tension and compression sides. European Journal of Oral Sciences. 2006;**114**:416-422

[48] Kim T, Handa A, Iida J, Yoshida S. RANKL expression in rat periodontal ligament subjected to a continuous orthodontic force. Archives of Oral Biology. 2007;**52**:244-250

[49] Yamaguchi M. RANK/RANKL/OPG during orthodontic tooth movement. Orthodontics & Craniofacial Research. 2009;**12**:113-119

[50] Brooks PJ, Nilforoushan D, Manolson MF, Simmons CA, Gong SG. Molecular markers of early orthodontic tooth movement. The Angle Orthodontist. 2009;**79**:1108-1113

[51] Uribe F, Kalajzic Z, Bibko J, Nanda R, Olson C, Rowe D, Wadhwa S. Early effects of orthodontic forces on osteoblast differentiation in a novel mouse organ culture model. The Angle Orthodontist. 2011;**81**:284-291

[52] Kanzaki H, Chiba M, Takahashi I, Haruyama N, Nishimura M, Mitani H. Local OPG gene transfer to periodontal tissue inhibits orthodontic tooth movement. Journal of Dental Research. 2004;**83**:920-925

[53] Di Domenico M, Ricciardi C, Fusco A, Pierantoni GM. Anti-VEGF therapy in breast and lung mouse models of cancer. Journal of Biomedicine and Biotechnology. 2011; **2011**:947928

[54] Miyagawa A, Chiba M, Hayashi H, Igarashi K. Compressive force induces VEGF production in periodontal tissues. Journal of Dental Research. 2009;**88**:752-756

[55] Kaku M, Motokawa M, Tohma Y, Tsuka N, Koseki H, Sunagawa H, Marquez Hernandes RA, Ohtani J, Fujita T, Kawara T, Tanne K. VEGF and M-CSF levels in periodontal tissue during tooth movement. Biomedical Research. 2008;**29**:181-187

[56] Kaku M, Kohno S, Kawata T, Fujita I, Tokimasa C, Tsutsui K, Tanne K. Effects of vascular endothelial growth factor on osteoclast induction during tooth movement in mice. Journal of Dental Research. 2001;**80**:1880-1183

[57] Masella RS, Meister M. Current concepts in the biology of orthodontic tooth movement. American Journal of Orthodontics and Dentofacial Orthopedics. 2006;**129**:458-468

[58] Kojima T, Yamaguchi M, Kasai K. Substance P stimulates release of RANKL via COX-2 expression in human dental pulp cells. Inflammation Research. 2006;**56**:78-84

[59] Yan X, Chen J, Hao Y, Wang Y, Zhu L. Changes of Caspase-1 after the application of orthodontic forces in the periodontal tissues of rats. The Angle Orthodontist 2009;**79**:1126-1132

[60] Stack J, Beaumont K, Larsen PD, Straley KS, Henkel GW, Randle JC, Hoffman HM. IL-converting enzyme/caspase-1 inhibitor VX-765 blocks the hypersensitive response to an inflammatory stimulus in monocytes from familial cold autoinflammatory syndrome patients. Journal of Immunology. 2005;**175**:2630-2634

[61] Rudolphi K, Gerwin N, Verzijl N, van der Kraan P, van den Berg W. Pralnacasan, an inhibitor of interleukin-1β converting enzyme, reduces joint damage in two murine models of osteoarthritis. Osteoarthritis Cartilage. 2003;**11**:738-746

[62] Tzannetou S, Efstratiadis S, Nicolay O, Grbic J, Lamster I. Comparison of levels of inflammatory mediators IL-1β and βG in gingival crevicular fluid from molars, premolars, and incisors during rapid palatal expansion. American Journal of Orthodontics and Dentofacial Orthopedics. 2008;**133**:699-707

[63] Perinetti G, Paolantonio M, D'Attilio M, D'Archivio D, Dolci M, Femminella B, Festa F, Spoto G. Aspartate aminotransferase activity in gingival crevicular fluid during orthodontic treatment. A controlled short-term longitudinal study. Journal of Periodontology. 2003;**74**:145-152

[64] Perinetti G, Serra E, Paolantonio M, , Bruè, Meo SD, Filippi MR, Festa F, Spoto G. Lactate dehydrogenase activity in human gingival crevicular fluid during orthodontic treatment: A controlled, short-term longitudinal study. Journal of Periodontology. 2005;**76**:411-417

[65] Lamster IB, Oshrain RL, Fiorello LA, Celenti RS, Gordon JM. A comparison of 4 methods of data presentation for lysosomal enzyme activity in gingival crevicular fluid. Journal of Clinical Periodontology. 1988;**15**:347-352

[66] Watts NB. Clinical utility of biochemical markers of bone remodeling. Clinical Chemistry. 1999;**45**:1359-1368

[67] Groeneveld MC. Alkaline phosphatase activity in the periodontal ligament and gingiva of the molar: Its relation to cementum formation. Journal of Dental Research. 1995;**74**:1374-1381

[68] Yamaguchi M, Shimizu N, Shibata Y, Abiko Y. Effects of different magnitudes of tension-force on alkaline phosphatase activity in periodontal ligament cells. Journal of Dental Research. 1996;**75**:889-894

[69] Insoft M, King GJ, Keeling SD. The measurement of acid and alkaline phosphatase in gingival crevicular fluid during orthodontic tooth movement. American Journal of Orthodontics and Dentofacial Orthopedics. 1996;**109**:287-296

[70] Perinetti G, Paolantonio M, Serra E, D'Archivio D, D'Ercole S, Festa F, Spoto G. Longitudinal monitoring of subgingival colonization by Actinobacillus actinomycetem-comitans, and crevicular alkaline phosphatase and aspartate aminotransferase activities around orthodontically treated teeth. Journal of Clinical Periodontology. 2004;**31**:60-67

[71] Batra P, Kharbanda OP, Duggal R, Singh N, Parkash H. Alkaline phosphatase activity in gingival crevicular fluid during canine retraction. Orthodontics and Craniofacial Research. 2006;**9**:44-51

[72] Perinetti G, Baccetti T, Contardo L, Di Lenarda R. Gingival crevicular fluid alkaline phosphatase activity as a non-invasive biomarker of skeletal maturation. Orthodontics and Craniofacial Research. 2011;**14**:44-50

[73] Matarese G, Isola G, Pio Anastasi G, Favaloro A, Milardi D, Vita G, Cordasco G, Cutroneo G, Luca Zizzari V, Teté S, Perillo L. Trasforming growth factor Beta1 and vascular epithelial growth factor in the pathogenesis of periodontal desease. European Journal of Inflammation. 2013;**11**(2):479-488

[74] Zainal Ariffin SH, Yamamoto Z, Zainol Abidin IZ, Abdul Wahab RM, Zainal Ariffin Z. Cellular and molecular changes in orthodontic tooth movement. Scientific World Journal. 2011;**11**:1788-1803

[75] Jamilian A, Perillo L, Rosa M. Missing upper incisors: A retrospective study of orthodontic space closure versus implant. Progress in Orthodontics. 2015;**16**:2

[76] Taba M, Kinney J, Kim AS, Giannobile WV. Diagnostic biomarkers for oral and periodontal diseases. Dental Clinics of North America. 2005;**49**:551-571

7

Polycaprolactone-Based Biomaterials for Guided Tissue Regeneration Membrane

Thanaphum Osathanon,
Phunphimp Chanjavanakul, Pattanit Kongdecha,
Panipuk Clayhan and Nam Cong-Nhat Huynh

Abstract

Guided tissue regeneration (GTR) is a clinical procedure promoting regeneration of periodontal tissues. In general, this technique provides spaces for periodontal cells to repopulate and regenerate in the periodontal defect by physically preventing an invasion of gingival tissues in the affected area. Although various reports certify clinical success of GTR, high variation of favourable outcome among studies leads to the investigation to improve clinical GTR efficiency for periodontal tissue regeneration. Recent development of GTR membrane aims to augment bioactivity for facilitating and enhancing tissue healing and regeneration. Various approaches are examined, for example, the release of growth factor, the incorporation of bioactive ceramics and the delivery of antimicrobial agents. Polycaprolactone (PCL) is widely used in biomedical application due to its acceptable biocompatibility and degradability. Physical characteristics are easy to manipulate. Various forms and shapes are simple to fabricate. PCL can be employed as GTR membrane and scaffold filling in the periodontal-defect area. Bioactive PCL could be fabricated by various techniques to enhance periodontal tissue regeneration. The present chapter reviews the bioactive approaches for GTR membrane, and the potential utilization of PCL for GTR application is described.

Keywords: guided tissue regeneration, periodontal tissues, polycaprolactone, biomaterials

1. Introduction

The guided tissue regeneration (GTR) aims to regenerate the periodontal tissue apparatus in its original architecture. GTR procedure is well established and has proven to be a successful clinical procedure to regenerate periodontal tissues [1]. Treatment is conducted by applying a membrane barrier over the affected area in order to exclude the gingival tissues, connective tissues and epithelial tissues from the defect area, allowing specific cells to regenerate in the affected site [1]. Various materials have been employed and investigated in both clinical and experimental setting [2]. However, the results from systemic review and meta-analysis demonstrated that guided tissue regeneration technique exhibited highly variable between and within the studies [3, 4]. In human, the weighted-average bone-filling ration in the infrabony defect treated by GTR alone ranges from 42 to 77%, implying the variety of response [5]. One possibility of this discrepancy is the different types of membrane employed in the studies [4]. Thus, it suggests that the clinical available membranes are still needed for further improvement to efficiently promote periodontal tissue regeneration.

In order to advance the healing capability of the periodontal tissues, the membrane modification is widely investigated. In this regard, the development of drug/bioactive agent-containing membrane has been developed. Various specific agents, such as bioactive ceramics, antimicrobials, growth factors and small molecules, have been added into the membrane aiming to facilitate and/or enhance periodontal tissue regeneration [2, 6]. Many studies have proven the incremental effect imposed by the combination of these agents with traditional guided tissue regeneration membranes [6].

Polycaprolactone (PCL) has been introduced as a candidate biomaterial for tissue regeneration. It has many properties that satisfied the criterion for GTR membrane. For example, it exhibits biocompatibility properties and is not toxic [7]. It has been widely investigated as a scaffold material for tissue-engineering application [8, 9]. In addition, it has been approved for clinical application, for example, suture materials, confirming the biocompatibility and safety in clinical use. Besides, the physical characteristics (e.g. strength and degradability) could be easily manipulated. Further, a precise control of membrane architecture could be simply fabricated. PCL also has less chance to induce immunological reaction. Together, it may imply the potential use of PCL as a material-based for GTR membrane.

2. Periodontal tissue healing and regeneration

Like healing processes of the other tissues, periodontal tissue-healing processes are divided into four phases: inflammation, proliferation, matrix formation, and remodelling [10]. First, the stability of blood clot at the defect site is crucial for periodontal tissue regeneration as it supports cell migration and proliferation in the affected area [10, 11]. However, periodontal tissue healing requires a unique healing process due to the complex nature of periodontal apparatus, which composes of cementum, periodontal ligament and alveolar bone. In addition, the distinctive periodontal ligament character requires the formation of collagen fibril embedding on the root surface of the teeth and alveolar bone. This contributes as another unique factor for periodontal tissue healing [10]. It is postulated that connective tissues recognize the exposed root dentin as a foreign body. Therefore, the formation of parallel collagen fibres is noted along the root surface [10]. The exposed root dentin provides a substrate for cementoblast-like cells to attach and differentiate. Further, cementoblasts form extracellular matrix where collagen fibres are anchored [10].

There are several cell types involved in periodontal regeneration/healing, for example, periodontal fibroblasts, osteoblasts, gingival fibroblasts and epithelial cells. A majority of cells in periodontal tissues is fibroblasts [12]. Fibroblastic cell population contains stem/progenitor cells that can differentiate into fibroblast, osteoblast and cementoblasts, depending on the stimulator [13–15]. These cells further participate in the regeneration and healing of periodontal tissues. However, it has been reported that gingival fibroblasts exhibited significantly higher *in vitro* wound-healing rate than periodontal ligament cells [16], implying that the speed of periodontal tissue healing is relatively slower than gingival tissues. Further, the bone healing is relatively slower than epithelium [15, 17]. Thus, normal periodontal tissue healing results in the formation of long junctional epithelium rather than the organized periodontal tissue formation [17]. This information indicates the complex and distinct regeneration/healing process of periodontal tissues. The control of specific time for each cell type to migrate into periodontal defect area is critical in the success of periodontal tissue regeneration/healing.

3. Guided tissue regeneration

GTR is one of the procedures that could ultimately regenerate the damaged periodontal tissues and restore them to a functional state [18]. GTR procedure is accomplished by placing the GTR membrane over the defect. This membrane acts as a physical barrier separating the gingival tissues and epithelium from the periodontal defect, allowing the required cell population (periodontal ligament cells and osteoblasts) to formulate a new attachment apparatus and functional periodontal tissues (**Figure 1**) [1, 17–19]. At the same time, the migration of epithelial cells and gingival fibroblasts is prevented. Thus, the formation of long junctional epithelium healing is attenuated [12].

GTR is well known for its successful clinical uses in an intrabony and furcation defect treatment [1, 18]. A systematic review of literature reports that GTR treatment results in better clinical outcomes than open-flap debridement procedure, for example, the improvement of clinical attachment levels, the reduction of probing depth and gingival recession [4, 20, 21]. Although other benefits of GTR for other types of periodontal defects are not as recognizable, GTR remains a beneficial treatment [1]. In this regard, GTR therapy results in a higher amount of clinical attachment gain than a therapy of accessing flap alone [22]. The disadvantage of GTR is that the result of the treatment varies due to the difference of host response, patient's oral hygiene, surgical technique and the lack of biological property to facilitate periodontal healing [1, 23–27].

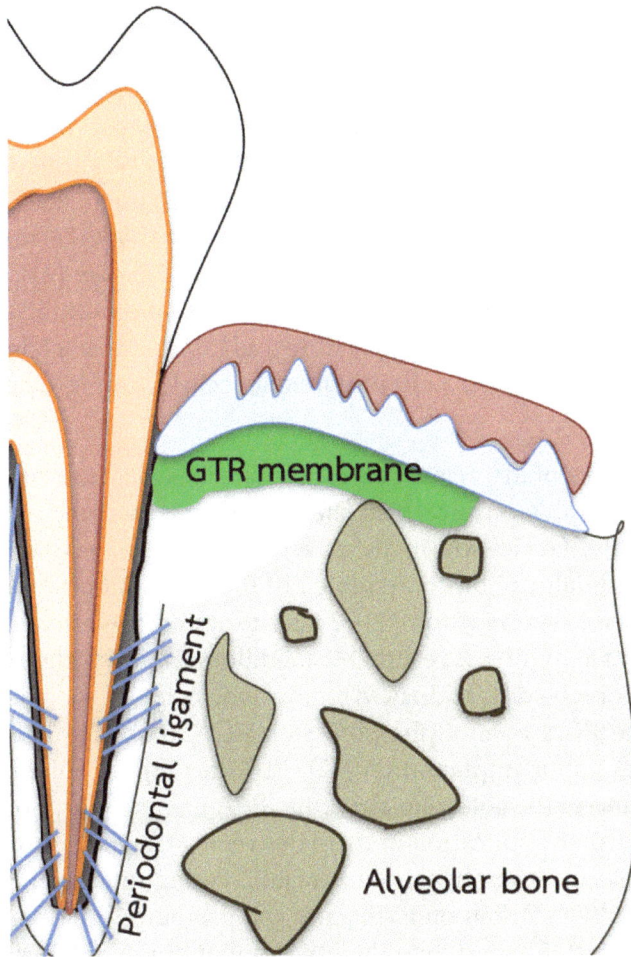

Figure 1. GTR membrane is positioned over the periodontal defect to separate gingival tissues and epithelium from the affected area, allowing the regeneration of periodontal tissues.

4. Guided tissue regeneration membrane materials

In general, like other biomaterials, GTR membrane should exhibit a biocompatibility. The degradation ability should match with the rate of new tissue formation, and the degradation product should not elicit host-inflammatory response. GTR should have the suitable mechanical and physical properties to maintain its shape *in vivo* and to easily manipulate. In this regard, GTR should have the adequate strength to maintain its form as a separating barrier and the clinical manageability [2, 6]. Materials for GTR membrane can be roughly categorized into two groups according to their degradation property, namely non-resorbable and resorbable materials. Both types of GTR materials exert similar clinical results [28, 29]. The non-biodegradable material currently available is polytetrafluoroethylene (PTFE) and methylcellulose acetate [1]. Major disadvantage of non-resorbable-guided tissue regeneration membranes is owing to the need for re-entering into the surgical site in order to remove the placed membranes, thus creating extra pain and discomfort to patients [2, 6, 29, 30].

Due to the disadvantage of the non-resorbable membrane, the resorbable membranes are created in order to eliminate the second surgery to remove the membrane [28]. The bioresorbable membranes can be further grouped into two categories: the natural and the synthetic membranes. The advantage of the natural membrane is that these can be degraded by normal physiological or pathological process in vivo [6]. In addition, the natural-derived membranes inherit biological properties that can induce or maintain biological activity of local cells and tissues. Collagen is widely used as a resorbable GTR membrane as it is an abundant structural protein in various types of connective tissues [31]. Although collagen exhibits low immunogenicity, the antigenic response and autoimmunization are noted [29, 31]. Another drawback of collagen is the fast degradation period leading to the failure of GTR treatment due to the downgrowth of epithelial cells, forming long junctional epithelium [6].

A resorbable membrane made from synthetic materials has the advantage in several aspects. Firstly, the desirable physical and chemical properties can be altered with simple methods [32]. Secondly, fabrication methods are controllable, easy and reproducible. In general, synthetic materials are biocompatible but the degradation products of some synthetic materials induce tissue reaction [33]. Many types of polyester-based material have been clinically utilized as synthetic resorbable membranes [2]. Synthetic materials for GTR membrane include polyglycolic acid (PGA), polylactic acid (PLA), polydioxanone (PDS), and polycaprolactone PGA is an alpha-polyester. PGA is able to hold their mechanical strength for 2–4 weeks after implantation [32]. PLA has higher solubility in organic solvents than PGA because of its molecular structure. PLA has an amorphous poly(D,L-lactide) which is useful for further application in drug delivery. PGA and PLA can be copolymerized to form high-molecular weight copolymers [32]. Periodontal ligament cells attach better on PLA and co-PLA-PGA than on PTFE, and cell proliferation is observed on PLA and co-PLA-PGA but not on PTFE, implying their biocompatibility [34]. PDS is a homopolymer of p-dioxanone. PDS can maintain its strength for 4–8 weeks and completely resorb in 4–6 months [32]. PDS membrane treatment for human infrabony defects demonstrated the reduction of probing depth and the increase of vertical clinical attachment levels as well as bony filling in the defect sites [35]. These results are similar to those defects treated with polylactide acetyltributyl citrate [35].

5. Bioactive-guided tissue regeneration membrane

With the evolution of tissue-engineering approach, the recent development of GTR membranes is not only used as a physical barrier but also used as a delivery device of specific agents such as antimicrobials, growth factors and stem cells [6]. This development of bioactive GTR membranes aims for facilitating the regeneration and healing of periodontal tissues [6]. This type of membrane is considered as bioactive-guided tissue regeneration membrane. The first approach is to incorporate antimicrobial agents with GTR membrane to attenuate the risk of bacterial infection, leading to the reduction of inflammation process [36]. The bacterial contamination and infection could effect on the healing and regeneration outcome and it has been shown that bacterial infection may be associated with gingival recession and impediment

Subjects	Materials	Agents	Results	Reference
Human	ePTFE	Tetracycline (3%)	Additional gain of clinical periodontal attachment	Zarkesh et al. [45]
Dog	PGA and PLA copolymer	Doxycycline (25%)	More pronounced new bone formation and less crestal bone resorption	Chang and Yamada [46]
Human	Collagen	Minocycline	Not significantly beneficial	Minabe et al. [47]
Dog	Polytetrafluoroethylene (ePTFF)	Platelet-derived growth factor-BB (PDGF-BB)	Effectively promoted periodontal regeneration	Cho et al. [48]
Dog	Polytetrafluoroethylene (ePTFF) (GORE-TFX)	Platelet-derived growth factor-BB (PDGF-BB)	Effectively promoted periodontal regeneration with reproducibility	Park et al. [49]
Rat	Poly L-lactide (PLLA)	Platelet-derived growth factor-BB (PDGF-BB)	Enhanced regenerative efficacy	Park et al. [50]
Human	Collagen	1. Recombinant human platelet-derived growth factor-BB (rhPDGF-BB) 2. Platelet-rich plasma (PRP) 3. Commercially available enamel matrix derivative (cEMD) 4. Peptide P-15 (P-15)	1. cEMD effectively used to treat intra-osseous defects 2. The combined use of rhPDGF-BB and P-15 has shown beneficial effects in intra-osseous defects 3. PRP and graft combinations are not beneficial	Trombelli and Farina [51]
Dog	Polytetrafluoroethylene (ePTFF) (GORE-TFX)	Recombinant human transforming growth factor-beta1 (rhTGF-β1)	Restricted potential to enhance alveolar bone regeneration in conjunction with guided tissue regeneration	Wikesjö et al. [52]
Dog	Collagen	Basic fibroblast growth factor (bFGF)	Enhance periodontal regenerative results, both mineralized and non-mineralized tissues	Rossa et al. [53]
Dog	Sandwich membrane: collagen and gelatin	Basic fibroblast growth factor (bFGF)	Active vascularization and osteogenesis Successful regeneration of the periodontal tissues in a short period of time	Nakahara et al. [54]
Human	Cellulose	human fibroblast growth factor-2 (FGF-2)	Efficacious in the regeneration of human periodontal tissue	Kitamura et al. [55]
Rat	Alginate/nanofibre	Recombinant bone morphogenetic protein-2 (rhBMP-2)	Effective in repair of critical-sized segmental defect	Kolambkar et al. [56]

Table 1. Studies on the bioactive-guided tissue regeneration membrane.

of attachment gain [37, 38]. Local minocycline application in combination with GTR treatment results in the significant higher clinical attachment gain [39]. In addition, GTR loaded with metronidazole reduces inflammatory response in vivo [40]. Further, the antimicrobial-incorporated GTR membrane has been shown to improve the attachment of periodontal ligament cells by effective oral pathogen eradication [41]. The second approach is to incorporate bioactive calcium phosphate in GTR membrane [6]. The addition of hydroxyapatite improves the biocompatibility and osteoconductivity of GTR membrane [42, 43]. These composite membranes also enhance osteoblast cell proliferation *in vitro* [42, 44]. In addition, the different response could be obtained by varying the concentration of calcium phosphate in the composite membrane [42].

The last approach is to incorporate with growth factor. Growth factors regulate various biological processes, for example, cell differentiation, cell proliferation, angiogenesis and chemotaxis, resulting in the promotion of tissue healing and regeneration. Various growth factors have been identified as factors enhancing periodontal tissue healing. The exemplification of these growth factors is platelet-derived growth factor (PDGF), insulin-like growth factor-1 (IGF-I), fibroblast growth factor-2 (FGF-2), transforming growth factor β-1 (TGFβ-1), bone morphogenetic protein-2 (BMP-2), bone morphogenetic protein-4 (BMP-4), bone morphogenetic protein-7 (BMP-7), bone morphogenetic protein-12 (BMP-12) and enamel matrix derivative (EMD). The example of the development of bioactive GTR membrane is demonstrated in **Table 1**.

6. Polycaprolactone in guided tissue regeneration

PCL is a semi-crystalline, aliphatic polyester [57]. The structure of PCL comprises a repeating unit of one ester group and five methylene groups (**Figure 2**). PCL has an excellent biocompatibility and slow degradation rate [7, 58]. In regard to many studies, there is no evidence revealing that PCL could potentially induce any cytotoxic effects nor accumulate in human

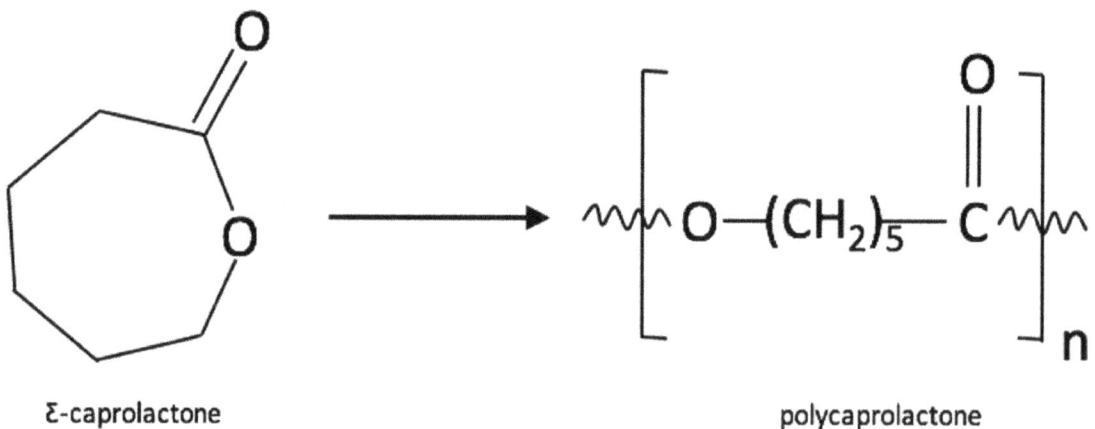

ε-caprolactone   polycaprolactone

Figure 2. Structure of polycaprolactone.

body [59]. Its ester linkages can be hydrolysed and excreted under normal physiological conditions. The degradation rate of PCL is slower than other aliphatic polyester [60]. In this regard, the degradation of PCL and its copolymers can be altered with different form and molecular weight of the materials. The high-molecular-weight (≥50,000 g/mol) PCL requires 3 years to degrade in host [60].

Therefore, PCL is a practicable option for many applications in tissue-engineering approaches. PCL been approved by the Food and Drug Administration (FDA) for several medical applications, for example, suture materials and subdermal contraceptive implants [57, 61, 62]. It has been applied as a beneficial biomaterial for drug delivery devices [63, 64]. The drug-releasing property is able to be controlled [64]. Thus, the biological activity could be lengthened [8]. For example, PCL was employed as wound-dressing materials, which released chemical antiseptic agent [65]. In dentistry, PCL has been introduced as root canal-filling materials. It was noted that PCL-filled root canal gave a predictable seal in an aqueous environment [66]. PCL is also employed as materials for bone tissue-engineering scaffolds that could be used for bone augmentation [58, 67–69]. Furthermore, PCL composites are recognized for its significant uses in tissue-engineering scaffolds in order to regenerate bone, ligament, cartilage, skin, nerve and vascular tissues [57]. PCL-based biomaterials have demonstrated the osteoconductive properties as they support various cell proliferations and differentiations, including bone marrow-derived mesenchymal stem cells (BMSCs), dental pulp stem cells (DPSCs) and adipose-derived mesenchymal stem cells (ADSCs) in PCL scaffold which was confirmed [68, 69]. Further, PCL implantation in murine calvarial defect model does not significantly increase the total IgG levels as compared with sham surgery group, demonstrating the immune compatibility of PCL-based materials [70].

As aforementioned, there has been a development in manufactured membrane used for GTR in order to meet its basic requirements. PCL is considered as satisfactory candidate for GTR due to its useful properties such as biocompatibility, proper mechanical strength, biodegradability and ease of fabrication [71–73]. Many studies investigated on the effectiveness of PCL membrane in GTR reveals an improvement of bone formation in the presence of noticeable bone cell attachment and proliferation [74, 75]. PCL and hydroxyapatite-incorporated PCL membrane were biocompatible and able to support human periodontal ligament cell attachment, spreading and proliferation (**Figure 3**). It was also shown that nano-apatite-incorporated PCL membrane facilitates osteoblast-like cell proliferation and differentiation [76]. Moreover, hydroxyapatite and gelatin nanocomposite-incorporated PCL supported osteoblast proliferation, induced alkaline phosphatase activity and enhanced mineralization [77]. For further study, the researcher has invented a new polymer/calcium phosphate composite for guided tissue regeneration use. Osteoblast alkaline phosphatase activity and expression of osteoblast marker gene, which indicates the promotion in bone maturation, have been recorded as the result [78]. The basic fibroblast growth factor-releasing heparin-conjugated PCL membrane has been successfully developed and exhibits biocompatibility. This basic fibroblast growth factor-releasing PCL membrane promotes human osteoblast-like cell attachment, proliferation and differentiation as compared

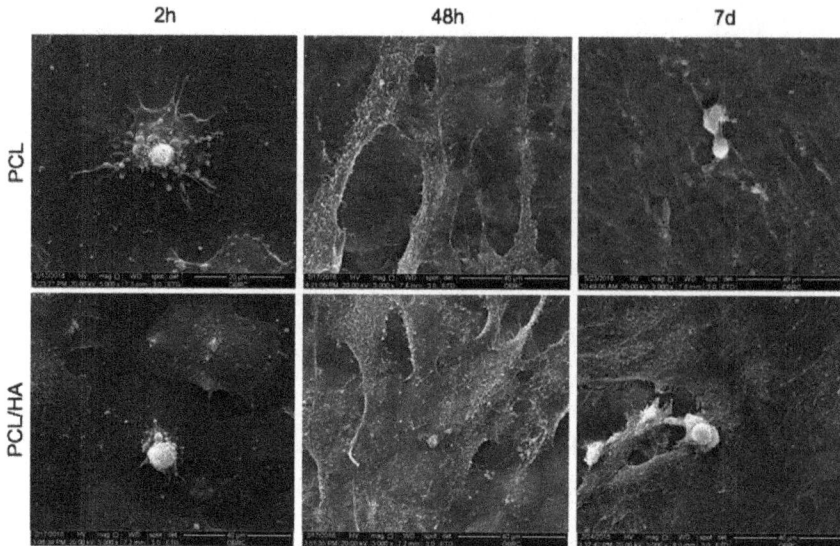

Figure 3. Scanning electron micrographs demonstrated the morphology of human periodontal ligament cell attachment, spreading and proliferation on polycaprolactone (PCL) and hydroxyapatite-incorporated PCL (PCL/HA) membrane. At 2 h, cells exhibited lamellipodia extension and completed cell spreading covering the surface was noted at 48 h after seeding. Cell monolayer was observed on the membrane at day 7.

with the naïve PCL membrane [79]. Metronidazole-incorporated PCL-based membranes decrease inflammatory response, determined in subcutaneous implantation model as compared to the unmodified PCL membrane [40, 80]. According to these studies, PCL become an appropriate material for the use of GTR membrane and advantageous prototype for further clinical membrane invention [76].

Beside GTR membrane, PCL has been developed as bone-defect-filling materials aiming to promote bone regeneration in periodontal defects. The scaffolds aim to support periodontal ligament and alveolar bone cell migration and repopulation in the affected site, facilitating the regeneration process. Three-dimensional PCL scaffolds can be fabricated by a modified solvent casting and particulate-leaching techniques, resulting in the highly porous and interconnected structure in PCL scaffolds [81]. Hydroxyapatite incorporation in PCL scaffolds exhibited biocompatibility and degradability [67]. These scaffolds have osteoconductive property which enhanced primary human osteoblast response *in vitro* and promoted bone formation in rat calvarial defect *in vivo* [67]. The incorporation of hydrophilic polyethylene glycol into hydrophobic PCL enhanced the overall hydrophilicity and cell culture performance of PCL/PEG copolymer as an optimal guided tissue regeneration material [82]. PCL/PEG scaffolds supported growth and osteogenic differentiation of human periodontal ligament cells *in vitro* [70]. Huynh et al. demonstrated that PCL/PEG scaffolds incorporated with epigenetic-modified human periodontal ligament cells could promote bone formation in calvarial defect [70]. Together, these findings strongly support the potential application of PCL as the potential guided scaffold in periodontal tissue regeneration therapy.

7. Notch signalling as a potential bioactive molecule in guided tissue regeneration of periodontal tissues

Notch ligands, Jagged1, promote cell differentiation towards osteoblast lineages of human periodontal ligament stem cells and bone marrow-derived mesenchymal stem cells [83–85]. Other studies also demonstrated that Jagged1-immobilized surface could reduce epithelial cell proliferation and enhanced epithelial cell differentiation [86, 87]. In addition, in rafted organ culture model, Jagged1-coated porous biomaterial significantly reduced the formation of epithelial tongue [87]. In other words, Jagged1 could prevent epithelial cells migration down into the dermis. For this reason, Jagged1 is considered as a beneficial molecule to be coated on a guided tissue regeneration membrane to enhance periodontal tissue formation. The schematic diagram of the propose idea is demonstrated in **Figure 4**. The Jagged1-coated PCL membrane firstly acts as a physical barrier to prevent epithelial down-growth into periodontal-defect site. In biological events, Jagged1 inhibits proliferation and induced the differentiation of epithelial cells. Further, Jagged1 promoted osteogenic differentiation of periodontal ligament cells and alveolar osteoblast cells. Together, these effects prevent the epithelium downgrowth in the lesion and promote the formation of alveolar bone, leading to the achievement of successful guided tissue regeneration.

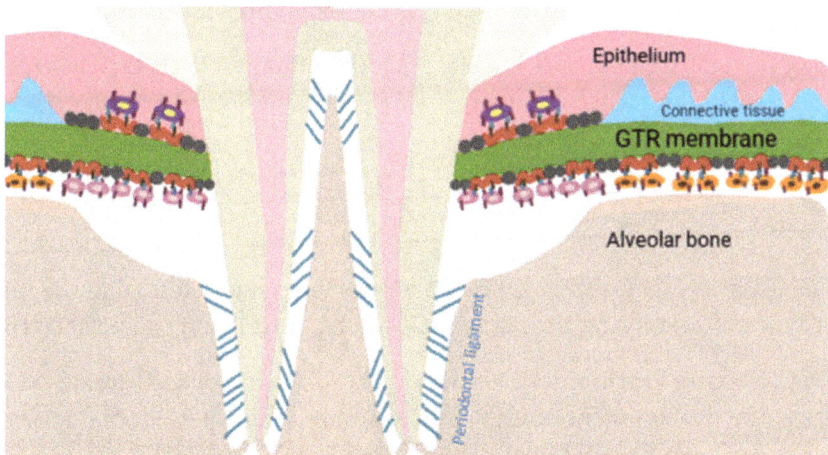

Figure 4. Schematic diagram of Jagged1-coated PCL membrane for GTR therapy.

8. Conclusion

The present chapter reviews the biological basis of GTR membrane in periodontal tissue healing and regeneration. In the past, GTR acts as a physical barrier to allow required cells to facilitate periodontal tissue formation. Recently, bioactive GTR membrane has been investigated and developed aiming to fabricate membrane that not only act as a physical barrier but also induce biological events to enhance periodontal tissue regeneration. PCL has been introduced as candidate materials for bioactive GTR membrane due to its biocompatibility and simple fabrication procedure. The modification with other agents/biomolecules could be easily constructed. With the use of proposed Notch ligands, PCL-decorated Jagged1 could be beneficial to promote periodontal tissue formation. However, further investigations are indeed required.

Acknowledgements

The authors are supported by the Faculty of Dentistry Research Fund, Chulalongkorn University.

Author details

Thanaphum Osathanon[1,2]*, Phunphimp Chanjavanakul[1], Pattanit Kongdecha[1], Panipuk Clayhan[1] and Nam Cong-Nhat Huynh[3]

*Address all correspondence to: thanaphum.o@chula.ac.th

1 STAR in Craniofacial Genetics and Stem Cells Research, Faculty of Dentistry, Chulalongkorn University, Bangkok, Thailand

2 Department of Anatomy, Faculty of Dentistry, Chulalongkorn University, Bangkok, Thailand

3 Department of Dental Basic Sciences, Faculty of Odonto-Stomatology, University of Medicine and Pharmacy, Ho Chi Minh City, Vietnam

References

[1] Villar CC, Cochran DL. Regeneration of periodontal tissues: Guided tissue regeneration. Dental Clinics of North America. 2010;**54**:73-92. DOI: 10.1016/j.cden.2009.08.011

[2] Bottino MC, Thomas V, Schmidt G, Vohra YK, Chu TM, Kowolik MJ, Janowski GM. Recent advances in the development of GTR/GBR membranes for periodontal regeneration—A materials perspective. Dental Materials. 2012;**28**:703-721. DOI: 10.1016/j.dental.2012.04.022

[3] Needleman I, Tucker R, Giedrys-Leeper E, Worthington H. Guided tissue regeneration for periodontal intrabony defects—A cochrane systematic review. Periodontology 2000. 2005;**37**:106-123. DOI: 10.1111/j.1600-0757.2004.37101.x

[4] Murphy KG, Gunsolley JC. Guided tissue regeneration for the treatment of periodontal intrabony and furcation defects. A systematic review. Annals of Periodontology. 2003;**8**:266-302. DOI: 10.1902/annals.2003.8.1.266

[5] Yen CC, Tu YK, Chen TH, Lu HK. Comparison of treatment effects of guided tissue regeneration on infrabony lesions between animal and human studies: A systematic review and meta-analysis. Journal of Periodontology Research. 2014;**49**:415-424. DOI: 10.1111/jre.12130

[6] Sam G, Pillai BR. Evolution of barrier membranes in periodontal regeneration-"Are the third generation membranes really here?" Journal of Clinical and Diagnostic Research. 2014;8:ZE14-ZE17. DOI: 10.7860/JCDR/2014/9957.5272

[7] Shi R, Xue J, He M, Chen D, Zhang L, Tian W. Structure, physical properties, biocompatibility and in vitro/vivo degradation behavior of anti-infective polycaprolactone-based electrospun membranes for guided tissue/bone regeneration. Polymer Degradation and Stability. 2014;109:293-306. DOI: http://dx.doi.org/10.1016/j.polymdegradstab.2014.07.017

[8] Dash TK, Konkimalla VB. Polymeric modification and its implication in drug delivery: Poly-epsilon-caprolactone (PCL) as a model polymer. Molecular Pharmaceutical. 2012;9:2365-2379. DOI: 10.1021/mp3001952

[9] Vieira A, Medeiros R, Guedes RM, Marques A, Tita V, editors. Visco-Elastic-Plastic Properties of Suture Fibers made of PLA-PCL. Materials Science Forum. Trans Tech Publ; 2013. Zurich, Switzerland

[10] Wikesjo UM, Selvig KA. Periodontal wound healing and regeneration. Periodontology 2000. 1999;19:21-39

[11] Baker DL, Stanley Pavlow SA, Wikesjo UM. Fibrin clot adhesion to dentin conditioned with protein constructs: An in vitro proof-of-principle study. Journal of Clinical Periodontology. 2005;32:561-566. DOI: 10.1111/j.1600-051X.2005.00714.x

[12] Bowers GM, Chadroff B, Carnevale R, Mellonig J, Corio R, Emerson J, Stevens M, Romberg E. Histologic evaluation of new attachment apparatus formation in humans. Part III. Journal of Periodontology. 1989;60:683-693. DOI: 10.1902/jop.1989.60.12.683

[13] Yin X, Li Y, Li J, Li P, Liu Y, Wen J, Luan Q. Generation and periodontal differentiation of human gingival fibroblasts-derived integration-free induced pluripotent stem cells. Biochemical and Biophysical Research Communication. 2016;473:726-732. DOI: 10.1016/j.bbrc.2015.10.012

[14] Kim BC, Bae H, Kwon IK, Lee EJ, Park JH, Khademhosseini A, Hwang YS. Osteoblastic/cementoblastic and neural differentiation of dental stem cells and their applications to tissue engineering and regenerative medicine. Tissue Engineering Part B: Reviews. 2012;18:235-244. DOI: 10.1089/ten.TEB.2011.0642

[15] Listgarten MA, Rosenberg MM. Histological study of repair following new attachment procedures in human periodontal lesions. Journal of Periodontology. 1979;50:333-344. DOI: 10.1902/jop.1979.50.7.333

[16] Lackler KP, Cochran DL, Hoang AM, Takacs V, Oates TW. Development of an in vitro wound healing model for periodontal cells. Journal of Periodontology. 2000;71:226-237. DOI: 10.1902/jop.2000.71.2.226

[17] Xu C, Lei C, Meng L, Wang C, Song Y. Chitosan as a barrier membrane material in periodontal tissue regeneration. Journal of Biomedical Materials Research Part B: Applied Biomaterials. 2012;100:1435-1443. DOI: 10.1002/jbm.b.32662

[18] Laurell L, Gottlow J. Guided tissue regeneration update. International Dental Journal. 1998;**48**:386-398

[19] Nyman S, Gottlow J, Karring T, Lindhe J. The regenerative potential of the periodontal ligament. An experimental study in the monkey. Journal of Clinical Periodontology. 1982;**9**:257-265. DOI: 10.1111/j.1600-051X.1982.tb02065.x

[20] Needleman IG, Worthington HV, Giedrys-Leeper E, Tucker RJ. Guided tissue regeneration for periodontal infra-bony defects. Cochrane Database of Systematic Reviews. 2006;**19**(2):CD001724. DOI: 10.1002/14651858.CD001724.pub2

[21] Parrish LC, Miyamoto T, Fong N, Mattson JS, Cerutis DR. Non-bioabsorbable vs. bioabsorbable membrane: Assessment of their clinical efficacy in guided tissue regeneration technique. A systematic review. Journal of Oral Science. 2009;**51**:383-400

[22] Tonetti MS, Cortellini P, Suvan JE, Adriaens P, Baldi C, Dubravec D, Fonzar A, Fourmousis I, Magnani C, Muller-Campanile V, Patroni S, Sanz M, Vangsted T, Zabalegui I, Pini Prato G, Lang NP. Generalizability of the added benefits of guided tissue regeneration in the treatment of deep intrabony defects. Evaluation in a multi-center randomized controlled clinical trial. Journal of Periodontology. 1998;**69**:1183-1192. DOI: 10.1902/jop.1998.69.11.1183

[23] Abou Neel EA, Chrzanowski W, Salih VM, Kim HW, Knowles JC. Tissue engineering in dentistry. Journal of Dentistry. 2014;**42**:915-928. DOI: 10.1016/j.jdent.2014.05.008

[24] Machtei EE, Oettinger-Barak O, Peled M. Guided tissue regeneration in smokers: Effect of aggressive anti-infective therapy in Class II furcation defects. Journal of Periodontology. 2003;**74**:579-584. DOI: 10.1902/jop.2003.74.5.579

[25] Rosenberg ES, Cutler SA. The effect of cigarette smoking on the long-term success of guided tissue regeneration: A preliminary study. Annals of the Royal Australasian College of Dental Surgeons. 1994;**12**:89-93

[26] Machtei EE, Cho MI, Dunford R, Norderyd J, Zambon JJ, Genco RJ. Clinical, microbiological, and histological factors which influence the success of regenerative periodontal therapy. Journal of Periodontology. 1994;**65**:154-161. DOI: 10.1902/jop.1994.65.2.154

[27] Verma PK, Srivastava R, Gupta KK, Chaturvedi TP. Treatment strategy for guided tissue regeneration in various class II furcation defect: Case series. Dental Research Journal. 2013;**10**:689-694

[28] Wolff LF, Mullally B. New clinical materials and techniques in guided tissue regeneration. International Dental Journal. 2000;**50**:235-244

[29] Bottino MC, Thomas V. Membranes for periodontal regeneration—A materials perspective. Frontiers in Oral Biology. 2015;**17**:90-100. DOI: 10.1159/000381699

[30] Jovanovic SA, Nevins M. Bone formation utilizing titanium-reinforced barrier membranes. International Journal of Periodontics and Restorative Dentistry. 1995;**15**:56-69

[31] Sheikh Z, Qureshi J, Alshahrani AM, Nassar H, Ikeda Y, Glogauer M, Ganss B. Collagen based barrier membranes for periodontal guided bone regeneration applications. Odontology. 2017;**105**:1-12. DOI: 10.1007/s10266-016-0267-0

[32] Hutmacher D, Hürzeler MB, Schliephake H. A review of material properties of biodegradable and bioresorbable polymers and devices for GTR and GBR applications. The International Journal of Oral & Maxillofacial Implants. 1995;**11**:667-678

[33] Schmidmaier G, Baehr K, Mohr S, Kretschmar M, Beck S, Wildemann B. Biodegradable polylactide membranes for bone defect coverage: Biocompatibility testing, radiological and histological evaluation in a sheep model. Clinical Oral Implants Research. 2006;**17**:439-444. DOI: 10.1111/j.1600-0501.2005.01242.x

[34] Takata T, Wang HL, Miyauchi M. Attachment, proliferation and differentiation of periodontal ligament cells on various guided tissue regeneration membranes. Journal of Periodontal Research. 2001;**36**:322-327

[35] Eickholz P, Kim TS, Steinbrenner H, Dorfer C, Holle R. Guided tissue regeneration with bioabsorbable barriers: Intrabony defects and class II furcations. Journal of Periodontology. 2000;**71**:999-1008. DOI: 10.1902/jop.2000.71.6.999

[36] Machtei EE, Dunford RG, Norderyd OM, Zambon JJ, Genco RJ. Guided tissue regeneration and anti-infective therapy in the treatment of class II furcation defects. Journal of Periodontology. 1993;**64**:968-973. DOI: 10.1902/jop.1993.64.10.968

[37] Gottlow J, Nyman S. Barrier membranes in the treatment of periodontal defects. Current Opinion in Periodontology. 1996;**3**:140-148

[38] Selvig KA, Kersten BG, Chamberlain ADH, Wikesjö UM, Nilvúus RE. Regenerative surgery of intrabony periodontal defects using ePTFE barrier membranes: Scanning electron microscopic evaluation of retrieved membranes versus clinical healing. Journal of Periodontology. 1992;**63**:974-978

[39] Yoshinari N, Tohya T, Kawase H, Matsuoka M, Nakane M, Kawachi M, Mitani A, Koide M, Inagaki K, Fukuda M, Noguchi T. Effect of repeated local minocycline administration on periodontal healing following guided tissue regeneration. Journal of Periodontology. 2001;**72**:284-295. DOI: 10.1902/jop.2001.72.3.284

[40] Xue J, He M, Niu Y, Liu H, Crawford A, Coates P, Chen D, Shi R, Zhang L. Preparation and in vivo efficient anti-infection property of GTR/GBR implant made by metronidazole loaded electrospun polycaprolactone nanofiber membrane. International Journal of Pharmaceuticals. 2014;**475**:566-577. DOI: 10.1016/j.ijpharm.2014.09.026

[41] Hung SL, Lin YW, Chen YT, Ling LJ. Attachment of periodontal ligament cells onto various antibiotics-loaded GTR membranes. International Journal of Periodontics and Restorative Dentistry. 2005;**25**:265-275

[42] Talal A, McKay IJ, Tanner KE, Hughes FJ. Effects of hydroxyapatite and PDGF concentrations on osteoblast growth in a nanohydroxyapatite-polylactic acid composite for guided

tissue regeneration. Journal of Material Science: Materials in Medicine. 2013;**24**:2211-2221. DOI: 10.1007/s10856-013-4963-9

[43] Liao S, Wang W, Uo M, Ohkawa S, Akasaka T, Tamura K, Cui F, Watari F. A three-layered nano-carbonated hydroxyapatite/collagen/PLGA composite membrane for guided tissue regeneration. Biomaterials. 2005;**26**:7564-7571. DOI: 10.1016/j.biomaterials.2005.05.050

[44] Hurt AP, Getti G, Coleman NJ. Bioactivity and biocompatibility of a chitosan-tobermorite composite membrane for guided tissue regeneration. International Journal of Biological Macromolecules. 2014;**64**:11-16. DOI: 10.1016/j.ijbiomac.2013.11.020

[45] Zarkesh N, Nowzari H, Morrison JL, Slots J. Tetracycline-coated polytetrafluoroethylene barrier membranes in the treatment of intraosseous periodontal lesions. Journal of Periodontology. 1999;**70**:1008-1016. DOI: 10.1902/jop.1999.70.9.1008

[46] Chang CY, Yamada S. Evaluation of the regenerative effect of a 25% doxycycline-loaded biodegradable membrane for guided tissue regeneration. Journal of Periodontology. 2000;**71**:1086-1093. DOI: 10.1902/jop.2000.71.7.1086

[47] Minabe M, Kodama T, Kogou T, Fushimi H, Sugiyama T, Takeuchi K, Miterai E, Nishikubo S. Clinical significance of antibiotic therapy in guided tissue regeneration with a resorbable membrane. Periodontal Clinical Investigations. 2001;**23**:20-30

[48] Cho MI, Lin WL, Genco RJ. Platelet-derived growth factor-modulated guided tissue regenerative therapy. Journal of Periodontology. 1995;**66**:522-530. DOI: 10.1902/jop.1995.66.6.522

[49] Park JB, Matsuura M, Han KY, Norderyd O, Lin WL, Genco RJ, Cho MI. Periodontal regeneration in class III furcation defects of beagle dogs using guided tissue regenerative therapy with platelet-derived growth factor. Journal of Periodontology. 1995;**66**:462-477. DOI: 10.1902/jop.1995.66.6.462

[50] Park YJ, Ku Y, Chung CP, Lee SJ. Controlled release of platelet-derived growth factor from porous poly(L-lactide) membranes for guided tissue regeneration. Journal of Controlled Release. 1998;**51**:201-211

[51] Trombelli L, Farina R. Clinical outcomes with bioactive agents alone or in combination with grafting or guided tissue regeneration. Journal of Clinical Periodontology. 2008;**35**:117-135. DOI: 10.1111/j.1600-051X.2008.01265.x

[52] Wikesjo UME, Razi SS, Sigurdsson TJ, Tatakis DN, Lee MB, Ongpipattanakul B, Nguyen T, Hardwick R. Periodontal repair in dogs: Effect of recombinant human transforming growth factor-beta1 on guided tissue regeneration. Journal of Clinical Periodontology. 1998;**25**:475-481. DOI: 10.1111/j.1600-051X.1998.tb02476.x

[53] Rossa Jr C, Marcantonio Jr E, Cirelli JA, Marcantonio RA, Spolidorio LC, Fogo JC. Regeneration of Class III furcation defects with basic fibroblast growth factor (b-FGF) associated with GTR. A descriptive and histometric study in dogs. Journal of Periodontology. 2000;**71**:775-784

[54] Nakahara T, Nakamura T, Kobayashi E, Inoue M, Shigeno K, Tabata Y, Eto K, Shimizu Y. Novel approach to regeneration of periodontal tissues based on in situ tissue engineering: Effects of controlled release of basic fibroblast growth factor from a sandwich membrane. Tissue Engineering. 2003;9:153-162. DOI: 10.1089/107632703762687636

[55] Kitamura M, Akamatsu M, Machigashira M, Hara Y, Sakagami R, Hirofuji T, Hamachi T, Maeda K, Yokota M, Kido J, Nagata T, Kurihara H, Takashiba S, Sibutani T, Fukuda M, Noguchi T, Yamazaki K, Yoshie H, Ioroi K, Arai T, Nakagawa T, Ito K, Oda S, Izumi Y, Ogata Y, Yamada S, Shimauchi H, Kunimatsu K, Kawanami M, Fujii T, Furuichi Y, Furuuchi T, Sasano T, Imai E, Omae M, Yamada S, Watanuki M, Murakami S. FGF-2 stimulates periodontal regeneration: Results of a multi-center randomized clinical trial. Journal of Dental Research. 2011;90:35-40. DOI: 10.1177/0022034510384616

[56] Kolambkar YM, Dupont KM, Boerckel JD, Huebsch N, Mooney DJ, Hutmacher DW, Guldberg RE. An alginate-based hybrid system for growth factor delivery in the functional repair of large bone defects. Biomaterials. 2011;32:65-74. DOI: 10.1016/j.biomaterials.2010.08.074

[57] Ulery BD, Nair LS, Laurencin CT. Biomedical applications of biodegradable polymers. Journal of Polymer Science Part B: Polymer Physics. 2011;49:832-864. DOI: 10.1002/polb.22259

[58] Woodruff MA, Hutmacher DW. The return of a forgotten polymer--Polycaprolactone in the 21st century. Progress in Polymer Science. 2010;35:1217-1256. DOI: 10.1016/j.progpolymsci.2010.04.002

[59] Lo HY, Kuo HT, Huang YY. Application of polycaprolactone as an anti-adhesion biomaterial film. Artificial Organs. 2010;34:648-653. DOI: 10.1111/j.1525-1594.2009.00949.x

[60] Rezwan K, Chen QZ, Blaker JJ, Boccaccini AR. Biodegradable and bioactive porous polymer/inorganic composite scaffolds for bone tissue engineering. Biomaterials. 2006;27:3413-431. DOI: 10.1016/j.biomaterials.2006.01.039

[61] Darney PD, Monroe SE, Klaisle CM, Alvarado A. Clinical evaluation of the Capronor contraceptive implant: Preliminary report. American Journal of Obstetrics & Gynecology. 1989;160:1292-1295

[62] Bezwada RS, Jamiolkowski DD, Lee IY, Agarwal V, Persivale J, Trenka-Benthin S, Erneta M, Suryadevara J, Yang A, Liu S. Monocryl suture, a new ultra-pliable absorbable monofilament suture. Biomaterials. 1995;16:1141-1148

[63] Wang Q, Jiang J, Chen W, Jiang H, Zhang Z, Sun X. Targeted delivery of low-dose dexamethasone using PCL-PEG micelles for effective treatment of rheumatoid arthritis. Journal of Controlled Release. 2016;230:64-72. DOI: 10.1016/j.jconrel.2016.03.035

[64] Pohlmann AR, Fonseca FN, Paese K, Detoni CB, Coradini K, Beck RC, Guterres SS. Poly(ε-caprolactone) microcapsules and nanocapsules in drug delivery. Expert Opinion on Drug Delivery. 2013;10:623-638. DOI: 10.1517/17425247.2013.769956

[65] Scaffaro R, Botta L, Sanfilippo M, Gallo G, Palazzolo G, Puglia AM. Combining in the melt physical and biological properties of poly(caprolactone) and chlorhexidine to

obtain antimicrobial surgical monofilaments. Applied Microbiology and Biotechnology. 2013;**97**:99-109. DOI: 10.1007/s00253-012-4283-x

[66] Álvarez AL, Espinar FO, Méndez JB. The application of microencapsulation techniques in the treatment of endodontic and periodontal disease. Pharmaceutics. 2011;**3**:538-571. DOI: 10.3390/pharmaceutics3030538

[67] Chuenjitkuntaworn B, Inrung W, Damrongsri D, Mekaapiruk K, Supaphol P, Pavasant P. Polycaprolactone/hydroxyapatite composite scaffolds: Preparation, characterization, and in vitro and in vivo biological responses of human primary bone cells. Journal of Biomedical Materials Research Part A. 2010;**94**:241-251. DOI: 10.1002/jbm.a.32657

[68] Chuenjitkuntaworn B, Osathanon T, Nowwarote N, Supaphol P, Pavasant P. The efficacy of polycaprolactone/hydroxyapatite scaffold in combination with mesenchymal stem cells for bone tissue engineering. Journal of Biomedical Materials Research Part A. 2016;**104**:264-271. DOI: 10.1002/jbm.a.35558

[69] Osathanon T, Chuenjitkuntaworn B, Nowwarote N, Supaphol P, Sastravaha P, Subbalekha K, Pavasant P. The responses of human adipose-derived mesenchymal stem cells on polycaprolactone-based scaffolds: An in vitro study. Tissue Engineering and Regenerative Medicine. 2014;**11**:239-246. DOI: 10.1007/s13770-014-0015-x

[70] Huynh NC, Everts V, Nifuji A, Pavasant P, Ampornaramveth RS. Histone deacetylase inhibition enhances in-vivo bone regeneration induced by human periodontal ligament cells. Bone. 2017;**95**:76-84. DOI: 10.1016/j.bone.2016.11.017

[71] Fecek C, Yao D, Kacorri A, Vasquez A, Iqbal S, Sheikh H, Svinarich DM, Perez-Cruet M, Chaudhry GR. Chondrogenic derivatives of embryonic stem cells seeded into 3D polycaprolactone scaffolds generated cartilage tissue in vivo. Tissue Engineering Part A. 2008;**14**:1403-1413. DOI: 10.1089/tea.2007.0293

[72] Li WJ, Tuli R, Okafor C, Derfoul A, Danielson KG, Hall DJ, Tuan RS. A three-dimensional nanofibrous scaffold for cartilage tissue engineering using human mesenchymal stem cells. Biomaterials. 2005;**26**:599-609. DOI: 10.1016/j.biomaterials.2004.03.005

[73] Li WJ, Jiang YJ, Tuan RS. Cell-nanofiber-based cartilage tissue engineering using improved cell seeding, growth factor, and bioreactor technologies. Tissue Engineering Part A. 2008; **14**:639-648. DOI: 10.1089/tea.2007.0136

[74] Zhang LJ, Webster TJ. Nanotechnology and nanomaterials: Promises for improved tissue regeneration. Nano Today. 2009;**4**:66-80. DOI: 10.1016/j.nantod.2008.10.014

[75] Basile MA, d'Ayala GG, Malinconico M, Laurienzo P, Coudane J, Nottelet B, Ragione FD, Oliva A. Functionalized PCL/HA nanocomposites as microporous membranes for bone regeneration. Materials Science & Engineering C Materials for Biological Applications. 2015;**48**:457-468. DOI: 10.1016/j.msec.2014.12.019

[76] Yang F, Both SK, Yang X, Walboomers XF, Jansen JA. Development of an electrospun nano-apatite/PCL composite membrane for GTR/GBR application. Acta Biomaterial. 2009;**5**:3295-304. DOI: 10.1016/j.actbio.2009.05.023

[77] Venugopal JR, Low S, Choon AT, Kumar AB, Ramakrishna S. Nanobioengineered electrospun composite nanofibers and osteoblasts for bone regeneration. Artificial Organs.
2008;**32**:388-397. DOI: 10.1111/j.1525-1594.2008.00557.x

[78] Osathanon T, Linnes ML, Rajachar RM, Ratner BD, Somerman MJ, Giachelli CM.
Microporous nanofibrous fibrin-based scaffolds for bone tissue engineering. Biomaterials.
2008;**29**:4091-4099. DOI: 10.1016/j.biomaterials.2008.06.030

[79] Cao C, Song Y, Yao Q, Yao Y, Wang T, Huang B, Gong P. Preparation and preliminary
in vitro evaluation of a bFGF-releasing heparin-conjugated poly(epsilon-caprolactone)
membrane for guided bone regeneration. Journal of Biomaterials Science, Polymer
Edition. 2015;**26**:600-616. DOI: 10.1080/09205063.2015.1049044

[80] Xue J, He M, Liu H, Niu Y, Crawford A, Coates PD, Chen D, Shi R, Zhang L. Drug
loaded homogeneous electrospun PCL/gelatin hybrid nanofiber structures for anti-
infective tissue regeneration membranes. Biomaterials. 2014;**35**:9395-405. DOI: 10.1016/j.
biomaterials.2014.07.060

[81] Thadavirul N, Pavasant P, Supaphol P. Development of polycaprolactone porous
scaffolds by combining solvent casting, particulate leaching, and polymer leaching
techniques for bone tissue engineering. Journal of Biomedical Materials Research A.
2014;**102**:3379-3392. DOI: 10.1002/jbma.35010

[82] Hoque ME, San WY, Wei F, Li S, Huang MH, Vert M, Hutmacher DW. Processing of polycaprolactone and polycaprolactone-based copolymers into 3D scaffolds, and their cellular
responses. Tissue Engineering Part A. 2009;**15**:3013-3024. DOI: 10.1089/ten.TEA.2008.0355

[83] Osathanon T, Nowwarote N, Manokawinchoke J, Pavasant P. bFGF and JAGGED1 regulate alkaline phosphatase expression and mineralization in dental tissue-derived mesenchymal stem cells. Journal of Cell Biochemistry. 2013;**114**:2551-2561. DOI: 10.1002/jcb.24602

[84] Osathanon T, Ritprajak P, Nowwarote N, Manokawinchoke J, Giachelli C, Pavasant P.
Surface-bound orientated Jagged-1 enhances osteogenic differentiation of human peri-
odontal ligament-derived mesenchymal stem cells. Journal of Biomedical Materials
Research A. 2013;**101**:358-367. DOI: 10.1002/jbm.a.34332

[85] Dishowitz MI, Zhu F, Sundararaghavan HG, Ifkovits JL, Burdick JA, Hankenson KD.
Jagged1 immobilization to an osteoconductive polymer activates the Notch signaling
pathway and induces osteogenesis. Journal of Biomedical Materials Research A.
2014;**102**:1558-1567. DOI: 10.1002/jbm.a.34825

[86] Beckstead BL, Santosa DwM, Giachelli CM. Mimicking cell-cell interactions at the
biomaterial-cell interface for control of stem cell differentiation. Journal of Biomedical
Materials Research A. 2006;**79**:94-103. DOI: 10.1002/jbm.a.30760

[87] Beckstead BL, Tung JC, Liang KJ, Tavakkol Z, Usui ML, Olerud JE, Giachelli CM.
Methods to promote Notch signaling at the biomaterial interface and evaluation in a
rafted organ culture model. Journal of Biomedical Materials Research A. 2009;**91**:436-
446. DOI: 10.1002/jbm.a.32214

8

Anaerobic Bacteria Associated with Periodontitis

Ahmed Zuhair Jasim Alwaeli

Abstract

Oral bacteria are highly associated with oral diseases, and periodontitis is a strongly prevalent disease, presenting a substantial economical burden. Furthermore, there is a strong association between periodontal bacteria and other diseases, such as cardiovascular disease, rheumatoid arthritis, or diabetes, so it becomes clear that efficient periodontal cure would be of good medical benefit to general health. Periodontally, Healthy loci show a low number of bacteria which are cultivable by individual sulcus, 10^2–10^3 microorganisms with almost Gram-positive microbiota, including *Streptococcus* and *Actinomyces* species. In gingivitis, it is characterized by an increased bacterial number, 104–105 microorganisms by periodontal sulcus, besides an increased diffusion of Gram negative bacteria (15–50%).The increased number of oral bacteria could be associated with the decreased role of the innate and adaptive immunity; so, this chapter will focus on the most prevalent bacteria associated with the oral disease on the one hand and the role of innate immunity and adaptive immunity (Interleukin 1 Beta Il-1β and Tumor necrosis factor-alpha TNF-α) in oral diseases on the other hand.

Keywords: anaerobic bacteria, oral bacteria, oral diseases, periodontitis, oral immunity

1. Introduction

Oral bacteria are highly associated with oral diseases; periodontitis is a strongly prevalent disease, presenting substantial economic problem [1]; and oral disease are associated with other diseases, such as cardiovascular, rheumatoid arthritis, or diabetes, so it becomes clear that good periodontal cure would be of excellent medical interest to general health [2]. Periodontally, healthy sites show a low number of bacteria which are cultivable by individual sulcus, 10^2–10^3 microorganisms with almost Gram-positive microbiota, including

Streptococcus and *Actinomyces* species. In gingivitis, it is characterized by an increased bacterial number, 10^4–10^5 microorganisms by periodontal sulcus besides an increased diffusion of Gram-negative bacteria (15–50%) [3]. The increased number of oral bacteria could be associated with the decreased role of the innate and adaptive immunity; so, this chapter will focus on the most prevalent bacteria associated with the oral disease on the one hand and the role of innate immunity and adaptive immunity (interleukin-1 beta (IL-1β) and tumor necrosis factor-alpha (TNF-α)) in oral diseases on the other hand.

2. Historical review on the classification and identification of oral bacteria

The initial date for the identification of oral bacteria belongs to 1680, when Antonie van Leeuwenhoek noticed, described, and isolated the microorganisms from his teeth plaque by using a primitive microscope. He drawn the noticed microbes and, when he established with the current knowledge, these drawings represented the most plentiful bacteria found within the oral cavity, including fusiform, spirochetes, and cocci bacteria [4].

Record research, a wide range of clinical studies on animals, engaged these oral bacteria with two common diseases, periodontitis, and dental caries. Even long before the visual observations of microorganisms, about 5000 BC, the Sumerians accused certain form of living (called as tooth worm) as a causative agent of caries on teeth [5]. Limited microbiological cultivation procedures and isolation techniques beginning of the nineteenth century forbid scientists to identify the exact causative agent of the disease. But this finding was partially done in 1925, by Clarke [6]. Unlike dental caries, another human oral disease is called periodontitis, and it is considered as the second most common disease worldwide. The early studies including oral bacteria in the pathogenesis of periodontitis were done on a hamster. Administration of penicillin inhibited-periodontitis in hamster gives a clear evidence of a bacterial agent [7]. Some studies isolated bacteria from dental caries, called *Streptococcus mutans* and described its ability to ferment many sugars and produce acids in glucose broth (pH of 4.3). However, he was not able to prove that *S. mutans* actually produces dental caries, but this finding was experimentally proven later in 1960 [8]. Whereas the infectious case of periodontitis appeared by demonstration of its transmissibility during infection from a person to another [9]. For a long time, periodontal disease researchers aimed to determine specific bacteria from a complex microbial plaque that may be considered a sole causative agent of periodontitis. The big problem was the cultivation of oral bacteria in laboratory. Most of the oral bacteria are anaerobic that died by air and considered fastidious microbes. This was recognized by researchers at that time. Major progress in the anaerobic culture was done in 1960 by designation of anaerobic glove boxes (a primitive form of now widely used anaerobic chambers), and it was used for the first time by Socransky [10]. This invention improved anaerobic cultivation techniques and was combined with optimized complex culture media; it allowed the invention of a pure and a good culture of more than 300 oral bacteria types in the period of 40 years ago, including clinical samples from supragingival and subgingival dental plaque taken from diseased and healthy subjects [11].

The studies on healthy subjects who agreed to take toothbrushing for a prolonged period appeared direct association between assembly of dental plaque and the initiation of gingiva diseases, mild form of oral diseases [12, 13]. After 28 days without basic oral hygiene in periodontally healthy subjects, there was a rapid assembly of bacterial plaque on the surface of teeth, and gingivitis was developed in all subjects within 10–21 days. These damages were reversible when toothbrushing was reintroduced. The researchers analyzed the smear of dental plaque specimen taken during the 28th day, and they found, at first, colonizing bacteria on the surface of the teeth, bacteria which belonged to the Gram-positive cocci and rods, Gram-negative cocci and rods, filaments, and fusobacteria, respectively, while finally spirochetes and spirilla were taken place in some times during colonizing. The outside of clinical gingivitis linked with the manifestation of the Gram-negative bacteria, and other studies on the microbial rotation in oral plaque formation confirmed these outcomes [14]. Through the years' progress, many other culture-based and molecular methods were given a huge information about the type of species included in periodontitis. A passionate dentist, W. D. Miller, studied hard for a long time in the of Robert Koch's laboratory trying to discover the microorganisms which were responsible for teeth decay; he published his research in 1980, with a book called *Microorganisms of the Human Mouth*; and in the same book, he suggested a chemoparasitic theory. According to that theory, in a sensitive host, carbohydrates fermentable oral microorganisms convert carbohydrates into acid, then the acid demineralizes tooth structure specially enamel [15, 16].

The classification of periodontal pathogens was tried to figure out by many researchers. The most understanding classification divided the periodontal pathogens into color-coded clusters published by Socransky and his team in 1998. This division resolves and identifies many problems and complexes of bacteria and clears their series of infection in the oral plaque and their role in periodontitis. Biofilm structure, which extends away from the tooth surface, was essential in this classification, and the bacteria responsible for dental plaque were classified into six clusters (red, orange, yellow, green, blue, and purple). *Actinomyces odontolyticus* and *Veillonella parvula* represented the "purple" form, while species of *Streptococci* including *S. sanguinis* and *S. oralis* refer to the "yellow" form [17].

The first colonizers of the surface of the teeth with *Actinomyces* species are purple and yellow form of this classification. The next complex, designated with green, included *Capnocytophaga* spp., *Campylobacter concisus*, *Eikenella corrodens*, and *Actinobacillus actinomycetemcomitans*, the bacteria contributing to the primary changes in the host. The "bridging species" formed the orange cluster are as follows: *Prevotella* spp., *Micromonas micros*, *Fusobacterium* spp., *Eubacterium* spp., and *Streptococcus constellatus*. That cluster included the species capable of using and secreting nutrients in the biofilm, in addition to expressing cell surface molecules facilitating binding to early colonizers, and the individual of the red complex. Finally, *P. gingivalis* and *T. denticola* in addition to *Tannerella forsythia* refer to the red cluster, and these are considered the prevalent pathogens in periodontitis progression; however, there is a clear association between the prevalence, number of these bacteria, and periodontitis clinical parameters [17, 18]. These three bacteria (in particular *P. gingivalis*), besides individuals of the orange cluster also linked with periodontal lesions, have been heavily studied in vitro, aiming to the identification of their key virulence mechanisms [18].

3. Most prevalent diseases caused by oral bacteria

Many major periopathogens can be seen in healthy individuals of all ages, indicating the coexistence of these bacteria as a normal flora in the host. These bacteria increase their numbers over time, and this change depends on the conditions of the internal or external environment, and it induces chronic periodontal inflammation that can cause the teeth loss as an outcome destroying the alveolar bone [19]. The inflammation of the tissues around the tooth due to accumulation of dental plaque is considered the main characteristic of acute and chronic periodontitis. The current classification of oral disease included the following [20]:

- Gingivitis: Plaque triggers inflammation in the gingivae that are characterized by red, swollen tissues and bleeding while brushing or probing.

- Chronic periodontitis: The connective tissue attachment of the teeth and destruction of junctional epithelium are damaged. Periodontal pockets and alveolar bone destruction occurred, and this state leads to chronic periodontitis.

- Aggressive periodontitis: It is a severe condition that represented the high proportion of younger cohort patients, the progression of disease is rapid, and the degree of destruction of the tissue (connective tissue) is high. The higher the level of the plaque, the higher the level of the disease.

- Necrotizing ulcerative gingivitis (NUG): Painful ulceration of the tips of the interdental papillae. Grey necrotic tissue is visible and there is an associated halitosis. The condition is termed necrotizing ulcerative periodontitis (NUP).

- Periodontal abscess: Inside the periodontal pocket is a different species of bacteria when the immune system responded to infection, and the periodontal abscess is form. Acute or chronic condition may occur, and in some time, the condition is asymptomatic.

- Perio-endo lesions: Lesions may be coalescing or independent, and the periodontal pathogen source originates either in the root canal system or in the periodontium.

- Gingival enlargement: The thickness occurs in response to irritation caused by plaque or calculus, and the other responses are repeated friction or trauma changes in hormone levels or in some time the effect of a drug.

The most common periodontopathogen correlated with aggressive forms of periodontitis is *Aggregatibacter* (previously *Actinobacillus*) *actinomycetemcomitans*. This small Gram-negative coccobacillus, capnophilic and non-motile have been determined as the most causative factor of aggressive periodontitis in young individuals and adults [21]. *A. actinomycetemcomitans* has been divided into six serotypes, and it has been postulated that some serotypes are correlated with periodontitis more frequently than periodontal health. Exemplifying this relationship, serotype C has appeared more repeatedly from healthy subjects and serotypes A and B more frequently in periodontitis [22]. But differences are pointed in *A. actinomycetemcomitans* serotype distribution when ethnicity and geographic location are taken into account; still, 3–8% of strains have remained nonserotypeable [23].

Gram-negative obligate anaerobe asaccharolytic bacteria (*Porphyromonas gingivalis*, *Treponema denticola*, and *Tannerella forsythia*) have been extensively correlated with periodontitis [17]. *P. gingivalis* has been detected in correlation with periodontal damages and has an arsenal of virulent factors that can affectively stimulate the host responses [18]. *T. forsythia* was first described at the Forsyth Institute, and it became a recognized periodontopathogen because of its repeated detection from sites with periodontitis and its huge correlation with the formation of pocket with deep size [24]. *T. denticola* is also frequently presented in periodontitis subgingivally sites, and their number is decreased after appropriate treatment [25]. Other bacteria that have been related with periodontitis include *Prevotella intermedia*, *Prevotella nigrescens*, *Fusobacterium nucleatum*, *Selenomonas*, *Eubacteria*, *Eikenella corrodens*, *Campylobacter rectus*, and *Parvimonas micra* [26].

Molecular microbiological studies have shown that many of the bacteria species are recognized in correlation with periodontitis and expanded to include uncultivated and less-often-identified phylotypes [27].

4. Mechanisms of destruction in periodontal tissues

Bacteria can cause damage directly and indirectly. Various mechanisms are described in the steps below. Cytotoxic cellular immune responses to self- and pro-inflammatory responses involving release of interleukin-1 beta (IL-1β), tumor necrosis factor-α (TNF-α), and interleukin-6 (IL-6) could lead to tissue destruction [28].

- Crevicular epithelium is destroyed by Porphyromonas gingivalis, Treponema denticola, and Aggregatibacter actinomycetemcomitans.

- Leukotoxin is secreted by A. actinomycetemcomitans, and it is impaired with polymorphonuclear (PMN) function (chemotaxis, phagocytosis, and intracellular killing) and other leukocytes.

- P. gingivalis is dysregulated of cytokine networks by their R1 proteinase activity.

- Capnocytophaga spp. are degraded of immunoglobulins.

- P. gingivalis, *P. intermedia*, T. forsythia, and T. denticola increase the mucosal permeability and degradation of collagen by fibroblastic collagenase by volatile sulfur compounds from Gram-negative anaerobes in addition to disaggregation of proteoglycans by disrupting SH (sulphydryl) bonds or impaired host cell function.

- Destruction of periodontal tissues proteins by proteolytic enzymes (collagenases and trypsin-like proteinases) to peptides and amino acids provides nutrients for Gram-negative bacteria. While the extracellular matrix is destroyed by other type of enzymes that called hydrolytic enzymes.

- The complement is activated when infection occurs by bacteria in response to LPS.

- Lipoteichoic acid from Gram-positive bacterial cell walls stimulates bone resorption.

5. Immunopathological factor associated with periodontal pathogens

The pathogenesis of periodontal disease is categorized into four stages, based on histopathological examination of the development of periodontal inflammation due to plaque accumulation. These stages are called **(a)** the initial, **(b)** the early, **(c)** the established, and **(d)** the advanced lesions [28, 29]. The description of stages in periodontal damage progression is listed below:

(a) Initial lesion

Without normal oral hygiene measures, within 2–4 days of plaque accumulation, the first inflammatory response is observed histologically. It is characterized by vasodilatation, loss of perivascular collagen, and active migration of monocytes and neutrophils into the periodontal tissues and junctional epithelium mediated by endothelial leucocyte adhesion molecules (ELAM) and intercellular adhesion molecules (ICAM) that are observed. The exudation of serum proteins from the dilated capillaries leads to an increase in gingival crevicular fluid (GCF) flow.

(b) Early lesion

The early lesion presents after 4–7 days of plaque accumulation. This is clinically detectable as gingivitis, with more pronounced vascular changes and an increase in extravascular neutrophils. Histologically, the inflammatory infiltrate consists of numerous lymphocytes (predominantly T lymphocytes), immediately below the proliferating basal cells of the junctional epithelium. Destruction of the gingival connective tissue occurs through apoptosis of fibroblasts, and a reduction in the collagen fiber network of the marginal gingivae occurs via host- and pathogen-derived MMP.

(c) Established lesion

This is similar to the early lesion with a shift in the cell population in the inflammatory (2–3 weeks of plaque accumulation). Here, plasma cells are the main histological features in older patients, whereas in younger patients, the infiltrate continues to be dominated by lymphocytes. Clinically, inflammation will become more pronounced with an increase in swelling, and the false pocket will form. T and B lymphocytes, antibodies, and complement are found in the inflamed marginal gingival and gingival sulcus.

(d) Advanced lesion

At this stage the inflammatory lesion expands into the periodontal ligament and alveolar bone. There is a destruction of a tissue linked to the teeth. The junctional epithelium migrates down the root surface to form a true periodontal pocket. MMP has the ability to destroy periodontal ligament and the surrounding alveolar bone through enhanced osteolytic activity. The direct cytotoxicity of bacterial products leads to direct tissue damage. Proteinases, collagenases, epitheliotoxin, cytolethal distending toxin, hemolysin, hydrogen sulfide, and ammonia are examples of bacterial products. Moreover, dysregulation of the factor derived from the host such as proteinases and proteinase inhibitors; MMPs and tissue inhibitors to metalloproteinases (TIMPs); pro-inflammatory cytokines such as IL-1α, IL-1β, TNF-α, and others; prostaglandins; and the products of polymorphonuclear leukocytes leads to the damage of the connective tissue attachment.

5.1. Innate immunity response to periodontal pathogens

The innate host response primarily involves the recognition of microbial components such as LPS by the immune cells of the host, and the result of activation produced inflammatory mediators. The Toll-like receptors (TLRs), which are synthesized by leukocytes and resident cells in the periodontal tissues, can activate the innate immunity response by binding to numerous bacterial components [30–31]. The developing biofilm consists of initially Gram-positive cocci in health, changing to the increased numbers of motile Gram-negative anaerobes in gingivitis and periodontitis [17].

Endotoxin (LPS) of Gram-negative bacteria is considered a huge stimulator of TLR4. LPS from Gram-negative bacteria cell wall can be released through cell lysis. It becomes linked to the extracellular acute-phase protein LPS-binding protein before binding to the cluster of differentiation 14 (CD14). The outcome is transferred from LPS to the extracellular domain of the TLR4 receptor and subsequent TLR4 signaling [32]. Gram-negative bacteria also activate TLR2 through their cell membrane proteins, TLR5 through flagella, TLR9 through the determination of bacterial cytosine-phosphate-guanine (CpG) DNA, and nucleotide-binding oligomerization domain-containing proteins 1 and 2 (NOD 1, NOD 2) through peptidoglycan derivatives [32, 33].

Periodontal pathogens have been reported to stimulate TLRs in vitro, such as LPS of *P. gingivalis*, and fimbriae is a potent TLR2 agonists [34–36]. *A. actinomycetemcomitans* and whole *P. gingivalis* will stimulate TLRs [37–40]. Moreover, many bacteria can initiate an immune response via TLR9, which also detects viable bacterial DNA [41]. It is therefore clear that the myriad of bacteria that are found in both health and increasing hardness of periodontitis will present a challenge to the response innate immunity. Following TLR activation, an intracellular signaling cascade occurs which can result in stimulation of transcription factors, subsequent inflammatory cytokine expression, leukocyte migration to the infection locus, and tissue damaging [42, 43]. The nucleotide-binding oligomerization domain (NOD) and the inflammation system have been submitted as possible accessory molecules in the induction of response of innate immunity against periodontopathogens [44–46]. The junctional epithelium is the front line between the oral normal flora and the host. It is well equipped to recognize invading pathogens, some studies showed that the present of mRNA encoding TLR2, TLR3, TLR4, TLR5, TLR6, and TLR9 in gingival epithelial cells is a clear indication of the existence of the infectious agent [47]. Within the gingival epithelium and between the connective tissue, Langerhans cells and tissue dendritic cells are also found. TLRs are produced by antigen-presenting cells and appear on their surface including TLR1, TLR2, TLR3, TLR4, TLR5, TLR6, TLR8, and TLR10. The response of adaptive immunity against bacterial products is monitored by these receptors [30, 33].

The alveolar bone is the supporting structure into which the periodontal ligament inserts that is ultimately destroyed by the inflammatory lesion of periodontitis. Osteoblasts and osteoclasts included in bone turnover also express TLR1, TLR4, TLR5, TLR6, and TLR9 [35] and TLR1, TLR2, TLR3, TLR4, TLR5, TLR6, TLR7, TLR8, and TLR9, respectively [48]. It is therefore possible that TLR signaling within the bone can generate an inflammatory response to invading pathogens, leading to pathological resorption of the bone through excessive or prolonged production of osteolytic host molecules, including IL-1, tumor necrosis factor-α (TNF-α), and prostaglandin E2 (PGE2), which stimulate osteoblast inhibition and osteoclast activation and maturation through the receptor activator of nuclear factor kappa-B ligand/osteoprotegerin (RANKL/OPG). Many biological events in periodontal disease are obligatory regulated by cell–cell interactions, which may be grouped into two forms: cognate (adhesive) interaction, achieved by mutual recognition between membrane-bound cell surface molecules, and cytokine-mediated interactions [49].

Intercellular adhesion molecule-1 (ICAM- 1, CD54) and ITGB2 (integrin beta 2, CD18), which stabilize cell–cell interactions and facilitation of leukocyte migration across the endothelial barrier, are achieved by ICAM-1 (intercellular adhesion molecule-1, CD54) and ITGB2 (integrin beta 2, CD18); therefore, they are called adhesion molecules [22].

5.1.1. Adaptive immunity cytokine (pro-inflammatory cytokines) response to periodontal pathogens

Cytokines are a large and diverse family of soluble mediators including interleukins. Cytokines play a major role in various biological activities such as differentiation, proliferation, regeneration, development, repair inflammation, and homeostasis. Cytokine networks are an important side of periodontal inflammation and subject to several excellent reviews [50].

The IL-1 family of cytokines (IL-1α and IL-1β) has different roles in immunity, tissue homeostasis, tissue breakdown, and inflammation. Monocytes and macrophages are released TNF-α in huge amount in responses for infection. It induces the production of collagenase and is secreted by fibroblasts to make damages on the cartilage and bone, and it has been involved in the damage of the periodontal tissue in periodontitis [51].

5.1.2. Interleukin-1α and interleukin-1β (IL-1α/IL-1β) role in periodontal pathogens

IL-1 is a polypeptide, which has diverse activities and roles in immunity, inflammation, tissue breakdown, and tissue homeostasis [52]. IL-1 is synthesized by various cell types, such as fibroblasts, lymphocytes, skin cells, macrophages, monocytes, vascular cells, and osteocytes, following its activation. IL-1α and IL-1β belong to the IL-1 family of cytokines which have similar biological functions and bind to the same receptors found on many cell types. Fibroblast cells in periodontal ligament are triggered by IL-1 to stimulate them to release cellular mediators, prostaglandin E2 (PGE2), and matrix-degrading enzymes which destroyed the connective tissue and lead to attachment loss [53]. Some studies refer that IL-1 is involved in the pathogenesis of periodontitis and also associated with bone destruction. Together, IL-1α and IL-1β have appeared to stimulate bone resorption and bone inhibition in cooperation with TNF-α. IL-1β has appeared to be significantly more potent in mediating bone resorption compared with IL-1α and TNF-α. IL-1 can also stimulate elevated production of matrix metalloproteinases (MMPs), procollagenase, and plasminogen activator [54].

5.1.3. Tumor necrosis factor-alpha (TNF-α) role against periodontal pathogens

TNF-α is a pro-inflammatory cytokine released by activated monocytes and macrophages [55]. TNF-α functions include the upregulation of attachment molecules and chemokines which are involved in the cell migration to inflamed and infected sites [56]. Collagenase secreted by fibroblasts, resorption of the cartilage and bone, and damaging of the periodontal tissue all are stimulated by cytokine production [57]. Both GCF and periodontitis tissues have shown high levels of TNF-α, and it has shown positive correlation to MMP and RANKL expression [58, 59]. Animal studies also demonstrated that TNF-α plays a key role in inflammation and periodontal tissue damaging including bone resorption and loss of connective tissue attachment [58, 60]. Pro-inflammatory cytokines produced during infection (IL-1β and IL-6) are upregulated by TNF-α, this production linked with cell migration into the site of infection, and finally bone resorption occurred [55, 61]. New studies was done by Alwaeli and Abd [62, 63] who tried to interpret the relation between concentration of TNF-α and IL-1β and polymorphism of their genes, and they found some of SNPs (single-nucleotide polymorphisms) that trigger the production of TNF-α and IL-1β, by increasing the activity of their genes so the high concentration level of TNF-α and IL-1β leads to additional damage in periodontal tissue, while the other SNPs decrease the production of TNF-α and IL-1β, for this reason the termed "SNP-genotype combination principal" for this phenomena by Alwaeli and Abd (62–63).

List of abbreviation

BC	Before Christ
CD	cluster of differentiation
CpG	cytosine-phosphate-guanine
ELAM	endothelial leukocyte adhesion molecules
GCF	gingival crevicular fluid
ICAM	intercellular adhesion molecules
IL-1β	interleukin-1 beta
ITGB2	integrin beta 2
LPS	lipopolysaccharide
MMP	matrix metalloproteinases
NOD	nucleotide-binding oligomerization domain
NUG	necrotizing ulcerative gingivitis
NUP	necrotizing ulcerative periodontitis
OPG	osteoprotegerin
PGE2	prostaglandin E2
PMN	polymorphonuclear
RANKL	receptor activator nuclear factor kappa-B ligand

SNP	single-nucleotide polymorphism
TIMP	tissue inhibitors to metalloproteinases
TLRs	toll-like receptors
TNF-α	tumor necrosis factor-alpha

Author details

Ahmed Zuhair Jasim Alwaeli

Address all correspondence to: ahmed_z85j@yahoo.com

Department of Pathological Analysis Technique, University of Altoosi college, An-Najaf, Iraq

References

[1] Brown LJ, Johns BA, Wall TP. The economics of periodontal diseases. Periodontology 2000. 2002;**29**:223-234

[2] Kuo LC, Polson AM, Kang T. Associations between periodontal diseases and systemic diseases: A review of the inter-relationships and interactions with diabetes, respiratory diseases, cardiovascular diseases and osteoporosis. Public Health. 2008;**122**:417-433

[3] Darveau RP. Periodontitis: A polymicrobial disruption of host homeostasis. Nature Reviews. Microbiology. 2010;**8**:481-490

[4] Gest H. The discovery of microorganisms by Robert Hooke and Antoni van Leeuwenhoek, fellows of the Royal Society. Notes and Records of the Royal Society of London. 2004;**58**:187-201

[5] Suddick RP, Harris NO. Historical perspectives of oral biology: A series. Critical Reviews in Oral Biology and Medicine. 1990;**1**:135-151

[6] Clarke JK. On the bacterial factor in the etiology of dental caries. British Journal of Experimental Pathology. 1924;**5**:141-147

[7] Mitchell DF, Johnson M. The nature of the gingival plaque in the hamster: Production, prevention, and removal. Journal of Dental Research. 1956;**35**:651-655

[8] Fitzgerald RJ, Keyes PH. Demonstration of the etiologic role of streptococci in experimental caries in the hamster. Journal of the American Dental Association (1939). 1960;**61**:9-19

[9] Keyes PH, Jordan HV. Periodontal lesions in the Syrian Hamster.Iii. Findings related to an infectious and transmissible component. Archives of Oral Biology. 1964;**9**:377-400

[10] Socransky S, Macdonald JB, Sawyer S. The cultivation of Treponema microdentium as surface colonies. Archives of Oral Biology. 1959;**1**:171-172

[11] Kolenbrander PE. Oral microbial communities: Biofilms, interactions, and genetic systems. Annual Review of Microbiology. 2000;**54**:413-437

[12] Loe H, Theilade E, Jensen SB. Experimental gingivitis in man. Journal of Periodontology. 1965;**36**:177-187

[13] Theilade E, Wright WH, Jensen SB, Loe H. Experimental gingivitis in man. II. A longitudinal clinical and bacteriological investigation. Journal of Periodontal Research. 1966;**1**:1-13

[14] Listgarten MA. Structure of the microbial flora associated with periodontal health and disease in man. A light and electron microscopic study. Journal of Periodontology. 1976;**47**:1-18

[15] Tanner AC, Haffer C, Bratthall GT, Visconti RA, Socransky SS. A study of the bacteria associated with advancing periodontitis in man. Journal of Clinical Periodontology. 1979;**6**:278-307

[16] Moore WE, Holdeman LV, Smibert RM, Good IJ, Burmeister JA, Palcanis KG, Ranney RR. Bacteriology of experimental gingivitis in young adult humans. Infection and Immunity. 1982;**38**:651-667

[17] Socransky SS, Haffajee AD. Periodontal microbial ecology. Periodontology 2000. 2005;**38**:135-187

[18] Holt SC, Ebersole JL. *Porphyromonas gingivalis, Treponema denticola, and Tannerella forsythia*: The "red complex", a prototype polybacterial pathogenic consortium in periodontitis. Periodontology 2000. 2005;**38**:72-122

[19] Hajishengallis G, Lamont RJ. Beyond the red complex and into more complexity: The polymicrobial synergy and dysbiosis (PSD) model of periodontal disease etiology. Molecular Oral Microbiology. 2012;**27**:409-419

[20] Young. Practitioners guide to periodontology. In: British Society of Periodontology Scotland. 2nd ed. 2012

[21] Fine DH, Kaplan JB, Kachlany SC, Schreiner HC. How we got attached to *Actinobacillus actinomycetemcomitans*: A model for infectious diseases. Periodontology 2000. 2006;**42**:114-157

[22] Yang L, Froio RM, Sciuto TE, Dvorak AM, Alon R, Luscinskas FW. ICAM-1 regulates neutrophil adhesion and transcellular migration of TNF-alpha-activated vascular endothelium under flow. Blood. 2005;**106**:584-592

[23] Doğan B, Antinheimo J, Cetiner D, Bodur A, Emingil G, Buduneli E, Uygur C, Firatli E, Lakio L, Asikainen S. Subgingival microflora in Turkish patients with periodontitis. Journal of Periodontology. 2003;**74**(6):803-814

[24] Tanner AC, Izard J. Tannerella forsythia, a periodontal pathogen entering the genomic era. Periodontology 2000. 2006;**42**:88-113

[25] Feres M, Cavalca S, Figueredo LC, Haffajee AD, Socransky SS. Microbiological basis for periodontal therapy. Journal of Applied Oral Science. 2004;**12**(4):256-266

[26] Teles R, Teles F, Frias-Lopez J, Paster B, Haffajjee A. Lessons learned and unlearned in periodontal microbiology. Periodontology 2000. 2013;**62**(1):95-162

[27] Anne CR, Tannar. Anaerobic culture to detect periodontal and caries pathogens. Journal of Oral Biosciences. 2015;**25**:18-26

[28] Hasan A, Palmer RM. A clinical guide to periodontology: Pathology of periodontal disease. British Dental Journal. 2016;**216**(8):457-461

[29] Ohlrich EJ, Cullinan MP, Seymour GJ. The immunopathogenesis of periodontal disease. Australian Dental Journal. 2009;**54**(Suppl 1):S2-S10

[30] Mahanonda R, Pichyangkul S. Toll-like receptors and their role in periodontal health and disease. Periodontology 2000. 2007;**43**:41-55

[31] Garlet GP. Destructive and protective roles of cytokines in periodontitis: A re-appraisal from host defense and tissue destruction viewpoints. Journal of Dental Research. 2010;**89**(12):1349-1363

[32] Akira S. TLR signaling. Current Topics in Microbiology and Immunology. 2006;**311**:1-16

[33] Mogensen TH. Pathogen recognition and inflammatory signaling in innate immune defenses. Clinical Microbiology Reviews. 2009;**22**:240-273

[34] Hirschfeld M, Weis JJ, Toshchakov V, Salkowski CA, Cody MJ, Ward DC, Qureshi N, Michalek SM, Vogel SN. Signaling by toll-like receptor 2 and 4 agonists results in differential gene expression in murine macrophages. Infection and Immunity. 2001;**69**:1477-1482

[35] Asai Y, Ohyama Y, Gen K, Ogawa T. Bacterial fimbriae and their peptides activate human gingival epithelial cells through toll-like receptor 2. Infection and Immunity. 2001;**69**:7387-7395

[36] Erridge C, Pridmore A, Eley A, Stewart J, Poxton IR. Lipopolysaccharides of *Bacteroides fragilis*, *Chlamydia trachomatis* and *Pseudomonas aeruginosa* signal via toll-like receptor 2. Journal of Medical Microbiology. 2004;**53**:735-740

[37] Yoshimura A, Kaneko T, Kato Y, Golenbock DT, Hara Y. Lipopolysaccharides from periodontopathic bacteria *Porphyromonas gingivalis* and *Capnocytophaga ochracea* are antagonists for human toll like receptor 4. Infection and Immunity. 2002;**70**:218-225

[38] Darveau RP, Pham TT, Lemley K, Reife RA, Bainbridge BW, Coats SR, Howald WN, Way SS, Hajjar AM. *Porphyromonas gingivalis* lipopolysaccharide contains multiple lipid a species that functionally interact with both toll-like receptors 2 and 4. Infection and Immunity. 2004;**72**:5041-5051

[39] Kikkert R, Laine ML, Aarden LA, Van Winkelhoff AJ. Activation of toll-like receptors 2 and 4 by gram-negative periodontal bacteria. Oral Microbiology and Immunology. 2007;**22**:145-151

[40] Nussbaum G, Ben-Adi S, Genzler T, Sela M, Rosen G. Involvement of toll-like receptors 2 and 4 in the innate immune response to *Treponema denticola* and its outer sheath components. Infection and Immunity. 2009;**77**:3939-3947

[41] Bauer S, Kirschning CJ, Hacker H, Redecke V, Hausmann S, Akira S, Wagner H, Lipford GB. Human TLR9 confers responsiveness to bacterial DNA via species-specific CpG motif recognition. Proceedings of the National Academy of Sciences of the United States of America. 2001;**98**:9237-9242

[42] Gelani V, Fernandes AP, Gasparoto TH, Garlet TP, Cestari TM, Lima HR, Ramos ES, De Souza Malaspina TS, Santos CF, Garlet GP, Da Silva JS, Campanelli AP. The role of toll-like receptor 2 in the recognition of *Aggregatibacter actinomycetemcomitans*. Journal of Periodontology. 2009;**80**:2010-2019

[43] Lima HR, Gelani V, Fernandes AP, Gasparoto TH, Torres SA, Santos CF, Garlet GP, Da Silva JS, Campanelli AP. The essential role of toll like receptor-4 in the control of *Aggregatibacter actinomycetemcomitans* infection in mice. Journal of Clinical Periodontology. 2010;**37**:248-254

[44] Uehara A, Takada H. Functional TLRs and NODs in human gingival fibroblasts. Journal of Dental Research. 2007;**86**:249-254

[45] Bostanci N, Emingil G, Saygan B, Turkoglu O, Atilla G, Curtis MA, Belibasakis GN. Expression and regulation of the NALP3 inflammasome complex in periodontal diseases. Clinical and Experimental Immunology. 2009;**157**:415-422

[46] Okugawa T, Kaneko T, Yoshimura A, Silverman N, Hara Y. NOD1 and NOD2 mediate sensing of periodontal pathogens. Journal of Dental Research. 2010;**89**:186-191

[47] Kusumoto Y, Hirano H, Saitoh K, Yamada S, Takedachi M, Nozaki T, Ozawa Y, Nakahira Y, Saho T, Ogo H, Shimabukuro Y, Okada H, Murakami S. Human gingival epithelial cells produce chemotactic factors interleukin-8 and monocyte chemoattractant protein-1 after stimulation with *Porphyromonas gingivalis* via toll-like receptor 2. Journal of Periodontology. 2004;**75**:370-379

[48] Itoh K, Udagawa N, Kobayashi K, Suda K, Li X, Takami M, Okahashi N, Nishihara T, Takahashi N. Lipopolysaccharide promotes the survival of osteoclasts via toll-like receptor 4, but cytokine production of osteoclasts in response to lipopolysaccharide is different from that of macrophages. Journal of Immunology. 2003;**170**:3688-3695

[49] Beutler BA. TLRs and innate immunity. Blood. 2009;**113**:1399-1407

[50] Preshaw PM, Taylor JJ. How has research into cytokine interactions and their role in driving immune responses impacted our understanding of periodontitis? Journal of Clinical Periodontology. 2011;**38**(Suppl 11):60-84

[51] Kinane DF, Preshaw PM, Loos BG. Host-response: Understanding the cellular and molecular mechanisms of host microbial interactions--consensus of the seventh European workshop on periodontology. Journal of Clinical Periodontology. 2011;**38**(Suppl 11):44-48

[52] Ozbabacan SEA, Gursoy A, Nussinov R, Keskin O. The structural pathway of interleukin 1 (IL-1) initiated signaling reveals mechanisms of oncogenic mutations and SNPs in inflammation and cancer. PLOS Computational Biology. 2014;**10**(2):1-14

[53] Nazeer AM. Biological response at the cellular level within the periodontal ligament on application of orthodontic force – An update. Journal of Orthodontic Science. 2012;**1**(1):2-10

[54] Stefan AH, Sweta P, Saso I. Mechanisms of bone resorption in periodontitis. Journal of Immunology Research. 2015;**615486**:1-10

[55] George DK, Lionel BI. TNF biology, pathogenic mechanisms and emerging therapeutic strategies. Nature Reviews Rheumatology. 2016;**12**:49-62

[56] Wajant H, Pfizenmaier K, Scheurich P. Tumor necrosis factor signaling. Cell Death and Differentiation. 2003;**10**:45-65

[57] Kindle L, Rothe L, Kriss M, Osdoby P, Collin-Osdoby P. Human microvascular endothelial cell activation by IL-1 and TNF-alpha stimulates the adhesion and transendothelial migration of circulating human CD14+ monocytes that develop with RANKL into functional osteoclasts. Journal of Bone and Mineral Research. 2006;**21**:193-206

[58] Graves DT, Cochran D. The contribution of interleukin-1 and tumor necrosis factor to periodontal tissue destruction. Journal of Periodontology. 2003;**74**:391-401

[59] Garlet GP, Martins W Jr, Fonseca BA, Ferreira BR, Silva JS. Matrix metalloproteinases, their physiological inhibitors and osteoclast factors are differentially regulated by the cytokine profile in human periodontal disease. Journal of Clinical Periodontology. 2004;**31**:671-679

[60] Graves DT, Fine D, Teng YT, Van Dyke TE, Hajishengallis G. The use of rodent models to investigate host-bacteria interactions related to periodontal diseases. Journal Of Clinical Periodontology. 2008;**35**:89-105

[61] Fonseca JE, Santos MJ, Canhao H, Choy E. Interleukin-6 as a key player in systemic inflammation and joint destruction. Autoimmunity Reviews. 2009;**8**:538-542

[62] Alwaeli AZJ, Abd FJ. The association between periodontitis and polymorphism of tumor necrosis factor-α −308 in Iraqi population. International Journal of PharmTech Research. 2016a;**9**(9):331-340

[63] Alwaeli AZJ, Abd FJ. New term (SNPs-genotypes combination principal) gives better understanding about effect of SNPs on the concentration of IL-1β and TNFα in clinical samples of periodontitis. Journal of Chemical and Pharmaceutical Sciences. 2016b;**9**(4):3239-3244

9

Cellular Response Mechanisms in *Porphyromonas gingivalis* Infection

Hazem Khalaf, Eleonor Palm and
Torbjörn Bengtsson

Abstract

The pathogenicity of the periodontal biofilm is highly dependent on a few key species, of which *Porphyromonas gingivalis* is considered to be one of the most important pathogens. *P. gingivalis* expresses a broad range of virulence factors, of these cysteine proteases (gingipains) are of special importance both for the bacterial survival/proliferation and for the pathological outcome. Several cell types, for example, epithelial cells, endothelial cells, dendritic cells, osteoblasts, and fibroblasts, reside in the periodontium and are part of the innate host response, as well as platelets, neutrophils, lymphocytes, and monocytes/macrophages. These cells recognize and respond to *P. gingivalis* and its components through pattern recognition receptors (PRRs), for example, Toll-like receptors and protease-activated receptors. Ligation of PRRs induces downstream-signaling pathways modifying the activity of transcription factors that regulates the expression of genes linked to inflammation. This is followed by the release of inflammatory mediators, for example, cytokines and reactive oxygen species. Periodontal disease is today considered to play a significant role in various systemic conditions such as cardiovascular disease (CVD). The mechanisms by which *P. gingivalis* and its virulence factors interact with host immune cells and contribute to the pathogenesis of periodontitis and CVD are far from completely understood.

Keywords: host-microbe interaction, immune cells, pathogen recognition receptors, intracellular signaling, inflammatory responses, *Porphyromonas gingivalis*, gingipains, LPS, cardiovascular disease, treatment

1. Introduction

Evidence suggests that it is the early host-inflammatory and immune responses to the oral microbiota that changes the subgingival environment and favors the emergence of periodontal opportunistic pathogens during the development of periodontitis. Substances released from the dental biofilm, such as lipopolysaccharides, proteolytic enzymes, and other virulence factors, activate the innate immune system and initiate an inflammatory response, which disrupts the host-microbe homeostasis. The activation of immune cells leads to a release of an array of inflammatory mediators, for example, cytokines, chemokines, proteases, reactive oxygen species (ROS), and eicosanoids, which struggle against the bacterial burden. However, the complexity of the microbial biofilm of the subgingival dental plaque and the failure of the acute inflammation to resolve lead to an accumulation of mediators of the innate and adaptive immune systems that collectively promote chronic inflammation and tissue destruction. How host cells discriminate commensal from pathogenic microbial species and why this ability seems to differ between individuals is currently unknown. The variation in individual susceptibility to develop periodontal disease appears to be determined by the magnitude of the inflammatory response to a dysbiotic microbial community and whether only the innate or also the adaptive immune pathways are activated.

2. *Porphyromonas gingivalis* in periodontitis

There are a number of bacterial species that are associated to periodontitis, based on their detection in periodontal pockets, their pathogenicity, and the immunological responses they evoke [1]. The red complex is a consortium of three periodontal bacterial species, *Treponema denticola*, *Tannarella forsythia*, and *Porphyromonas gingivalis*, which are linked to each other and to diseased sites [2]. The development and progression of periodontitis is believed to be due to a synergistic and dysbiotic polymicrobial community, and the oral biofilm (dental plaque) [3]. A biofilm is a highly structured, three-dimensional matrix with a simple circulatory system. The biofilm provides physical protection and a gradient of oxygen, allowing anaerobic species to grow in the deeper pocket, and aerobic species near the surface. Furthermore, metabolic by-products from one species can be used as nutrients by other species in the biofilm, the so-called cross-feeding [4]. The keystone species hypothesis suggests that some species, like *P. gingivalis*, exerts a disproportionally large effect in the biofilm. *P. gingivalis* can turn from a natural low-abundance microorganism residing in the oral cavity to an opportunistic pathogen that interferes with the host immune system and from a normal, symbiotic microbiota, and enables the transition and emergence into a dysbiotic bacterial society that drives the progress of periodontitis [2, 5]. *P. gingivalis* is a late colonizer usually found in a rather low number in the dental plaque, and interestingly, *P. gingivalis* is not able to induce periodontitis in germ-free mice, suggesting that *P. gingivalis* is dependent on the complex microbial community. Through synergistic interactions, the biofilm promotes colonization, nutrition acquisition and subvert, and evades host immune responses [4, 6].

P. gingivalis is a non-motile, proteolytic, and Gram-negative rod that expresses several virulence factors that are related to colonization of oral tissues, periodontal tissue destruction, and evasion of the host responses [7]. *P. gingivalis* exhibits genotypic and phenotypic diversity, which results in differences in virulence and in the capacity of individual strains to colonize and induce destruction of periodontal tissues. Certain strains may therefore exhibit a higher pathogenic potential than others and may be linked to a more severe form of periodontitis [8–12]. The asaccharolytic bacterium *P. gingivalis* grows under anaerobic conditions and acquires metabolic energy by fermenting amino acids. *P. gingivalis* also uses micronutrients, such as metal ions for anabolic and catabolic purposes, as well as vitamin K. *P. gingivalis* expresses a broad range of virulence factors, all of which add to enhanced growth and survival in a hostile environment [7]. However, the virulence of *P. gingivalis* is affected by its surroundings, including other bacterial species in the biofilm and host-derived factors. By altering the gene expression of virulence factors, *P. gingivalis* can adjust to a more or less virulent phenotype depending on the environment [13].

Fimbriae are hair-like protrusions emanating from the outer cell surface that facilitate the adherence and colonization of the bacterium. Indeed, fimbriae are critical for mediating the initial bacterial interaction with the host tissue. *P. gingivalis* expresses major and minor fimbriae, encoded by the *fimA* and *mfa1* genes, respectively. Today, six *fimA* allele types are known (fimA I, Ib, II, III, IV, and V). These variants are more or less associated to periodontitis [14]. *P. gingivalis* isolated from periodontally healthy persons more often expresses type I, II, or V. Types Ib, II, and IV, on the other hand, are more associated to diseased periodontal pockets [9, 15]. Major fimbriae can attach and bind to host cells, extracellular matrix (ECM), as well as salivary proteins. Major fimbriae can also facilitate binding to other bacteria, both *P. gingivalis* itself and other species. Minor fimbriae have a role in biofilm formation [14, 16].

As a Gram-negative species, *P. gingivalis* possesses lipopolysaccharides (LPS). Intriguingly, the lipid A part of *P. gingivalis* LPS has a structure that is heterogeneous. The number of associated fatty acids coupled to the disaccharide core varies, resulting in penta- or tetra-acylated lipid A moieties that allows interaction with both Toll-like receptors (TLR) 2 and TLR4 [17]. It is the availability of hemin in the microenvironment that defines which lipid A form that *P. gingivalis* expresses, enabling the bacteria to determine how it interacts with the host to elicit various inflammatory responses [8, 18].

Gingipains are cysteine proteases which probably are the most vital virulence factor expressed by *P. gingivalis*. Gingipains are membrane-bound, as well as secreted from the bacterium, thus, *P. gingivalis* can exert all the various gingipain activities at distant sites. *P. gingivalis* possesses arginine-specific gingipains, Rgp (RgpA and RgpB), encoded by *rgpA* and *rgpB*, respectively, and the lysine-specific gingipain, Kgp, encoded by *kgp*. *P. gingivalis* expresses numerous proteolytic enzymes, but the gingipains are by far the most important ones, accounting for at least 85% of the total proteolytic activity. Furthermore, they are implicated and play key roles in adherence and colonization of the host, in nutrition acquisition by cleaving host proteins, in neutralization of host defense mechanisms, and in manipulation of the host inflammatory response. In summary, gingipains are vital for bacterial survival and proliferation *in vivo* [7]. In the process of adherence and colonization, *P. gingivalis* utilizes fimbrial adhesions, but nevertheless, gingipains are also necessary in these steps. RgpA and Kgp contain hemagglutinin-adhesin domains, which are directly involved in conjugation with other bacterial species, thereby promoting the construction of the bacterial biofilm. These domains also enable binding to ECM, as well as interaction with host cells [19–21]. Rgp is also important for processing various *P. gingivalis*-derived proteins. For instance, Rgp is necessary for the modification of major fimbriae to the mature form [22]. Gingipains are also key mediators in dysregulation of the host immune response [23, 24].

Some *P. gingivalis* strains possess a capsule. Encapsulated strains are more virulent since they have been shown to be more invasive and more resistant to phagocytosis [25–27]. *P. gingivalis* also releases outer membrane vesicles, small cargos that are shed from the outer bacterial membrane that are loaded with LPS, gingipains and other proteases, fimbriae, and capsule (encapsulated strains). The shedding of outer membrane vesicles occurs at a higher rate during colonization and biofilm formation, enabling immune modulation at sites distant from the actual site of infection [28].

3. Mechanisms of *P. gingivalis* interaction with host cells

P. gingivalis, as a keystone pathogen, has the ability to interfere with the host in such ways that the growth and survival of the entire biofilm is promoted and enhanced. It is vital for *P. gingivalis* in a hostile environment to be able to counteract, modify, and manipulate the host immune response in order to survive and evade the various host defense mechanisms. Although it is important to evade the host defense mechanisms, it is also of essential importance to induce inflammation to secure a constant delivery of nutrients to the biofilm through the formation of the nutrient-rich-inflammatory exudate that constitutes the gingival crevicular fluid. *P. gingivalis* has indeed evolved elaborated strategies to diminish as well as promote inflammation [5]. The complement system, which targets microbes, is itself a target for proteolysis by gingipains. In fact, *P. gingivalis* can both inhibit and stimulate the complement system [29]. Also, depending on the type of lipid A expressed, *P. gingivalis* can act as both a TLR4 agonist and an antagonist and regulate the TLR4-dependent immune responses [10, 18]. Realizing all the clever ways of escaping, it may not come as a surprise that *P. gingivalis*, as an additional function on the repertoire, also is resistant to oxidative killing by phagocytes and can survive phagocytosis by macrophages [26, 30]. Furthermore, *P. gingivalis* is able to activate the coagulation cascade and the kallikrein/kinin cascade, thereby enhancing inflammation [31–33]. *P. gingivalis* can invade host cells and replicate within the cell [34]. *P. gingivalis* is also able to protect itself from neutrophil-released reactive oxygen species, leaving the oxidative burst effortless and instead contributing to the destruction of the periodontium [13, 30].

The interactions between the host immune system and the oral microbial flora involve complex cellular and molecular mechanisms. Several cell types, for example, epithelial cells, dendritic cells, osteoblasts, and fibroblasts that reside in the periodontium, are part of the innate host response, as well as platelets, neutrophils, and monocytes/macrophages. Cells of the innate immune system recognize and respond to pathogens (e.g., LPS, fimbriae, DNA, and proteases) through pathogen recognition receptors (PRRs). Important PRRs are TLRs and protease-activated receptors

(PARs). Ligation of PRRs induces downstream signaling pathways that modify the activity of transcription factors that regulates the expression of genes linked to inflammation. Early cellular events leading to a phosphorylation cascade of mitogen-activated protein kinase (MAPK) signaling include the activation of Protein kinase C (PKC) by diacylglycerol and calcium. Signals transduced via MAPK pathways lead to the assembly and activation of the transcription factor AP-1. TLR activation results in the recruitment of an adaptor protein, which in many cases involves MyD88, followed by a signaling cascade that phosphorylates, polyubiquitylates, and degrades IκB. This allows the transcription factor NFκB to translocate to the nucleus and induces gene expression (**Figure 1**). AP-1, NFκB, and other transcription factors cooperatively regulate genes, such as inflammatory mediators and growth factors that are important in many biological processes [35, 36]. This is followed by the release of inflammatory mediators such as CXCL8 and interleukin (IL)-6. The chemokine CXCL8 attracts and recruits neutrophils to the site of infection and promotes monocyte adhesion to the vessel wall. The infiltrating neutrophils, as well as resident cells and macrophages, release cytokines, such as tumor necrosis factor-α (TNF-α), IL-1,

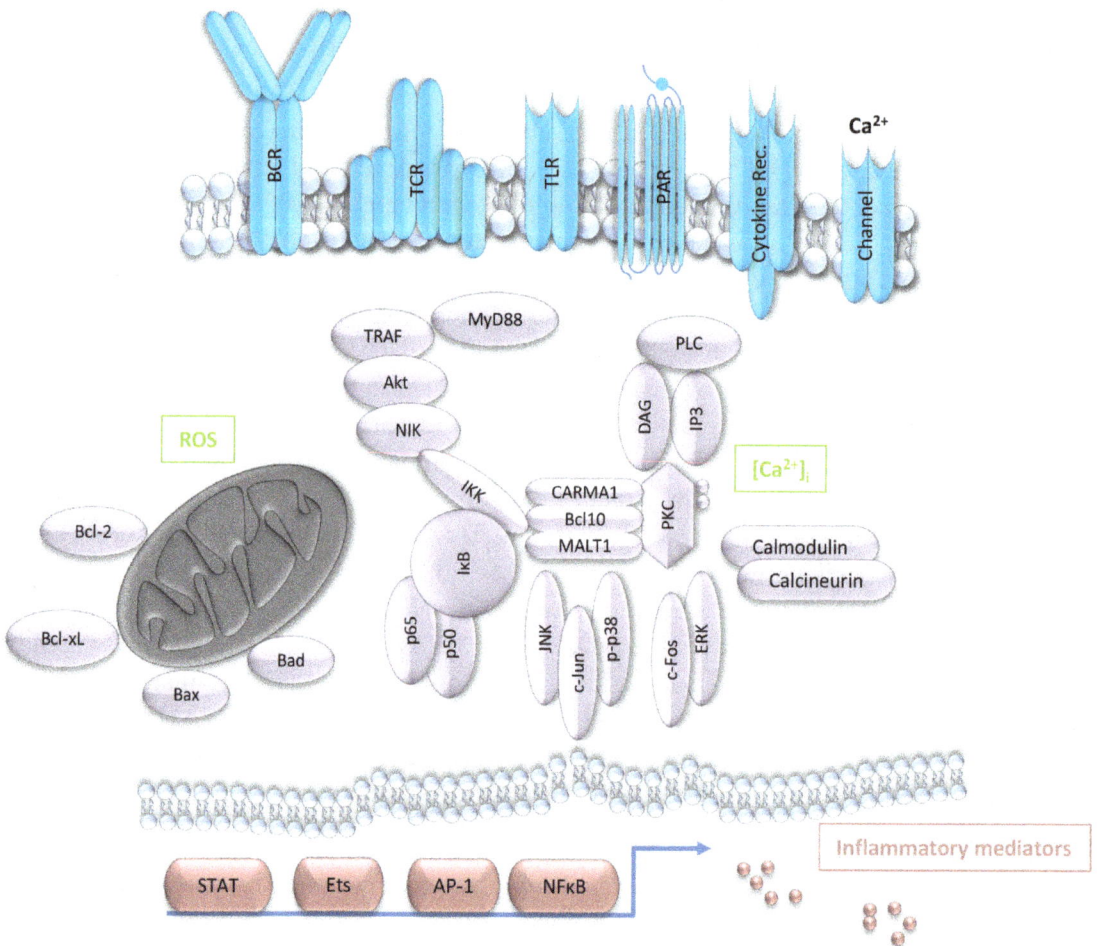

Figure 1. Overview of receptors and intracellular signaling pathways in response to virulence factors of *P. gingivalis*. See text for details.

and IL-6. These inflammatory mediators will eventually contribute to tissue destruction with alveolar bone loss and a sustained chronic inflammation. In addition, the innate immune system will in turn also activate the adaptive immune system with the involvement of lymphocytes [1, 2, 5].

How host-derived factors such as cytokines, hormones, and reactive oxygen species affect periodontal biofilm formation and bacterial virulence is poorly studied and thus not well understood. A recent study suggests that the host-inflammatory responses affect the physiology of bacteria, for example, by utilizing inflammatory mediators as transcription factors [37]. It thus seems quite reasonable that bacteria have evolved mechanisms to sense their environment and to respond to their surrounding by using inflammatory mediators as regulators to be able to adjust and adapt to a changing environment. Consequently, it is possible that early host-inflammatory and immune responses affect and modulate the composition and function of the oral biofilm and the progression of periodontitis.

TLRs are a family of receptors which are of high importance in the innate immune response in sensing pathogens and other danger-associated signals. LPS and fimbriae originate from *P. gingivalis* signals mainly through TLR2, which mediates the release of inflammatory mediators like CXCL8 [38–40]. *P. gingivalis*-mediated activation of TLR2 has been demonstrated to stimulate differentiation and formation of osteoclasts [40]. A study showed that TLR2−/− mice more rapidly cleared *P. gingivalis* infection, had a more efficient phagocytosis of *P. gingivalis*, and also resisted alveolar bone loss despite being repeatedly infected with *P. gingivalis* [41]. TLR2 expression has also been found to be upregulated by *P. gingivalis* [42]. During inflammation, the hemin concentration in the gingival crevicular fluid is high and the tetra-acylated lipid A form is expressed. The tetra-acylated lipid A is acting as a TLR4 antagonist, suppressing TLR4-mediated inflammatory events. The TLR4 antagonist also competitively blocks the binding of TLR4; hence, TLR4 is unable to respond to other bacterial species as well. In addition, since the outer membrane vesicles contain LPS, and can penetrate through the gingival tissue, *P. gingivalis* can dampen the TLR4 effects for the entire oral microbial community. When the hemin concentration is low, inflammation is promoted by expressing penta-acylated lipid A, which works as a TLR4 agonist [10, 18, 43].

PARs have been found to be activated by proteolytic cleaving by gingipains, leading to increased inflammatory response with the release of inflammatory chemokines [39, 44]. PAR2 activation has been demonstrated to induce alveolar bone loss in rats. Since PAR2 is expressed by the cells in the periodontium, *P. gingivalis* and its gingipains are able through PAR2 activation to significantly contribute to the release of several pro-inflammatory mediators that cause degradation of the periodontal tissue [45]. Furthermore, *P. gingivalis* per se has been demonstrated to upregulate the PAR2 expression in gingival fibroblasts [39].

A gradient of CXCL8 is normally established in the healthy periodontal tissue with the highest concentration at the border of the symbiotic dental plaque. This gradient establishes a "wall" of neutrophils, a continuous flow of migrating neutrophils that transit from the vasculature into the periodontium and the gingival crevice. *P. gingivalis* can interact with CXCL8 and this gradient in several ways [2]. In contact with gingival epithelial cells,

P. gingivalis expresses phosphoserine phosphatase SerB, which contributes to CXCL8 inhibition [46]. Gingipains are well known to cleave CXCL8, as well as other cytokines and chemokines, such as IL-6, IL-6 receptor, CXCL10, TNF-α, CD14, IL-4, and IL-12 [23, 24, 44, 47–52]. By targeting inflammatory mediators such as CXCL8, the resulting chemokine paralysis leads to inhibited neutrophil recruitment, thereby promoting the growth of the biofilm. Consequently, *P. gingivalis* undermines innate immunity [2]. Furthermore, CXCL8 is secreted in two different isoforms, as a 72 amino acid (CXCL8-72aa) variant from immune cells and as a 77 amino acid variant (CXCL8-77aa) from non-immune cells such as fibroblasts. CXCL8-72aa is a stronger chemoattractant than CXCL8-77aa, but after cleavage of CXCL8-77aa by gingipains, this is shifted so that the CXCL8-77a has a higher chemotactic potential. This could be a mechanism whereby *P. gingivalis*, by creating a gradient of gingipains across the periodontal tissue can suppress neutrophilic response in the periodontal pocket where the concentration of gingipains is the highest. At a more distant site, with lower concentrations of gingipains, the chemotactic function of CXCL8-77aa is increased, enhancing the inflammatory response and thereby promoting leaky vessels and a constant delivery of nutrients to the biofilm [47, 53].

4. Host cell responses in the oral cavity

4.1. Gingival epithelial cells

The first line of host defense in the gingiva consists of the epithelial cells forming a physical barrier against mechanical stress, exogenous substances, and pathogenic bacteria. This is achieved through different cell-cell junctions, including tight junction and gap junction. *P. gingivalis* uses different strategies to survive and persist in the oral cavity, and invasion of epithelium is one tactical approach in its lifestyle. The advantages of intracellular translocation of *P. gingivalis* into the cells include evasion from immune responses and antibiotics, and accessibility to disseminate to other sites, which collectively leads to persistence and proliferation [4]. The mechanism by which *P. gingivalis* enters epithelial cells is initiated by fimbriae that bind to $\alpha5\beta1$-integrin, followed by the formation of cellular pseudopodia and entry through early endosomes. Intracellular bacteria are then either sorted to late endosomes followed by lysosomes for degradation, or fused with autophagosomes and subsequently degraded in autolysosomes. However, a large number of bacteria are able to escape through recycling pathways for exocytosis and are able to infect new cells, which facilitate deeper penetration into the host tissue [54]. While in other cell types, such as endothelial and smooth muscle cells, *P. gingivalis* has been reported to reside and persist within autophagosomes, followed by the prevention of lysosomal fusion and formation of autolysosomes [55, 56]. Interestingly, $\alpha5\beta1$-integrin on epithelial cells has recently been shown to positively correlate with cells in S phase of the cell cycle, and *P. gingivalis* persistence may be associated with the ability to preferentially target dividing cells [57]. The virulence of intracellular *P. gingivalis* is associated with its ability to degrade paxillin and focal adhesion kinase, and may explain the significant periodontal tissue degradation and lack of wound healing and tissue regeneration processes in periodontitis [58, 59].

Epithelial cells also participate in innate immune responses by secreting a variety of cytokines and chemokines, such as TNF, IL-6, and CXCL8 [60]. *P. gingivalis* suppresses cytokine and chemokine accumulation below basal levels *in vitro*. These effects are most probably due to the potent enzymatic action of proteinases. Indeed, leukocytes are manipulated by *P. gingivalis* to express a limited repertoire of inflammatory mediators, while suppressing CXCL8 release, which is termed "local chemokine paralysis" [61]. Interestingly, *P. gingivalis* significantly increased TGF-β1 expression from gingival epithelial cells. TGF-β1 functions as a growth factor with anti-inflammatory characteristics. Besides TGF-β1, *P. gingivalis* was observed to induce the expression of a wide array of different growth factors, including Insulin-like growth factor (IGF), Platelet-derived growth factor (PDGF), endothelial growth factor (EGF), and Hepatocyte growth factor (HGF). We have previously shown that *P. gingivalis* induces high levels of HGF in clinical samples from patients with periodontitis. However, the activity of HGF was significantly reduced in patients compared to healthy controls [62].

4.2. Gingival fibroblasts

Gingival and periodontal ligament fibroblasts are the main cell types found in the connective tissue of the periodontium, and they are exposed to pathogens once the epithelial barrier is breached [2, 63]. Fibroblasts provide a structural tissue framework (stroma) and define the microanatomy of the tissue with the key function to regulate and maintain integrity of the connective tissue. Homeostasis of connective tissues is maintained through the production of ECM and by modifying existing ECM by secreting matrix metalloproteinases (MMPs) that cleave and degrade ECM components [64]. The ability of fibroblasts to secrete as well as respond to growth factors and cytokines/chemokines allows reciprocal communication with adjacent cells that facilitates homeostasis of the tissue. Considering the functions of fibroblasts makes it easy to realize that fibroblasts play a vital role in tissue development, differentiation, and repair. Fibroblasts are also of importance in tissue destruction by the release of MMPs and pro-inflammatory cytokines and chemokines [63–65]. PAR1 and TLR2 have been shown to be important in the interaction between gingival fibroblasts and *P. gingivalis*. Gingival fibroblasts can sense *P. gingivalis* through PAR1 and TLR2, and the activation of these receptors leads to the secretion of CXCL8 and IL-6, suggesting that fibroblasts could make a substantial contribution to the inflammatory process seen in periodontitis [38, 39, 66]. Furthermore, *P. gingivalis* is able to modify this response by cleaving fibroblast-derived cytokines through the proteolytic activity of the gingipains and thereby hampering the antimicrobial capacity of the fibroblasts [23, 24, 66].

4.3. Leukocytes

Periodontitis is characterized by interaction between a number of oral pathogens, such as *P. gingivalis*, and blood leukocytes. Neutrophils and monocytes are well equipped with PRRs, such as TLRs, nuclear-oligomerizing domains ½, and PARs. This arsenal of receptors enables the detection of invading pathogens and production of reactive oxygen species, cytokines, and chemokines. We have shown that *P. gingivalis* is capable of inducing ROS in isolated neutrophils and in whole blood, and stimulating the release of inflammatory mediators, such as IL-1β and CXCL8 [67]. Both these cytokines are capable of priming neutrophils, endothelial cells, and other vascular cells in an autocrine and paracrine manner. Studies have demonstrated that gingipains hydrolyze pro-inflammatory cytokines, but not growth factor/anti-inflammatory cytokines, which result in aberrant immune cell recruitment to the site of infection, ensuring a continued low-grade infection.

The critical balance of different T-cell subsets has previously been described to play an important role in the inflammatory process underlying periodontitis. The presence of specific antibodies for oral bacteria in patients with periodontitis indicates an involvement of adaptive immune responses [68], of which different T-cell subsets play a detrimental role in the pathogenesis of this inflammatory disease. The T-cell-associated cytokine profile in gingival tissue suggests an engagement of T-helper (Th) 1, Th2, and Th17 cells [69–71]. These T-cell subsets are associated with host-derived tissue destruction and bone loss, through, for example, Receptor activator of nuclear factor kappa-B ligand (RANKL) expression. Exaggerated pro-inflammatory responses from T-cells can be controlled by regulatory T-cells (Tregs) that display protective effects through the secretion of anti-inflammatory IL-10 and TGF-β1. Tregs have a central role in maintaining homeostasis by regulating other leukocyte functions and thereby avoiding extensive immune cell activation and its pathological consequences, for example, in periodontitis. Interestingly, we have previously shown that T-cell interaction with *P. gingivalis* leads to a gingipain-mediated inactivation of IL-2 [72], which may thus downregulate Tregs and support the process of periodontitis. Thus, the inhibition of gingipains and maintenance of a Treg-mediated beneficial homeostasis may be a successful strategy for the prevention and treatment of periodontitis.

5. Periodontitis, systemic inflammation, and cardiovascular disease

Periodontal disease is today considered to play a significant role in various systemic conditions and, in the past decade, the enhanced prevalence of cardiovascular disease (CVD) among patients with periodontitis has received increased attention [73, 74]. Several periodontal bacteria and their agents have been identified in atherosclerotic plaques, for example, *P. gingivalis, Fusobacterium nucleatum, T. forsythia, Prevotella intermedia, Aggregatibacter actinomycetecomitans*, and *T. denticola* [75–78]. The occurrence of periodontal bacteria in coronary artery plaques was found to be 5-fold greater in patients with severe periodontitis compared to those with medium periodontitis [79], and DNA from periodontal bacteria, including *P. gingivalis*, was identified in more than 70% of carotid plaque samples [80]. Furthermore, *P. gingivalis* has been shown to influence the development of abdominal aorta aneurysm, involving the activation of TLRs and MMPs [81]. Several animal experiments have demonstrated that oral and systemic infection with periodontal bacteria induces atherosclerosis [74]. Hokamura and Umemura [82] showed that the administration of *P. gingivalis* in a mouse model induces arterial intimal hyperplasia associated with upregulation of the calcium-binding protein S100A9.

When the periodontal disease develops, the gingival epithelium becomes ulcerated by proteolytic activity, for example, by *P. gingivalis*, leading to exposure of the underlying connective tissues and blood capillaries to the bacterial plaque biofilm. At medium periodontitis, the ulcerative area in the oral cavity ranges between 8 and 20 cm^2, which means that large amounts of periodontal bacteria and their toxins and metabolic products have a chance, during chewing and oral hygiene activities, to disseminate into the bloodstream and cause transient bacteremias and systemic inflammation [74]. By entering the circulation, the bacteria and/or their components (e.g., proteases, fimbrillin, and LPS) activate platelets and neutrophils, induce ROS production, and trigger inflammatory processes in coronary vessels.

Studies using knockout mice orally infected by *P. gingivalis*, demonstrate that atherosclerosis, involving the accumulation of macrophages and inflammatory mediators (CD40, IL-1ß, IL-6, and TNF-α) in atherosclerotic lesions, is highly dependent on TLR2 [41, 83]. In correlation, interaction between *P. gingivalis* and human blood cells, for example, platelets, neutrophils, monocytes, and T-cells, is mainly mediated by TLR2 and has dramatic inflammatory and immunomodulatory effects, including cellular aggregation, oxygen radical production, low-density lipoprotein (LDL) oxidation, and release and degradation of cytokines. Furthermore, *P. gingivalis* changes the expression of more than thousand genes in vascular smooth muscle cells [84]. For example, *P. gingivalis* upregulates genes involved in proliferation, for example, the TGFβ1 pathway and production of matrix proteins, but downregulates pro-inflammatory genes, such as those involved in IL-1β, IL-6, and CXCL8 production. *P. gingivalis* also caused a dramatic increase in the expression of angiopoietin2 (ANGPT2), which is highly correlated with inflammation and atherosclerosis, whereas ANGPT1, inhibitor of inflammation, was downregulated [85, 86]. These effects are mediated via gingipain R, possibly through PAR signaling. Furthermore, the level of another angiogenic factor, vascular endothelial

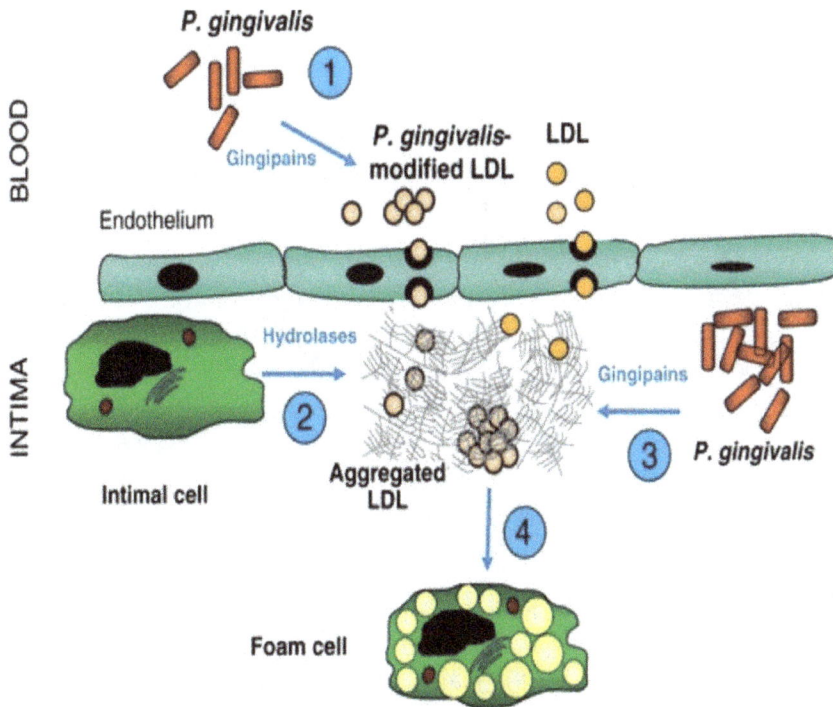

Figure 2. A novel biochemical link between periodontitis and cardiovascular disease.

growth factor (VEGF), increases in patients with periodontitis, and periodontal treatment reduces its concentration [87]. These data indicate that *P. gingivalis* causes a shift from contractile smooth muscle cells to proliferating and matrix-producing smooth muscle cells, which contributes to the growth of the fibrous atherosclerotic plaque, and promotes vascular inflammation and angiogenesis.

P. gingivalis has also been shown to modify LDL and promote phenotypic shift of monocytes to foam cells [75, 77, 88]. Our group has previously found fragmentation of the dominating apoprotein of LDL, apo B-100, by *P. gingivalis* and its Rgps [88]. Consequently, our findings together with others suggest that *P. gingivalis* during translocation in circulating blood modifies LDL to an atherogenic form which may represent a link between periodontal disease and atherosclerosis (**Figure 2**).

6. Host cell responses in the circulation and vascular wall

Endothelial cells possess secretory and immunological properties and play therefore important roles in the cardiovascular system. The association of periodontitis with cardiovascular complications includes the induction of endothelial dysfunction, oxidative stress, and systemic inflammation [89]. Furthermore, patients with periodontitis have increased levels of pro-inflammatory mediators, including C-reactive protein (CRP), IL-6, and TNF that may induce endothelial dysfunction [90]. Endothelial dysfunction, which is the initial step in the development and progression of atherosclerosis, is mediated by endotoxins and gingipains of periodontal bacteria. These toxins lead to an impairment of normal endothelial function, including vessel permeability and immune cell adhesion and function [91, 92]. Furthermore, *P. gingivalis* and other periodontal pathogens induce the expression of endothelin-1, a potent vasoconstrictor released by endothelial cells [93, 94]. Endothelin-1 expression has shown a positive correlation to pro-inflammatory cytokines TNF, IL-6, and IL-1β [95], and a negative correlation to anti-inflammatory mediators, for example, angiopoietin-1 [96, 97].

Platelets are key players in hemostasis and acute thrombosis and are initial actors in the development of atherosclerotic lesions often triggered by endothelial dysfunction [98]. However, they are also involved in the immune system and express a broad repertoire of immune cell features such as TLRs, the immunoglobulin γ-receptor FcγRIIA, complement receptors, inflammatory mediators, as well as microbicidal activities, for example, thrombocidins [99, 100]. Furthermore, platelets bind to and encapsulate bacteria, release ROS and recruit and activate leukocytes and regulate inflammatory processes of the vessel wall [101]. These characteristics make it possible for platelets to recognize and respond to pathogens, such as *P. gingivalis*, and engage other immune cells for enhanced bacterial clearance and inflammatory response.

Several studies suggest that platelet-leukocyte interaction is an essential underlying inflammatory process in atherosclerosis, and patients with cardiovascular disease have an increased number of neutrophil-platelet aggregates in the blood circulation [102, 103]. In correlation, we have shown that *P. gingivalis* markedly induces the formation of large aggregates of neutrophils and platelets, associated with ROS production and lipid peroxidation, in whole blood and that this effect is dependent on CD11b/CD18-fibrinogen-GpIIb/IIIa interaction, and Rac2 and Cdc42 activation [104, 105] (**Figure 3**). In addition, mice challenged with *P. gingivalis* were found to form platelet-neutrophil aggregates, whereas knockout TLR2$^{-/-}$ mice did not. Human platelets express TLRs (TLR 1, 2, 4, 6, and 9), which could be key molecules linking periodontal infection and CVD. For example, TLR2-mediated platelet activation involving the activation of GpIIb/IIIa and P-selectin contributes to the formation of platelet-leukocyte complexes and ROS production [99].

Platelets activation by TLR1/2 receptor ligands results in aggregation as well as secretion of inflammatory mediators such as RANTES, macrophage migration inhibitory factor (MIF), and plasminogen activator inhibitor-1 (PAI-1) [105]. Interestingly, these platelet-derived factors are degraded by gingipains from *P. gingivalis* [105]. Regulated on activation, normal T-cell expressed and secreted (RANTES) is induced by *P. gingivalis* and its lipopolysaccharides and is thus implicated in periodontitis, where elevated levels have been detected in the gingival crevicular fluid of patients with periodontitis [106]. It has been demonstrated that *P. gingivalis*, in addition to TLR2, also can trigger platelet activation via PAR receptors. Through the action of Rgp on PARs, *P. gingivalis* activates platelets by increasing intracellular-free calcium and induces aggregation [105]. In correlation, Lourbakos et al. and McNiol and Israels [107, 108] have demonstrated that gingipains activate PAR1 and PAR4 on platelets leading to aggregation and secretion. We have shown that *P. gingivalis* triggers platelet aggregation through

Bacteria-platelet hypothesis of atherosclerosis

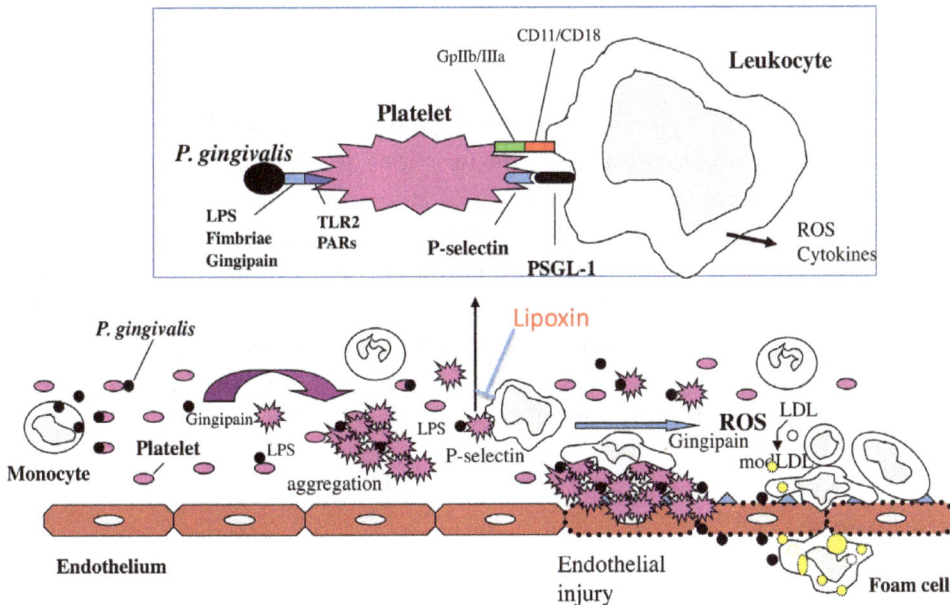

Figure 3. Model showing platelets as a linker between periodontal infection and innate immune response at the vessel wall.

gingipain interaction with PARs and sensitizes platelets for activation by epinephrine, which may explain the association between periodontitis, stress and CVD [109].

7. Preventive and treatment strategies

Periodontal pathogens reside in biofilms of subgingival dental plaque and form complex polymicrobial communities. The failure of the immune system to resolve bacterial biofilms results in an accumulation of inflammatory mediators that accelerates the disease state toward a chronic inflammatory condition. Bacterial biofilms are difficult to treat, and conventional methods, including mechanical removal and scaling and root planning (SRP), are still being used. These methods are less efficient and new preventive/treatment strategies are needed. A new approach includes the administration of adjunctive antibiotics systemically in combination with SRP. Different antibiotics have been applied, and a combination of metronidazole and amoxicillin was found to be effective at reducing pocket depth and clinical attachment gain compared to SRP alone, reviewed in [110]. Although antibiotic therapy is effective in modern medicine, microorganisms that are resistant to single or multiple antibiotics have emerged. The development of new families of antibiotics has significantly declined, which is associated with high costs and concerns for possible effects on the commensal microbiota and host health [111]. It is evident that new alternative strategies to traditional antibiotic therapy are needed. New approaches to combat bacterial infections include antibodies, vaccines, bacteriophages, probiotics, and antimicrobial peptides (host- and bacteria-derived) [111–114]. These strategies of promising candidates to traditional antibiotics deserve more consideration.

8. Concluding remarks

In summary, it is possible that *P. gingivalis* has a role in pathogenic oral biofilms to undermine important factors of innate immunity, by altering the functions of receptors and their intracellular signaling pathways and the levels of effector molecules, and thereby antagonizing an effective host response. These activities of key periodontal pathogens could contribute to an adaptation and maturation of dysbiotic biofilm communities and promote chronic inflammation and tissue destruction of periodontitis. Increased understanding of the interbacterial interactions that occur in the oral polymicrobial biofilm and its interplay with the host immune system is of uttermost importance for identifying novel targets for the prevention, diagnosis, and treatment of periodontitis and associated systemic disorders.

Acknowledgements

This work was supported by research grants from the Swedish Research Council (2016-04874), the Swedish Heart-Lung Foundation (20130576), the Knowledge Foundation (20150244, 20150086), and the foundation of Magnus Bergvall (201500823).

Author details

Hazem Khalaf*, Eleonor Palm and Torbjörn Bengtsson

*Address all correspondence to: hazem.khalaf@oru.se

School of Medical Sciences, Örebro University, Örebro, Sweden

References

[1] Haffajee AD, Socransky SS. Microbial etiological agents of destructive periodontal diseases. Periodontology. 2000. 1994 Jun;**5**:78-111. PubMed PMID: 9673164. Epub 1994/06/01. eng

[2] Darveau RP. Periodontitis: A polymicrobial disruption of host homeostasis. Nature Review Microbiology. 2010 Jul;**8**(7):481-490. PubMed PMID: 20514045. Epub 2010/06/02. eng

[3] Sanz M, Quirynen M. Advances in the aetiology of periodontitis. Group A consensus report of the 5th European Workshop in Periodontology. Journal of Clinical Periodontology. 2005;**32**(Suppl 6):54-56. PubMed PMID: 16128829. Epub 2005/09/01. eng

[4] Sakanaka A, Takeuchi H, Kuboniwa M, Amano A. Dual lifestyle of *Porphyromonas gingivalis* in biofilm and gingival cells. Microbial Pathogenesis. 2016 May;**94**:42-47. PubMed PMID: 26456558. Epub 2015/10/13. eng

[5] Hajishengallis G, Darveau RP, Curtis MA. The keystone-pathogen hypothesis. Nature Review Microbiology. 2012 Oct;**10**(10):717-725. PubMed PMID: 22941505. Pubmed Central PMCID: Pmc3498498. Epub 2012/09/04. eng

[6] Hajishengallis G, Liang S, Payne MA, Hashim A, Jotwani R, Eskan MA, et al. Low-abundance biofilm species orchestrates inflammatory periodontal disease through the commensal microbiota and complement. Cell Host & Microbe. 2011 Nov 17;**10**(5):497-506. PubMed PMID: 22036469. Pubmed Central PMCID: Pmc3221781. Epub 2011/11/01. eng

[7] Guo Y, Nguyen KA, Potempa J. Dichotomy of gingipains action as virulence factors: From cleaving substrates with the precision of a surgeon's knife to a meat chopper-like brutal degradation of proteins. Periodontology 2000. 2010 Oct;**54**(1):15-44. PubMed PMID: 20712631. Pubmed Central PMCID: Pmc2924770. Epub 2010/08/18. eng

[8] Herath TD, Wang Y, Seneviratne CJ, Lu Q, Darveau RP, Wang CY, et al. *Porphyromonas gingivalis* lipopolysaccharide lipid A heterogeneity differentially modulates the expression of IL-6 and IL-8 in human gingival fibroblasts. Journal of Clinical Periodontology. 2011 Aug;**38**(8):694-701. PubMed PMID: 21752043. Epub 2011/07/15. eng

[9] Missailidis CG, Umeda JE, Ota-Tsuzuki C, Anzai D, Mayer MP. Distribution of fimA genotypes of *Porphyromonas gingivalis* in subjects with various periodontal conditions.

Oral Microbiology and Immunology. 2004 Aug;**19**(4):224-229. PubMed PMID: 15209991. Epub 2004/06/24. eng

[10] Herath TD, Darveau RP, Seneviratne CJ, Wang CY, Wang Y, Jin L. Tetra- and penta-acylated lipid A structures of *Porphyromonas gingivalis* LPS differentially activate TLR4-mediated NF-kappaB signal transduction cascade and immuno-inflammatory response in human gingival fibroblasts. PloS One. 2013;**8**(3):e58496. PubMed PMID: 23554896. Pubmed Central PMCID: PMC3595299. Epub 2013/04/05. eng

[11] Al-Qutub MN, Braham PH, Karimi-Naser LM, Liu X, Genco CA, Darveau RP. Hemin-dependent modulation of the lipid A structure of *Porphyromonas gingivalis* lipopolysaccharide. Infection and immunity. 2006 Aug;**74**(8):4474-4485. PubMed PMID: 16861633. Pubmed Central PMCID: Pmc1539574. Epub 2006/07/25. eng

[12] Amano A, Nakagawa I, Kataoka K, Morisaki I, Hamada S. Distribution of *Porphyromonas gingivalis* strains with fimA genotypes in periodontitis patients. Journal of Clinical Microbiology. 1999 May;**37**(5):1426-1430. PubMed PMID: 10203499. Pubmed Central PMCID: PMC84792. Epub 1999/04/16. eng

[13] Hajishengallis G. *Porphyromonas gingivalis*-host interactions: Open war or intelligent guerilla tactics?. Microbes and infection. 2009 May–Jun;**11**(6-7):637-645. PubMed PMID: 19348960. Pubmed Central PMCID: PMC2704251. Epub 2009/04/08. eng

[14] Amano A. Molecular interaction of *Porphyromonas gingivalis* with host cells: Implication for the microbial pathogenesis of periodontal disease. Journal of Periodontology. 2003 Jan;**74**(1):90-96. PubMed PMID: 12593602. Epub 2003/02/21. eng

[15] Kristoffersen AK, Solli SJ, Nguyen TD, Enersen M. Association of the rgpB gingipain genotype to the major fimbriae (fimA) genotype in clinical isolates of the periodontal pathogen *Porphyromonas gingivalis*. Journal of Oral Microbiology. 2015;**7**:29124. PubMed PMID: 26387644. Pubmed Central PMCID: PMC4576663. Epub 2015/09/22. eng

[16] Inaba H, Nakano K, Kato T, Nomura R, Kawai S, Kuboniwa M, et al. Heterogenic virulence and related factors among clinical isolates of *Porphyromonas gingivalis* with type II fimbriae. Oral Microbiology and Immunology. 2008 Feb;**23**(1):29-35. PubMed PMID: 18173795. Epub 2008/01/05. eng

[17] Kumada H, Haishima Y, Umemoto T, Tanamoto K. Structural study on the free lipid A isolated from lipopolysaccharide of *Porphyromonas gingivalis*. Journal of Bacteriology. 1995 Apr;**177**(8):2098-2106. PubMed PMID: 7721702. Pubmed Central PMCID: Pmc176854. Epub 1995/04/01. eng

[18] Darveau RP, Pham TT, Lemley K, Reife RA, Bainbridge BW, Coats SR, et al. *Porphyromonas gingivalis* lipopolysaccharide contains multiple lipid A species that functionally interact with both Toll-like receptors 2 and 4. Infection and Immunity. 2004 Sep;**72**(9):5041-5051. PubMed PMID: 15321997. Pubmed Central PMCID: Pmc517442. Epub 2004/08/24. eng

[19] Chen T, Duncan MJ. Gingipain adhesin domains mediate *Porphyromonas gingivalis* adherence to epithelial cells. Microbial Pathogenesis. 2004 Apr;**36**(4):205-209. PubMed PMID: 15001226. Epub 2004/03/06. eng

[20] Pathirana RD, O'Brien-Simpson NM, Veith PD, Riley PF, Reynolds EC. Characterization of proteinase-adhesin complexes of *Porphyromonas gingivalis*. Microbiology (Reading, England). 2006 Aug;**152**(Pt 8):2381-2394. PubMed PMID: 16849802. Epub 2006/07/20. eng

[21] Pathirana RD, O'Brien-Simpson NM, Visvanathan K, Hamilton JA, Reynolds EC. The role of the RgpA-Kgp proteinase-adhesin complexes in the adherence of *Porphyromonas gingivalis* to fibroblasts. Microbiology (Reading, England). 2008 Oct;**154**(Pt 10):2904-2911. PubMed PMID: 18832297. Epub 2008/10/04. eng

[22] Kadowaki T, Nakayama K, Yoshimura F, Okamoto K, Abe N, Yamamoto K. Arg-gingipain acts as a major processing enzyme for various cell surface proteins in *Porphyromonas gingivalis*. The Journal of Biological Chemistry. 1998 Oct 30;**273**(44):29072-29076. PubMed PMID: 9786913. Epub 1998/10/24. eng

[23] Palm E, Khalaf H, Bengtsson T. Suppression of inflammatory responses of human gingival fibroblasts by gingipains from *Porphyromonas gingivalis*. Molecular Oral Microbiology. 2015 Feb;**30**(1):74-85. PubMed PMID: 25055828. Epub 2014/07/25. eng

[24] Palm E, Khalaf H, Bengtsson T. *Porphyromonas gingivalis* downregulates the immune response of fibroblasts. BMC Microbiology. 2013;**13**:155. PubMed PMID: 23841502. Pubmed Central PMCID: Pmc3717116. Epub 2013/07/12. eng

[25] Irshad M, van der Reijden WA, Crielaard W, Laine ML. In vitro invasion and survival of *Porphyromonas gingivalis* in gingival fibroblasts; role of the capsule. Archivum immunologiae et therapiae experimentalis. 2012 Dec;**60**(6):469-476. PubMed PMID: 22949096. Epub 2012/09/06. eng

[26] Singh A, Wyant T, Anaya-Bergman C, Aduse-Opoku J, Brunner J, Laine ML, et al. The capsule of *Porphyromonas gingivalis* leads to a reduction in the host inflammatory response, evasion of phagocytosis, and increase in virulence. Infection and Immunity. 2011 Nov;**79**(11):4533-4542. PubMed PMID: 21911459. Pubmed Central PMCID: PMC3257911. Epub 2011/09/14. eng

[27] Vernal R, Leon R, Silva A, van Winkelhoff AJ, Garcia-Sanz JA, Sanz M. Differential cytokine expression by human dendritic cells in response to different *Porphyromonas gingivalis* capsular serotypes. Journal of Clinical Periodontology. 2009 Oct;**36**(10):823-829. PubMed PMID: 19682172. Epub 2009/08/18. eng

[28] Gui MJ, Dashper SG, Slakeski N, Chen YY, Reynolds EC. Spheres of influence: *Porphyromonas gingivalis* outer membrane vesicles. Molecular Oral Microbiology. 2016 Oct;**31**(5):365-378. PubMed PMID: 26466922. Epub 2015/10/16. eng

[29] Popadiak K, Potempa J, Riesbeck K, Blom AM. Biphasic effect of gingipains from *Porphyromonas gingivalis* on the human complement system. Journal of Immunology (Baltimore, MD: 1950). 2007 Jun 01;**178**(11):7242-7250. PubMed PMID: 17513773. Epub 2007/05/22. eng

[30] Mydel P, Takahashi Y, Yumoto H, Sztukowska M, Kubica M, Gibson FC, 3rd, et al. Roles of the host oxidative immune response and bacterial antioxidant rubrerythrin during

Porphyromonas gingivalis infection. PLoS Pathogens. 2006 Jul;**2**(7):e76. PubMed PMID: 16895445. Pubmed Central PMCID: PMC1522038. Epub 2006/08/10. eng

[31] Imamura T, Tanase S, Hamamoto T, Potempa J, Travis J. Activation of blood coagulation factor IX by gingipains R, arginine-specific cysteine proteinases from *Porphyromonas gingivalis*. The Biochemical Journal. 2001 Jan 15;**353**(Pt 2):325-331. PubMed PMID: 11139397. Pubmed Central PMCID: PMC1221575. Epub 2001/01/05. eng

[32] Imamura T, Potempa J, Tanase S, Travis J. Activation of blood coagulation factor X by arginine-specific cysteine proteinases (gingipain-Rs) from *Porphyromonas gingivalis*. The Journal of Biological Chemistry. 1997 Jun 20;**272**(25):16062-16067. PubMed PMID: 9188512. Epub 1997/06/20. eng

[33] Imamura T, Potempa J, Travis J. Activation of the kallikrein-kinin system and release of new kinins through alternative cleavage of kininogens by microbial and human cell proteinases. Biological Chemistry. 2004 Nov;**385**(11):989-996. PubMed PMID: 15576318. Epub 2004/12/04. eng

[34] Houalet-Jeanne S, Pellen-Mussi P, Tricot-Doleux S, Apiou J, Bonnaure-Mallet M. Assessment of internalization and viability of *Porphyromonas gingivalis* in KB epithelial cells by confocal microscopy. Infection and Immunity. 2001 Nov;**69**(11):7146-7151. PubMed PMID: 11598091. Pubmed Central PMCID: PMC100107. Epub 2001/10/13. eng

[35] Zhao W, Wang L, Zhang M, Wang P, Zhang L, Yuan C, et al. NF-kappaB- and AP-1-mediated DNA looping regulates osteopontin transcription in endotoxin-stimulated murine macrophages. Journal of Immunology. 2011 Mar 01;**186**(5):3173-3179. PubMed PMID: 21257959. Pubmed Central PMCID: 4227538

[36] DebRoy A, Vogel SM, Soni D, Sundivakkam PC, Malik AB, Tiruppathi C. Cooperative signaling via transcription factors NF-kappaB and AP1/c-Fos mediates endothelial cell STIM1 expression and hyperpermeability in response to endotoxin. Journal of Biological Chemistry. 2014 Aug 29;**289**(35):24188-24201. PubMed PMID: 25016017. Pubmed Central PMCID: 4148850

[37] Mahdavi J, Royer PJ, Sjolinder HS, Azimi S, Self T, Stoof J, et al. Pro-inflammatory cytokines can act as intracellular modulators of commensal bacterial virulence. Open Biology. 2013 Oct 09;**3**(10):130048. PubMed PMID: 24107297. Pubmed Central PMCID: PMC3814720. Epub 2013/10/11. eng

[38] Morandini AC, Chaves Souza PP, Ramos-Junior ES, Brozoski DT, Sipert CR, Souza Costa CA, et al. Toll-like receptor 2 knockdown modulates interleukin (IL)-6 and IL-8 but not stromal derived factor-1 (SDF-1/CXCL12) in human periodontal ligament and gingival fibroblasts. Journal of Periodontology. 2013 Apr;**84**(4):535-544. PubMed PMID: 22680301. Epub 2012/06/12. eng

[39] Palm E, Demirel I, Bengtsson T, Khalaf H. The role of Toll-like and protease-activated receptors in the expression of cytokines by gingival fibroblasts stimulated with the periodontal pathogen *Porphyromonas gingivalis*. Cytokine. 2015 Dec;**76**(2):424-432. PubMed PMID: 26318255. Epub 2015/09/01. eng

[40]   Hiramine H, Watanabe K, Hamada N, Umemoto T. *Porphyromonas gingivalis* 67-kDa fimbriae induced cytokine production and osteoclast differentiation utilizing TLR2. FEMS Microbiology Letters. 2003 Dec 05;**229**(1):49-55. PubMed PMID: 14659542. Epub 2003/12/09. eng

[41]   Burns E, Bachrach G, Shapira L, Nussbaum G. Cutting edge: TLR2 is required for the innate response to *Porphyromonas gingivalis*: Activation leads to bacterial persistence and TLR2 deficiency attenuates induced alveolar bone resorption. Journal of Immunology (Baltimore, MD: 1950). 2006 Dec 15;**177**(12):8296-8300. PubMed PMID: 17142724. Epub 2006/12/05. eng

[42]   Wara-aswapati N, Chayasadom A, Surarit R, Pitiphat W, Boch JA, Nagasawa T, et al. Induction of Toll-like receptor expression by *Porphyromonas gingivalis*. Journal of Periodontology. 2013 Jul;**84**(7):1010-1018. PubMed PMID: 23003918. Epub 2012/09/26. eng

[43]   Coats SR, Jones JW, Do CT, Braham PH, Bainbridge BW, To TT, et al. Human Toll-like receptor 4 responses to P. gingivalis are regulated by lipid A 1- and 4'-phosphatase activities. Cellular Microbiology. 2009 Nov;**11**(11):1587-1599. PubMed PMID: 19552698. Pubmed Central PMCID: PMC3074576. Epub 2009/06/26. eng

[44]   Uehara A, Naito M, Imamura T, Potempa J, Travis J, Nakayama K, et al. Dual regulation of interleukin-8 production in human oral epithelial cells upon stimulation with gingipains from *Porphyromonas gingivalis*. Journal of Medical Microbiology. 2008 Apr;**57**(Pt 4):500-507. PubMed PMID: 18349372. Epub 2008/03/20. eng

[45]   Fagundes JA, Monoo LD, Euzebio Alves VT, Pannuti CM, Cortelli SC, Cortelli JR, et al. *Porphyromonas gingivalis* is associated with protease-activated receptor-2 upregulation in chronic periodontitis. Journal of Periodontology. 2011 Nov;**82**(11):1596-1601. PubMed PMID: 21513479. Epub 2011/04/26. eng

[46]   Bainbridge B, Verma RK, Eastman C, Yehia B, Rivera M, Moffatt C, et al. Role of *Porphyromonas gingivalis* phosphoserine phosphatase enzyme SerB in inflammation, immune response, and induction of alveolar bone resorption in rats. Infection and Immunity. 2010 Nov;**78**(11):4560-4569. PubMed PMID: 20805334. Pubmed Central PMCID: PMC2976320. Epub 2010/09/02. eng

[47]   Moelants EA, Loozen G, Mortier A, Martens E, Opdenakker G, Mizgalska D, et al. Citrullination and proteolytic processing of chemokines by *Porphyromonas gingivalis*. Infection and Immunity. 2014 Jun;**82**(6):2511-2519. PubMed PMID: 24686061. Pubmed Central PMCID: PMC4019151. Epub 2014/04/02. eng

[48]   Mikolajczyk-Pawlinska J, Travis J, Potempa J. Modulation of interleukin-8 activity by gingipains from *Porphyromonas gingivalis*: Implications for pathogenicity of periodontal disease. FEBS Letters. 1998 Dec 04;**440**(3):282-286. PubMed PMID: 9872387. Epub 1999/01/01. eng

[49]   Oleksy A, Banbula A, Bugno M, Travis J, Potempa J. Proteolysis of interleukin-6 receptor (IL-6R) by *Porphyromonas gingivalis* cysteine proteinases (gingipains) inhibits interleukin-6-mediated cell activation. Microbial Pathogenesis. 2002 Apr;**32**(4):173-181. PubMed PMID: 12079407. Epub 2002/06/25. eng

[50] Sugawara S, Nemoto E, Tada H, Miyake K, Imamura T, Takada H. Proteolysis of human monocyte CD14 by cysteine proteinases (gingipains) from *Porphyromonas gingivalis* leading to lipopolysaccharide hyporesponsiveness. Journal of Immunology (Baltimore, MD: 1950). 2000 Jul 01;**165**(1):411-418. PubMed PMID: 10861079. Epub 2000/06/22. eng

[51] Takayanagi H, Iizuka H, Juji T, Nakagawa T, Yamamoto A, Miyazaki T, et al. Involvement of receptor activator of nuclear factor kappaB ligand/osteoclast differentiation factor in osteoclastogenesis from synoviocytes in rheumatoid arthritis. Arthritis and Rheumatism. 2000 Feb;**43**(2):259-269. PubMed PMID: 10693864. Epub 2000/02/29. eng

[52] Yun PL, Decarlo AA, Collyer C, Hunter N. Hydrolysis of interleukin-12 by *Porphyromonas gingivalis* major cysteine proteinases may affect local gamma interferon accumulation and the Th1 or Th2 T-cell phenotype in periodontitis. Infection and Immunity. 2001 Sep;**69**(9):5650-5660. PubMed PMID: 11500441. Pubmed Central PMCID: PMC98681. Epub 2001/08/14. eng

[53] Dias IH, Marshall L, Lambert PA, Chapple IL, Matthews JB, Griffiths HR. Gingipains from *Porphyromonas gingivalis* increase the chemotactic and respiratory burst-priming properties of the 77-amino-acid interleukin-8 variant. Infection and Immunity. 2008 Jan;**76**(1):317-323. PubMed PMID: 18025101. Pubmed Central PMCID: PMC2223636. Epub 2007/11/21. eng

[54] Amano A, Chen C, Honma K, Li C, Settem RP, Sharma A. Genetic characteristics and pathogenic mechanisms of periodontal pathogens. Advances in Dental Research. 2014 May;**26**(1):15-22. PubMed PMID: 24736700

[55] Dorn BR, Dunn WA, Jr, Progulske-Fox A. *Porphyromonas gingivalis* traffics to autophagosomes in human coronary artery endothelial cells. Infection and Immunity. 2001 Sep;**69**(9):5698-5708. PubMed PMID: 11500446. Pubmed Central PMCID: 98686

[56] Ham H, Sreelatha A, Orth K. Manipulation of host membranes by bacterial effectors. Nature Reviews Microbiology. 2011 Jul 18;**9**(9):635-646. PubMed PMID: 21765451

[57] Al-Taweel FB, Douglas CW, Whawell SA. The periodontal pathogen *Porphyromonas gingivalis* preferentially interacts with oral epithelial cells in S phase of the cell cycle. Infection and Immunity. 2016 Jul;**84**(7):1966-1974. PubMed PMID: 27091929. Pubmed Central PMCID: 4936351

[58] Hintermann E, Haake SK, Christen U, Sharabi A, Quaranta V. Discrete proteolysis of focal contact and adherens junction components in *Porphyromonas gingivalis*-infected oral keratinocytes: A strategy for cell adhesion and migration disabling. Infection and Immunity. 2002 Oct;**70**(10):5846-5856. PubMed PMID: 12228316. Pubmed Central PMCID: 128337

[59] Kato T, Kawai S, Nakano K, Inaba H, Kuboniwa M, Nakagawa I, et al. Virulence of *Porphyromonas gingivalis* is altered by substitution of fimbria gene with different genotype. Cellular Microbiology. 2007 Mar;**9**(3):753-765. PubMed PMID: 17081195

[60] Groeger SE, Meyle J. Epithelial barrier and oral bacterial infection. Periodontology 2000. 2015 Oct;**69**(1):46-67. PubMed PMID: 26252401

[61] Darveau RP, Belton CM, Reife RA, Lamont RJ. Local chemokine paralysis, a novel pathogenic mechanism for *Porphyromonas gingivalis*. Infection and Immunity. 1998 Apr;**66**(4):1660-1665. PubMed PMID: 9529095. Pubmed Central PMCID: 108102. Epub 1998/04/07. eng

[62] Lonn J, Johansson CS, Nakka S, Palm E, Bengtsson T, Nayeri F, et al. High concentration but low activity of hepatocyte growth factor in periodontitis. Journal of Periodontology. 2014 Jan;**85**(1):113-122. PubMed PMID: 23594192

[63] Morandini AC, Sipert CR, Ramos-Junior ES, Brozoski DT, Santos CF. Periodontal ligament and gingival fibroblasts participate in the production of TGF-beta, interleukin (IL)-8 and IL-10. Brazilian Oral Research. 2011 Mar–Apr;**25**(2):157-162. PubMed PMID: 21537641. Epub 2011/05/04. eng

[64] Naylor AJ, Filer A, Buckley CD. The role of stromal cells in the persistence of chronic inflammation. Clinical Experimental Immunology. 2013 Jan;**171**(1):30-35. PubMed PMID: 23199320. Pubmed Central PMCID: Pmc3530092. Epub 2012/12/04. eng

[65] Filer A, Raza K, Salmon M, Buckley CD. Targeting stromal cells in chronic inflammation. Discovery Medicine. 2007 Feb;**7**(37):20-26. PubMed PMID: 17343801. Pubmed Central PMCID: PMC3160478. Epub 2007/03/09. eng

[66] Palm E, Demirel I, Bengtsson T, Khalaf H. The role of Toll-like and protease-activated receptors and associated intracellular signaling in *Porphyromonas gingivalis*-infected gingival fibroblasts. APMIS: Acta Pathologica, Microbiologica, et Immunologica Scandinavica. 2017 Feb;**125**(2):157-169. PubMed PMID: 28120492. Epub 2017/01/26. eng

[67] Jayaprakash K, Demirel I, Khalaf H, Bengtsson T. The role of phagocytosis, oxidative burst and neutrophil extracellular traps in the interaction between neutrophils and the periodontal pathogen *Porphyromonas gingivalis*. Molecular Oral Microbiology. 2015 Oct;**30**(5):361-375. PubMed PMID: 25869817

[68] Morozumi T, Nakagawa T, Nomura Y, Sugaya T, Kawanami M, Suzuki F, et al. Salivary pathogen and serum antibody to assess the progression of chronic periodontitis: A 24-mo prospective multicenter cohort study. Journal of Periodontal Research. 2016 Dec;**51**(6):768-778. PubMed PMID: 26791469

[69] Berglundh T, Liljenberg B, Lindhe J. Some cytokine profiles of T-helper cells in lesions of advanced periodontitis. Journal of Clinical Periodontology. 2002 Aug;**29**(8):705-709. PubMed PMID: 12390567

[70] Takeichi O, Haber J, Kawai T, Smith DJ, Moro I, Taubman MA. Cytokine profiles of T-lymphocytes from gingival tissues with pathological pocketing. Journal of Dental Research. 2000 Aug;**79**(8):1548-1555. PubMed PMID: 11023273

[71] Cheng WC, Hughes FJ, Taams LS. The presence, function and regulation of IL-17 and Th17 cells in periodontitis. Journal of Clinical Periodontology. 2014 Jun;**41**(6):541-549. PubMed PMID: 24735470

[72] Khalaf H, Bengtsson T. Altered T-cell responses by the periodontal pathogen *Porphyromonas gingivalis*. PLoS One. 2012;**7**(9):e45192. PubMed PMID: 22984628. Pubmed Central PMCID: 3440346. Epub 2012/09/18. eng

[73] Seymour GJ, Ford PJ, Cullinan MP, Leishman S, Yamazaki K. Relationship between periodontal infections and systemic disease. Clinical Microbiology and Infection. 2007 Oct;**13**(Suppl 4):3-10. PubMed PMID: 17716290

[74] Inaba H, Amano A. Roles of oral bacteria in cardiovascular diseases--from molecular mechanisms to clinical cases: Implication of periodontal diseases in development of systemic diseases. Journal of Pharmacological Sciences. 2010;**113**(2):103-109. PubMed PMID: 20501966

[75] Kozarov EV, Dorn BR, Shelburne CE, Dunn WA, Jr, Progulske-Fox A. Human atherosclerotic plaque contains viable invasive *Actinobacillus actinomycetemcomitans* and *Porphyromonas gingivalis*. Arteriosclerosis, Thrombosis, and Vascular Biology. 2005 Mar;**25**(3):e17-18. PubMed PMID: 15662025

[76] Rosenfeld ME, Campbell LA. Pathogens and atherosclerosis: Update on the potential contribution of multiple infectious organisms to the pathogenesis of atherosclerosis. Thrombosis and Haemostasis. 2011 Nov;**106**(5):858-867. PubMed PMID: 22012133

[77] Wada K, Kamisaki Y. Molecular dissection of *Porphyromonas gingivalis*-related arteriosclerosis: A novel mechanism of vascular disease. Periodontology 2000. 2010 Oct;**54**(1):222-234. PubMed PMID: 20712642

[78] Vongpatanasin W. Hydrochlorothiazide is not the most useful nor versatile thiazide diuretic. Current Opinion in Cardiology. 2015 Jul;**30**(4):361-365. PubMed PMID: 26049382. Pubmed Central PMCID: 4460599

[79] Koo J, Choe HK, Kim HD, Chun SK, Son GH, Kim K. Effect of mefloquine, a gap junction blocker, on circadian period2 gene oscillation in the mouse suprachiasmatic nucleus ex vivo. Endocrinology and Metabolism. 2015 Sep;**30**(3):361-370. PubMed PMID: 25491783. Pubmed Central PMCID: 4595362

[80] Reszec J, Szkudlarek M, Hermanowicz A, Bernaczyk PS, Mariak Z, Chyczewski L. N-cadherin, beta-catenin and connexin 43 expression in astrocytic tumours of various grades. Histology and Histopathology. 2015 Mar;**30**(3):361-371. PubMed PMID: 25386667

[81] Suzuki J, Aoyama N, Aoki M, Tada Y, Wakayama K, Akazawa H, et al. High incidence of periodontitis in Japanese patients with abdominal aortic aneurysm. International Heart Journal. 2014;**55**(3):268-270. PubMed PMID: 24806388

[82] Hokamura K, Umemura K. Roles of oral bacteria in cardiovascular diseases--from molecular mechanisms to clinical cases: *Porphyromonas gingivalis* is the important role of intimal hyperplasia in the aorta. Journal of Pharmacological Sciences. 2010;**113**(2):110-114. PubMed PMID: 20501963

[83] Hayashi C, Madrigal AG, Liu X, Ukai T, Goswami S, Gudino CV, et al. Pathogen-mediated inflammatory atherosclerosis is mediated in part via Toll-like receptor 2-induced inflammatory responses. Journal of Innate Immunity. 2010;2(4):334-343. PubMed PMID: 20505314. Pubmed Central PMCID: PMC2895755

[84] Zhang B, Elmabsout AA, Khalaf H, Basic VT, Jayaprakash K, Kruse R, et al. The periodontal pathogen *Porphyromonas gingivalis* changes the gene expression in vascular smooth muscle cells involving the TGFbeta/Notch signalling pathway and increased cell proliferation. BMC Genomics. 2013 Nov 09;14:770. PubMed PMID: 24209892. Pubmed Central PMCID: 3827841

[85] Zhang B, Khalaf H, Sirsjo A, Bengtsson T. Gingipains from the periodontal pathogen *Porphyromonas gingivalis* play a significant role in regulation of Angiopoietin1 and Angiopoietin 2 in human aortic smooth muscle cells. Infection and Immunity. 2015 Nov; 83(11):4256-65. PubMed PMID: 26283334

[86] Trollope AF, Golledge J. Angiopoietins, abdominal aortic aneurysm and atherosclerosis. Atherosclerosis. 2011 Feb;214(2):237-243. PubMed PMID: 20832800. Pubmed Central PMCID: 3012744

[87] Padma R, Sreedhara A, Indeevar P, Sarkar I, Kumar CS. Vascular endothelial growth factor levels in gingival crevicular fluid before and after periodontal therapy. Journal of Clinical and Diagnostic Research. 2014 Nov;8(11):ZC75–ZC79. PubMed PMID: 25584323. Pubmed Central PMCID: PMC4290334

[88] Bengtsson T, Karlsson H, Gunnarsson P, Skoglund C, Elison C, Leanderson P, et al. The periodontal pathogen *Porphyromonas gingivalis* cleaves apoB-100 and increases the expression of apoM in LDL in whole blood leading to cell proliferation. Journal of Internal Medicine. 2008 May;263(5):558-571. PubMed PMID: 18248365

[89] Higashi Y, Goto C, Jitsuiki D, Umemura T, Nishioka K, Hidaka T, et al. Periodontal infection is associated with endothelial dysfunction in healthy subjects and hypertensive patients. Hypertension. 2008 Feb;51(2):446-453. PubMed PMID: 18039979

[90] Bokhari SA, Khan AA, Butt AK, Azhar M, Hanif M, Izhar M, et al. Non-surgical periodontal therapy reduces coronary heart disease risk markers: A randomized controlled trial. Journal of Clinical Periodontology. 2012 Nov;39(11):1065-1074. PubMed PMID: 22966824

[91] Bhagat K, Moss R, Collier J, Vallance P. Endothelial "stunning" following a brief exposure to endotoxin: A mechanism to link infection and infarction? Cardiovascular Research. 1996 Nov;32(5):822-829. PubMed PMID: 8944812

[92] Maekawa T, Takahashi N, Honda T, Yonezawa D, Miyashita H, Okui T, et al. *Porphyromonas gingivalis* antigens and interleukin-6 stimulate the production of monocyte chemoattractant protein-1 via the upregulation of early growth response-1 transcription in human coronary artery endothelial cells. Journal of Vascular Research. 2010;47(4):346-354. PubMed PMID: 20016208

[93] Awano S, Ansai T, Mochizuki H, Yu W, Tanzawa K, Turner AJ, et al. Sequencing, expression and biochemical characterization of the *Porphyromonas gingivalis* pepO gene encoding a protein homologous to human endothelin-converting enzyme. FEBS Letters. 1999 Oct 22;**460**(1):139-144. PubMed PMID: 10571076

[94] Ansai T, Yamamoto E, Awano S, Yu W, Turner AJ, Takehara T. Effects of periodontopathic bacteria on the expression of endothelin-1 in gingival epithelial cells in adult periodontitis. Clinical Science. 2002 Aug;**103**(Suppl 48):327S–331S. PubMed PMID: 12193115

[95] Rikimaru T, Awano S, Mineoka T, Yoshida A, Ansai T, Takehara T. Relationship between endothelin-1 and interleukin-1beta in inflamed periodontal tissues. Biomedical Research. 2009 Dec;**30**(6):349-355. PubMed PMID: 20051644

[96] Lester SR, Bain JL, Serio FG, Harrelson BD, Johnson RB. Relationship between gingival angiopoietin-1 concentrations and depth of the adjacent gingival sulcus. Journal of Periodontology. 2009 Sep;**80**(9):1447-1453. PubMed PMID: 19722795

[97] McCarter SD, Lai PF, Suen RS, Stewart DJ. Regulation of endothelin-1 by angiopoietin-1: Implications for inflammation. Experimental Biology and Medicine. 2006 Jun;**231**(6):985-991. PubMed PMID: 16741035

[98] Gawaz M. Platelets in the onset of atherosclerosis. Blood Cells, Molecules & Diseases. 2006 Mar–Apr;**36**(2):206-210. PubMed PMID: 16476558

[99] Blair P, Rex S, Vitseva O, Beaulieu L, Tanriverdi K, Chakrabarti S, et al. Stimulation of Toll-like receptor 2 in human platelets induces a thromboinflammatory response through activation of phosphoinositide 3-kinase. Circulation Research. 2009 Feb 13;**104**(3):346-354. PubMed PMID: 19106411. Pubmed Central PMCID: 2732983

[100] Kerrigan SW. The expanding field of platelet-bacterial interconnections. Platelets. 2015;**26**(4):293-301. PubMed PMID: 25734214

[101] Hamzeh-Cognasse H, Damien P, Chabert A, Pozzetto B, Cognasse F, Garraud O. Platelets and infections—Complex interactions with bacteria. Frontiers in Immunology. 2015;**6**:82. PubMed PMID: 25767472. Pubmed Central PMCID: PMC4341565

[102] Klinger MH, Jelkmann W. Role of blood platelets in infection and inflammation. Journal of Interferon & Cytokine Research: The Official Journal of the International Society for Interferon and Cytokine Research. 2002 Sep;**22**(9):913-922. PubMed PMID: 12396713

[103] Blair P, Flaumenhaft R. Platelet alpha-granules: Basic biology and clinical correlates. Blood Review. 2009 Jul;**23**(4):177-189. PubMed PMID: 19450911. Pubmed Central PMCID: 2720568

[104] Borgeson E, Lonn J, Bergstrom I, Brodin VP, Ramstrom S, Nayeri F, et al. Lipoxin A(4) inhibits *Porphyromonas gingivalis*-induced aggregation and reactive oxygen species production by modulating neutrophil-platelet interaction and CD11b expression. Infection and Immunity. 2011 Apr;**79**(4):1489-1497. PubMed PMID: 21263017. Pubmed Central PMCID: 3067532

[105] Klarstrom Engstrom K, Khalaf H, Kalvegren H, Bengtsson T. The role of *Porphyromonas gingivalis* gingipains in platelet activation and innate immune modulation. Molecular Oral Microbiology. 2015 Feb;**30**(1):62-73. PubMed PMID: 25043711

[106] Gamonal J, Acevedo A, Bascones A, Jorge O, Silva A. Levels of interleukin-1 beta, -8, and -10 and RANTES in gingival crevicular fluid and cell populations in adult periodontitis patients and the effect of periodontal treatment. Journal of Periodontology. 2000 Oct;**71**(10):1535-1545. PubMed PMID: 11063385

[107] Lourbakos A, Yuan YP, Jenkins AL, Travis J, Andrade-Gordon P, Santulli R, et al. Activation of protease-activated receptors by gingipains from *Porphyromonas gingivalis* leads to platelet aggregation: A new trait in microbial pathogenicity. Blood. 2001 Jun 15;**97**(12):3790-3797. PubMed PMID: 11389018

[108] McNicol A, Israels SJ. Mechanisms of oral bacteria-induced platelet activation. Canadian Journal of Physiology and Pharmacology. 2010 May;**88**(5):510-524. PubMed PMID: 20555421

[109] Nylander M, Lindahl TL, Bengtsson T, Grenegard M. The periodontal pathogen *Porphyromonas gingivalis* sensitises human blood platelets to epinephrine. Platelets. 2008 Aug;**19**(5):352-358. PubMed PMID: 18791941

[110] Keestra JA, Grosjean I, Coucke W, Quirynen M, Teughels W. Non-surgical periodontal therapy with systemic antibiotics in patients with untreated aggressive periodontitis: A systematic review and meta-analysis. Journal of Periodontal Research. 2015 Dec;**50**(6):689-706. PubMed PMID: 25522248

[111] Czaplewski L, Bax R, Clokie M, Dawson M, Fairhead H, Fischetti VA, et al. Alternatives to antibiotics-a pipeline portfolio review. The Lancet Infectious Diseases. 2016 Feb;**16**(2):239-251. PubMed PMID: 26795692

[112] Bonifait L, Chandad F, Grenier D. Probiotics for oral health: Myth or reality? Journal. 2009 Oct;**75**(8):585-590. PubMed PMID: 19840501

[113] Cotter PD, Ross RP, Hill C. Bacteriocins—A viable alternative to antibiotics? Nature Reviews Microbiology. 2013 Feb;**11**(2):95-105. PubMed PMID: 23268227

[114] Khalaf H, Nakka SS, Sanden C, Svard A, Hultenby K, Scherbak N, et al. Antibacterial effects of Lactobacillus and bacteriocin PLNC8 alphabeta on the periodontal pathogen *Porphyromonas gingivalis*. BMC Microbiology. 2016 Aug 18;**16**(1):188. PubMed PMID: 27538539. Pubmed Central PMCID: 4990846

Periodontal Considerations in Adult Orthodontic Patients

10

Periodontal Considerations in Adult Orthodontic Patients

Zamira Kalemaj, Antonios D. Anastasiou,
Animesh Jha and Felice R. Grassi

Abstract

The relationship between periodontology and orthodontics consists of a highly complex, bidirectional and close interaction that is nowadays characterized by controversial scientific opinions and clinical approaches. The relevant increasing number of adult orthodontic patients which in most cases present already-compromised periodontal tissues has markedly highlighted the potential of orthodontic treatment in enhancing or deteriorating periodontal health and also the outmost relevance of peculiar periodontal planning prior and during orthodontic treatment. Since the progress in adult orthodontics trend is rapid, there is also an increasing need for evidence-based protocols that might guide clinicians through a comprehensive, interdisciplinary and successful treatment. This chapter has been compiled with the aim of providing orthodontists, periodontists and general practitioners with sound evidence-based protocols and valid clinical approaches that have proven to be successful for numerous patients over long follow-ups. It is structured following the steps for a correct therapy management, starting from comprehensive examination and diagnosis to before and during orthodontic treatment considerations, and finally analysing the present state of new adult orthodontic technologies.

Keywords: adult orthodontics, periodontal health, orthodontic therapy, interdisciplinary treatment, accelerated orthodontics, future orthodontics

1. Introduction

Over the past three decades, the number of adult orthodontic patients has increased markedly. Recent surveys have reported that orthodontic treatment contributes to significant improvements in both professional and personal life, especially in adult patients who generally have undergone substantial loss of sustaining tissues, resulting in compromised function and aesthetics. Based on the new-found self-confidence, the majority of these patients suggest orthodontic treatment to friends and relatives. Therefore, orthodontic treatment seems to be a promising emerging therapy to be integrated into a multidisciplinary dental treatment approach.

Apart from establishing a functional occlusion and improving dental and facial aesthetics, one of the major objectives of orthodontic therapy is enhancement and maintenance of periodontal health. In adult patients, the altered periodontal health might result in teeth loss, altered function and compromised aesthetics. Most of these patients present a variety of problems, which include teeth overeruption, migration, traumatic occlusion, irregular interdental spacing, consumed occlusal surfaces, irregular occlusal planes and loss of vertical dimension. In such complex and challenging clinical situations, an interdisciplinary treatment is mandatory. Unfortunately, in everyday orthodontic practice, insufficient emphasis is placed on comprehensive diagnosis prior to orthodontic therapy with particular attention to periodontal health and to its control and maintenance throughout the therapy. All attempts of limited treatment, with poor consideration of the whole picture will result in failure, relapse and very often aggravation of the pathology. The careful control of periodontal pathologies before, during and after orthodontic treatment, along with functional rehabilitation and patient's compliance can provide the most satisfactory results and long-term stability.

We present herein our step-by-step approach on pre-orthodontic and orthodontic treatment of periodontally compromised patients, through several detailed clinical cases and clear scientific protocols. Moreover, we consider several important issues concerning the bidirectional interaction of orthodontics and periodontology and discuss ways to optimize it. Potentials and limitations of such interaction are reflected. Furthermore, we summarize scientific evidence and clinical expertise on different techniques aiming enhancement and acceleration of adult orthodontic therapy, leading to conclusions of high relevance in terms of an effective and efficient therapy.

Guided by sound scientific principles and constructive clinical experience, it is vitally important to keep in mind that adult patients with orthodontic needs require individualized and tailored treatment plans to meet both clinical success and patient's expectations. The information presented in this chapter is gathered by considering these aspects and with the hope of providing investigators and clinicians with solid bases for the state of art and potential future directions of interdisciplinary treatments.

2. Periodontal considerations prior to orthodontic treatment

2.1. Comprehensive diagnosis

As all medical treatments, dental therapies might have two approaches, which are referred to as 'causal' and 'symptomatic'. It is of utmost importance that when possible, these approaches are considered complementary, not as an alternative to each other. Therefore, in all cases when causal factors can be identified, the treatment should focus on addressing them first. If these approaches are followed, the symptomatic spectrum might be easier to treat or even disappear.

In oral-related pathologies, many etiological factors are recognized and widely accepted, whereas sometimes their precise effects and multifactorial influences are difficult to quantify. Nevertheless, the identification of potential causal factors is the fundamental part of any diagnostic process and should be performed through an accurate clinical visit.

In case of particular malocclusions, such as severe deep bite or crowding, the direct causative relationships and influences on periodontal health are evident. Such influences are determined primarily by the pathological traumatic occlusion and unfavourable position of the tooth inside the bone envelope, and secondarily, by favouring the plaque accumulation which results in progression of plaque-induced periodontal breakdown.

This is not always the case for periodontal pathologies that trigger or predispose orthodontic problems. In the absence of a thorough clinical check and comprehensive causal diagnosis, numerous orthodontic symptoms might be wrongly treated without accounting for the underlying periodontal, often causative or predisposing factor. Such a situation is typically encountered in adult patient referring diastemas opening over time and teeth flaring (**Figure 1a**). If no detailed clinical and radiographic checks were performed, neglecting the periodontal health, the orthodontic treatment alone would have aggravated the periodontal state, resulting in an iatrogenic damage and the post-treatment stability would have been questionable.

The clinical check-up itself should always be preceded by a detailed anamnesis for identification of potential risk factors. Thereafter, it should include compilation of a periodontal chart including all relevant periodontal indexes, general radiographic estimation and, when deemed necessary, a detailed radiographic assessment through series of periapical radiographs (**Figure 1b**).

It is of utmost importance to consider the presence of highly compromised periodontal health in young patients as an indicator that might suggests need for further laboratory and genetic analysis in order to identify potential risk factors to periodontal pathology or important systemic pathologies (**Figure 1c**).

In terms of ethology, it is well established that periodontitis is a multifactorial condition and apart from microbial and environmental factors, its progression is determined also by genetic susceptibility [1]. Epidemiologic data suggest that approximately 10–15% of populations are susceptible to a quick progression from gingivitis to periodontitis which can hardly be explained by solely microbiological or external factors [2, 3]. Numerous genetic polymorphisms have been characterized and recognized to play a role here [4]. While the influence of genomic testing on non-surgical periodontal treatment outcomes has been recently questioned [5], it should be kept in mind that its consideration remains highly important for prevention measures, early diagnosis and better individualized treatment protocol. Moreover, when integrated into a multifactorial diagnostic scheme, it allows for a comprehensive estimation of risk factors. To-date epidemiological evidence is limited and further investigation is required in order to thoroughly understand the nature of this association and its clinical implications [3]. Nevertheless, since full genome sequencing is feasible, phenotypic and genotypic data can be used to improve 'personalized' treatment and public oral health [6]. Apart from genetic influences, other risk factors such as diabetes, smoking

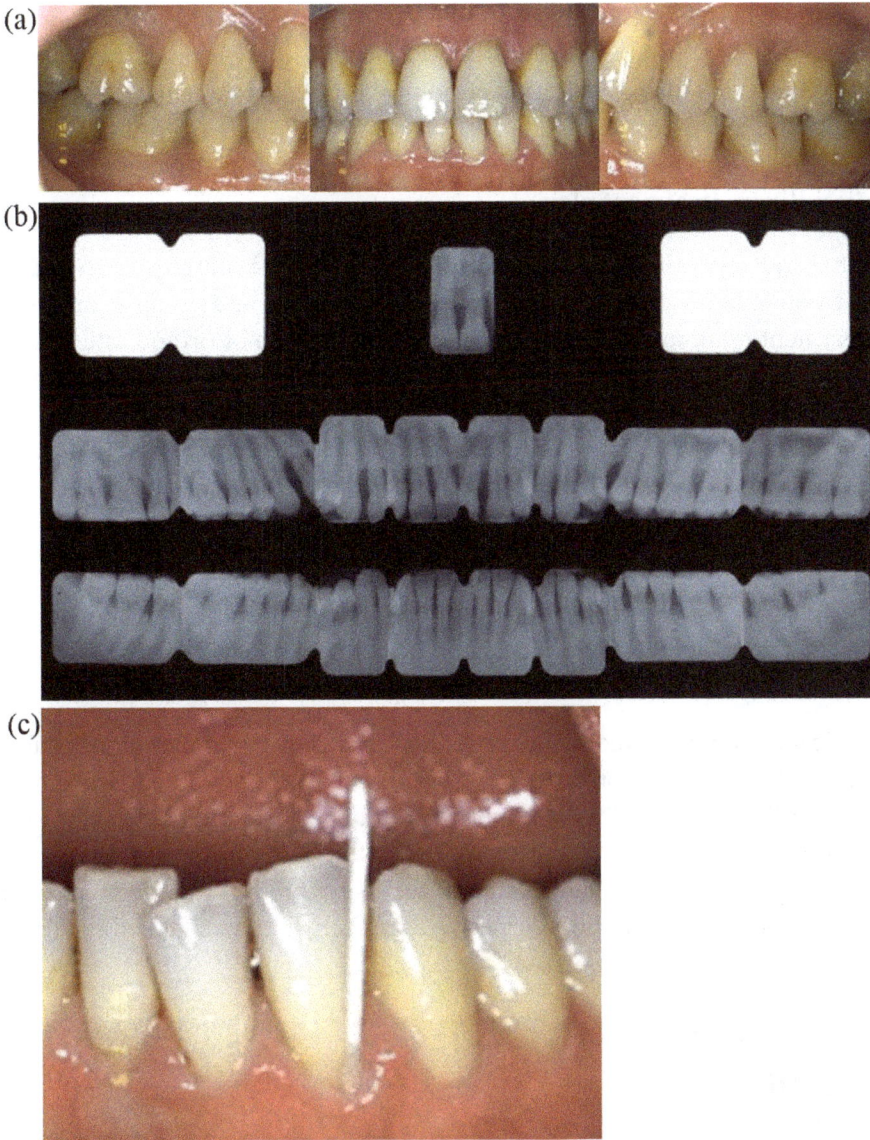

Figure 1. Twenty-eight-year-old female patient (FG), whose major requirement is diastema closure and teeth alignment. (a) Intraoral aspect; (b) during periodontal probing, it is noticed the presence of infrabony defects in multiple sites on both maxilla and mandible. A complete series of periapical radiographs is performed, showing a diffuse bone loss. (c) Bacteriological analysis on collected gingival cervicular fluid indicated high levels of actinobacillus actinomycetemcomitans, porphyromonas gingivalis and prevotella intermedia.

and stress should also be considered, controlled and integrated into the overall treatment plan. The destructive effects of smoking on periodontal tissues have long been recognized, and recent biochemical and genetic studies have clarified direct and indirect pathways of this association [7, 8]. Levels of matrix metalloproteinase-8 (MMP-8), which is involved in periodontal destructions, are significantly increased in smoking patients. Additionally, immune response is modified and the pathogenesis of the disease is negatively affected [8]. A similar pattern is present in patients affected by type 2 diabetes mellitus suggesting that diabetic-smoker patients have increased periodontal breakdown and are prone to a more severe periodontitis [9].

2.2. Multidisciplinary treatment plan

Oral functional and aesthetic rehabilitation in adult patients is a complex process that requires exhaustive scientific knowledge, extensive clinical experience and, in most cases, a multidisciplinary treatment planning. Independently of what the role of orthodontic therapy might be in the multidisciplinary frame, each tooth movement should initiate and be fulfilled in the presence of a healthy periodontium. It has already been demonstrated that if orthodontic treatment is conducted in the presence of periodontitis, it causes major bone destruction and clinical attachment loss (**Figure 2a, b**).

General treatment guidelines for orthodontic patients with chronic periodontitis suggest initial non-surgical therapy for adequate plaque control and then revaluation [10]. It is purported that critical pocket depth for maintaining periodontal health with no need for surgical intervention is 4–5 mm, but this should be carefully estimated considering patient compliance on adequate oral hygiene and specific needs for regenerative therapy [11].

The non-surgical periodontal treatment consisting of scaling a root planning results in gingival recession due to inflammation reduction (**Figure 3a**). It is advisable to inform the patient in advance regarding this effect as it might compromise aesthetics. Following the classical approach, in case of persistence of infrabony defects of 4–5 mm deep after the initial periodontal therapy, the open flap debridement and regenerative treatment are carried out (**Figure 3b–e**). Another more recent alternative approach at this stage is the performance of

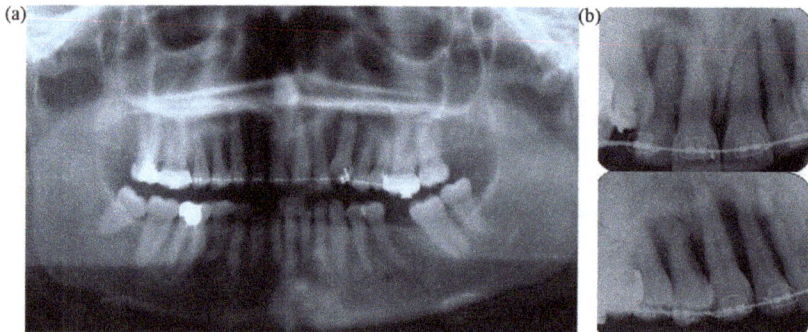

Figure 2. Twenty-two-year-old female patient having a fixed orthodontic appliance for 2 years. She was referred to us by an orthodontist who after one year of orthodontic therapy realised the gravity of the periodontal situation after performing a panoramic radiograph. The orthodontist refused to remove the orthodontic appliance, afraid that the patient would lose the teeth, being retained in their position only through the ligation to the archwire. (a) Panoramic radiograph showing the extensive bone loss in almost all maxillary teeth. (b) Periapical radiographs indicating the almost complete loss of periodontal support for multiple maxillary teeth.

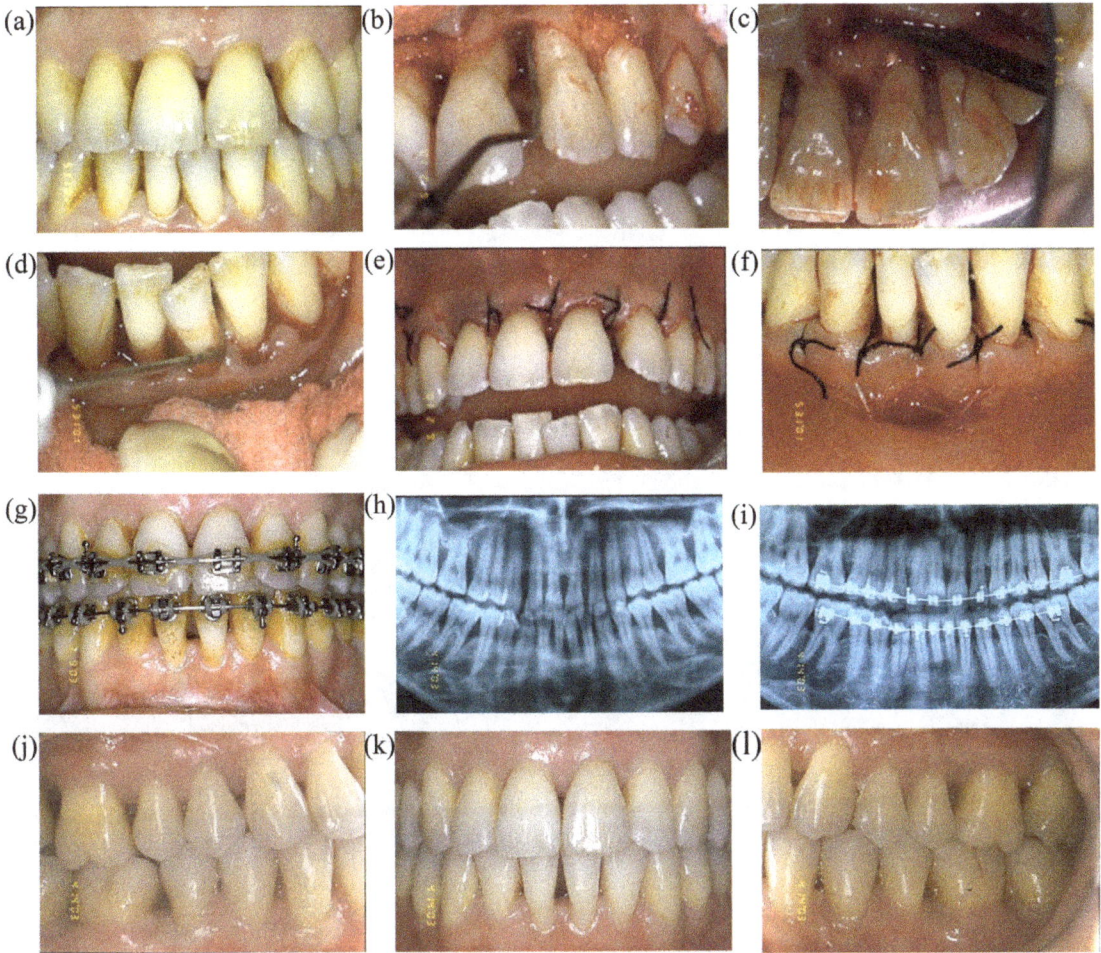

Figure 3. Patient F.G. (a) Intraoral aspect 2 weeks after completion of periodontal causal therapy (scaling and root planing). Notice the gingival recession that follows the reduction of inflammation; (b, c) open flap debridement on vestibular and palatal side; (d) injection of enamel matrix derivatives; (e, f) flap adaptation and suturing on the maxillary and mandibular arch. Because of the post-periodontal therapy recession, the flap adaptation results more challenging; (g) orthodontic therapy during space closure phase; (h) panoramic radiograph before periodontal therapy; (i) panoramic radiograph during orthodontic therapy. Please notice the overall enhancement of bone level and reduction of infrabony defects. (j, k, l) intraoral aspects at the day of orthodontic appliance removal. The patient showed great compliance during the entire treatment.

deep debridement and regeneration in a unique phase intra-surgically proceeded only by superficial debridement in order to avoid gingival recession and to have the possibility to reposition the soft tissues more coronally. This would allow for unaltered aesthetics and better root coverage, especially considering the fact that flap adaption is a crucial aspect of the healing quality (**Figures 4a–g** and **5a–g**). Despite the preferred approach, the surgical stage should be followed by a healing time before orthodontic therapy commencement. This period would allow for connective tissue stabilization and remodelling, restoration of health and evaluation of patient's compliance [12]. If the regenerative therapy is integrated into an ongoing orthodontic treatment, the compromised teeth should be immobilized through rigid splinting in order to stabilize the clot and the regenerative material throughout the healing phase.

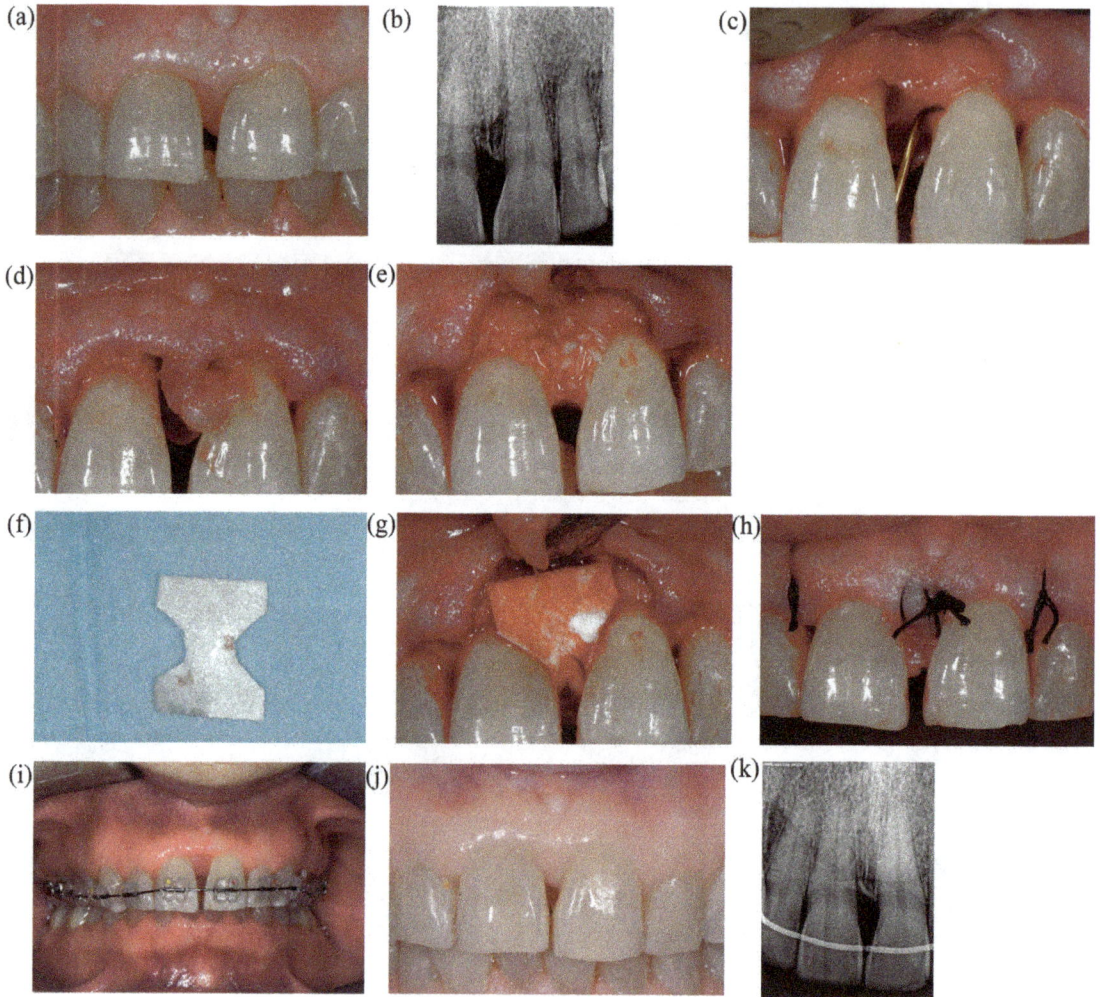

Figure 4. Thirty-eight-year-old female patient (T.A.), whose midline diastema was opened during the past 3 years. Major request was diastema closure. (a) Initial intraoral aspect; (b) initial radiograph; (c) deep manual debridement during surgical intervention. A supragingival debridement was previously performed; (d) sufficient gingival tissue for appropriate coverage of regenerative materials; (e) synthetic bone grafting; (f) membrane shaped extraorally following the area to be covered; (g) adaptation of the membrane in order to cover all grafting material; (h) suturing with coronal flap adaptation; (i) orthodontic treatment started 3 months after surgery; (j) clinical aspect at the end of orthodontic treatment; (k) radiograph at the end of orthodontic treatment with lingual fixed retainer.

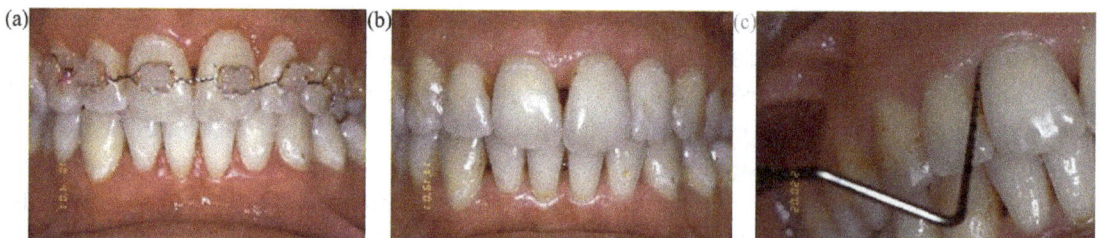

Figure 5. (a) Gingivitis present during orthodontic therapy. (b) when the inflammation is limited only at the gingival level and the deep periodontal tissue is not compromised, after orthodontic appliance removal the gingival inflammation disappears. (c) Periodontal probing after orthodontic appliance removal indicates healthy periodontal state.

The regenerative therapy might follow several approaches, including open flap debridement, guided tissue regeneration (GTR) associated or not with different types of bone grafting, growth factors and more recently also stem cell-based therapy [13–15]. Utilization of mesenchymal stem cells in periodontal regenerative therapy has already resulted in promising outcomes that need to be further elucidated especially in terms of cell survival and efficient expression of pro-grammed proliferative capacity to consent fully translation of mesenchymal stem cell-based therapy into clinical practice [15–22]. Irrespective of the chosen regenerative approach, the orthodontic treatment that follows should aim for elimination of occlusal traumatic contacts and establishment of a functional occlusion, which is one of the major factors for maintenance of periodontal health. Dental implant therapy for tooth replacement is incorporated after a thorough treatment planning followed by the positioning of teeth and roots into correct posi-tions. If implants are planned and inserted before the end of orthodontic therapy, they might also be used as an anchorage unit for facilitating the orthodontic treatment. Maintenance of periodontal health is of utmost importance also for implants success and survival. Patients sus-ceptible to periodontal pathologies are more prone to peri-implant inflammation and implant failure. Potential prosthetic restorations are usually performed at the end of orthodontic ther-apy, aiming reconstruction of lost tooth tissues or replacement of missing crowns.

Most of adult patients suffer also from enamel and dentine excessive consumption especially at the cervical area, which results in highly compromised aesthetics, hypersensitivity and impor-tant discomfort [23, 24]. Treatment of these cervical, non-carious defects is mainly focused on hypersensitivity reduction [25], whereas hard tissue reconstruction remains a controversial and challenging issue, especially considering the aetiology and progress of such pathology. Recent emerging technologies have proposed restoration of dental enamel using high repeti-tion rate femtosecond lasers and novel iron-doped calcium phosphate biomaterials. During this procedure, the irradiated mineral transforms into a densified layer of acid-resistant ion-doped β-pyrophosphate, which bonds with enamel and dentine surface of non-carious lesions [26, 27]. This promising technology is yet to be fully developed for optimal clinical usage.

Attempts in reducing duration of orthodontic treatment especially in adult patients have recently resulted in therapies combining surgical and non-surgical approaches to orthodon-tics. Even if surgical adjunctive therapies have been studied for many decades, their overall benefit is still questionable, whereas non-surgical approaches do not provide solid scien-tific bases for incorporation into everyday clinical practice [28, 29]. Careful consideration of patient-centred aspects, treatment time and overall cost-benefits must be performed for a thorough estimation of these approaches.

Each adult patient is a challenging situation that in the majority of cases requires the peri-odontal and orthodontic therapy for denture preparation and later prosthetic therapy for full rehabilitation. In almost all cases of mature patients, orthodontic treatment alone would not result in the best possible approach for oral functional and aesthetic rehabilitation and some-times it would also deteriorate the overall state of oral health.

It should be bared in mind that all orthodontic movements are guided by a periodontal dimension that should be of primary consideration during treatment planning and applica-tion of orthodontic biomechanics. On the other hand, correct functional occlusion and ideal tooth position are one of the major prerequisites for maintenance of periodontal health.

3. Interrelationship between periodontics and orthodontics in adult patients

3.1. Periodontal considerations during adult orthodontic treatment

The presence of healthy periodontal tissues is of vital importance for undertaking any kind of orthodontic or prosthetic therapy. In adult patients, even if periodontal tissues might be reduced and have compromised sustaining capacity, they should be free of inflammation. All attempts in applying an orthodontic treatment on inflamed periodontal tissues will aggravate the periodontal state and result in an iatrogenic damage [30].

Components of orthodontic appliances predispose aggregation of bacterial plaque which, if not properly controlled through accurate hygiene regimen, might trigger gingivitis or its conversion into periodontitis [31, 32]. On the other hand, when a thorough oral hygiene regimen is applied, gingivitis is easily controlled, and when no other periodontal tissues get involved, it seems to disappear in long term after appliance removal (**Figure 5**) [12, 33]. Periodontal short-term effects after orthodontic therapy remain controversial [34], which suggest that in all cases orthodontic patients are at a higher risk for periodontal disease development. The increasing demand for orthodontic treatment and the occurrence of biofilm-related complications has positioned orthodontic treatment as a potential public health threat [35].

Independent of whether the periodontal health is compromised or not, in all adult patients, particular attention should be paid to avoid when possible bulk elements such as bands or other orthodontic components placed close to gingival margin that apart from plaque retention might cause marginal gingival injury and attachment loss. In this respect, orthodontic treatments based on removable appliances or aligners permit unimpeded oral hygiene and result in better periodontal health [36]. Nonetheless, while these aligners behave superiorly in terms of oral hygiene maintenance and periodontal health, other important considerations, such as occlusal interferences, gnathologic effects and postural ones, must be made before applying them.

According to the 'bone envelope' theory, orthodontic tooth movement should be performed within an anatomically and functionally periodontal limited space which is in any case to be respected in order to obtain the desired movement. If the periodontal space is violated, its connective tissue might react through a series of mechanisms such as bone dehiscence and fenestration, gingival inflammation and gingival recession. Apical migration of the gingiva (gingival recession) has an unpleasant effect in both aesthetics and cervical dentinal hypersensitivity. It might be caused by periodontitis, gingival trauma and specific anatomical conditions such as tooth crowding or muscular inserts. It has been demonstrated that in cases of tooth movement beyond the 'alveolar envelope' such as uncontrolled orthodontic movement, the recession might arise immediately but also years after, resulting in unpleasant post-treatment effects [37, 38]. It has been reported that factors related to the development or progression of recessions in adult patients are the presence of pre-treatment recessions, thin gingival biotype, reduced width of keratinized gingiva and visual gingival inflammation [39]. Other features, such as gingival margin thickness smaller than 0.5 mm and vestibular incisor inclination (over 95°), have also been associated with higher incidence and severity of recession [40]. In cases of pre-existing recessions, it is recommended that mucogingival interceptive surgery be accomplished before orthodontic therapy to maintain the width of keratinized gingiva in the long term [41].

Every orthodontic movement induces remodelling and reorganization of periodontal tissues. It is demonstrated that light and continuous forces illicit non-destructive periodontal turn-over, whereas heavy forces might result in necrotic periodontal tissue and further irreversible periodontal damage. Another consequence of these uncontrolled and heavy forces might be the root resorption, which is of extreme importance in teeth with reduced periodontium as further loss of periodontal support results in increased crown-root ratio and in compromised stability and aesthetics. Peculiar control of force levels has been outlined especially for orthodontic intrusion where the surface of force application is reduced. Intrusion also requires absolute control of inflammation and bacterial biofilms in order to avoid any aggravation or creation of infrabony defect and loss of attachment [42–45].

In most adult patients, the already-compromised periodontal tissue would need particular care in order to avoid further destruction and when possible aim for periodontal health enhancement.

Professional cleaning and examination of periodontal tissues should be performed routinely during the entire orthodontic treatment, following a personalized schedule that is determined by the individual risk factors and the specific treatment plan.

In all cases, orthodontic treatment should be suspended if patient fails to comply in maintaining the appropriate level of oral hygiene.

3.2. Orthodontics as a tool for periodontal health enhancement

Orthodontic therapy on adult patients has become particularly popular in the last few decades, following the general trend of the modern life where overall aesthetic enhancement has become one of the major priorities. However, orthodontic treatment as a corrective tool that eliminates pathologic migration of teeth on periodontally compromised patients had been suggested long time ago in the literature, by authors such as Neustadt [46] Dummett [47] and Scoop [48]. Later studies conducted principally on animal models confirmed the beneficial effect of orthodontic therapy on periodontal health. The results of these animal studies demonstrated that movements of teeth with infrabony defects in an inflammation-free environment result in elimination of the bone defect through creation of a long epithelial junction [49, 50].

Extrapolation of animal studies' findings to human conditions has been questioned, mostly because of the specific pattern of attachment loss that occurs on humans [51]. However, it is well established that in the absence of periodontal inflammation, the biological process of bone resorption and apposition during orthodontic tooth movement might positively influence the healing of periodontal defects. Similarly, the positioning of teeth into correct occlusal relations, which allow for axial and physiological distribution of masticatory forces, results in reduced stress to periodontal tissues. Moreover, such an occlusal stability contributes in diminishing mesial migration of posterior teeth and related consequences such as incorrect interdental contact points, flaring of incisor teeth and diastema opening. All these clinical symptoms are typical in adult patients, in which the malocclusion is aggravated by chronic periodontitis, resulting in the establishment of a vicious cycle where the two pathologies contribute to the exacerbation of each other (**Figure 6**). If the therapeutic approach does not account for both pathologies and does not follow a correct protocol starting with periodontal therapy and stabilization, the final result and its maintenance are highly questionable.

The orthodontic therapy can contribute to the improvement of periodontal health through reduction of intraosseous defects or furcation lesions [52–56]. It can also help in reducing gingival recession, levelling uneven gingival margins or rebuilding missing interdental papilla [12, 57, 58].

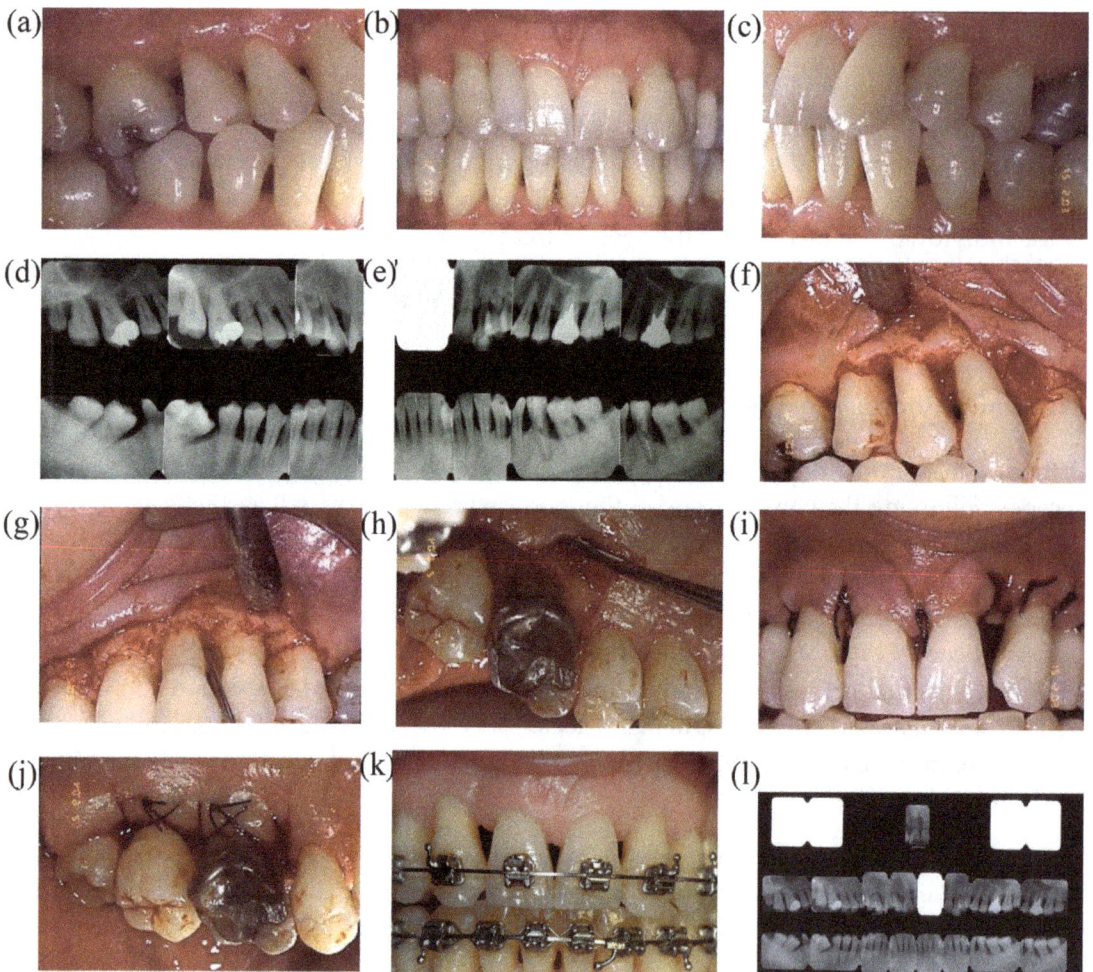

Figure 6. (a–e) The periodontal pathology has contributed in aggravating the malocclusion, characterized mainly by mesial tipping of posterior teeth, incisors flaring and diastema opening; (f–h) open flap debridement and regeneration; (i, j) soft tissue adaptation and suturing; (k) orthodontic therapy performed on a reduced periodontal tissue but with no active inflammation; (l) set of periapical radiographs after orthodontic alignment.

However, as reported by several recent systematic reviews, despite the major interest in trying to understand the beneficial effect of orthodontic therapy on periodontal health, the orthodontic scientific evidence still leaks solid protocols in this field and human studies are poor both qualitatively and quantitatively [44, 45, 54].

3.3. Post-orthodontic stability

Preservation of final orthodontic result is often considered as the third phase of overall orthodontic therapy and its major long-term goal. Post-orthodontic relapse has been mainly attributed to elasticity of gingival tissues that are compressed towards the direction of tooth movement. Considering this, the suggested retention period should exceed the time for remodelling of periodontal fibres, which usually ranges from 4 to 6 months [59, 60]. In order to enhance post-treatment stability attributed to soft periodontal fibres, many authors have suggested adjunctive interventions such as overcorrection, interproximal reduction or circumferential fibrotomy of supracrestal gingival fibres [61]. The variety of retainers is represented by the two big categories of fixed and removable ones. Scientific data report controversial opinions regarding the retentive method of choice for patients with reduced periodontal support. While the fixed retainer assures firm position and satisfying long-term stability, it does not allow for teeth to retain their physiological mobility, and in most cases, it impedes maintenance of good oral hygiene which is of fundamental importance for these patients [62]. In all cases, bulk fixed retentions that block easy access through interdental spaces should be avoided and patients should be given exhaustive instructions for appropriate oral hygiene maintenance (**Figure 7**).

Finally, despite the importance of considering all periodontal and mechanical features of retentive devices, the authors of the present manuscript consider of primarily importance for long term retention a final orthodontic result that assures occlusal stability, meaning correct teeth positioning, physiological movement with no interferences or dislocating pre-contacts [63]. It is extremely relevant to recognize the importance of a good balance between static and dynamic occlusion and all related craniofacial structures represented by temporomandibular joint (TMJ) and the neuromuscular system for both oral rehabilitation and long-term stability. A final orthodontic result that respects these parameters is the best tool for physiological retention, with no need for external mechanical elements (**Figure 8**).

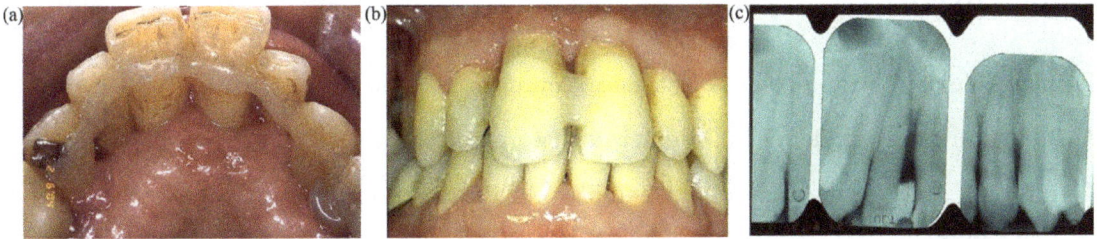

Figure 7. (a, b) Bulk lingual and vestibular splinting of teeth, which do not allow for appropriate oral hygiene maintenance. (c) Radiographic image showing the complete loss of periodontal support.

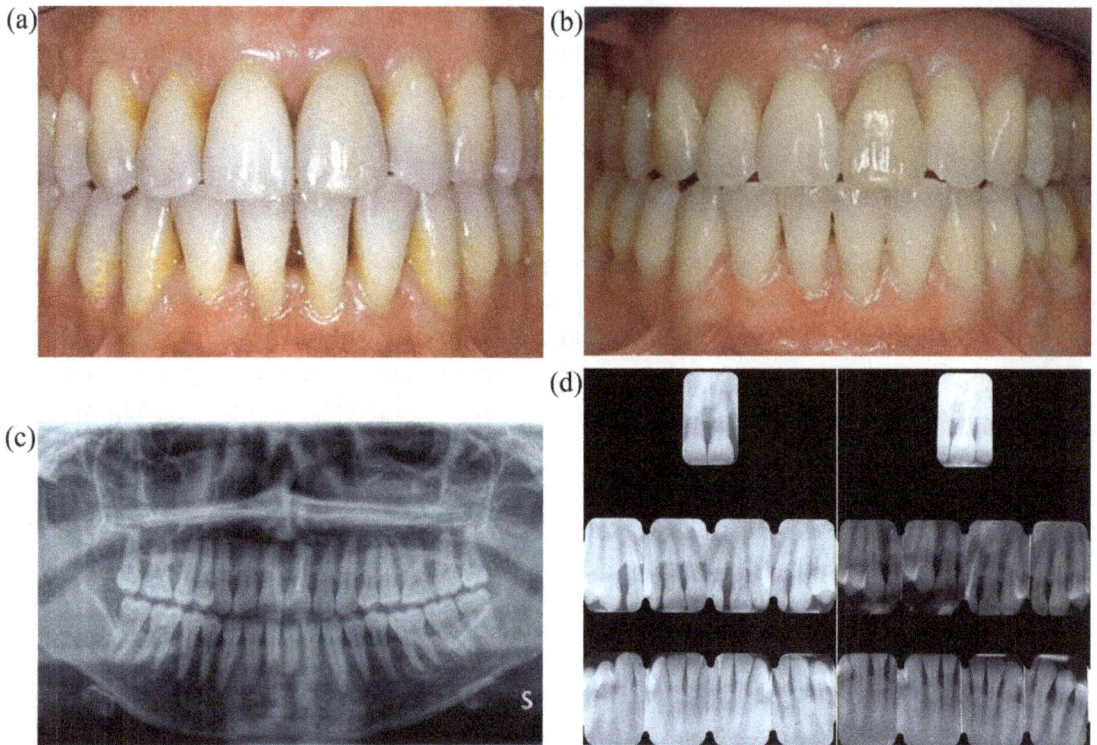

Figure 8. (a) Clinical check at 7 years of follow-up. (b) Clinical check at 13 years of follow-up. (c) Panoramic radiograph at 13 years of follow-up. (d) Periodontal radiographic status before the therapy and 13 years after the therapy with no fixed orthodontic retainer.

Acknowledgements

The authors acknowledge the financial support of EU-Marie-Curie-IAPP LUSTRE (324538) project.

Author details

Zamira Kalemaj[1]*, Antonios D. Anastasiou[1], Animesh Jha[1] and Felice R. Grassi[2]

*Address all correspondence to: kalemajzamira@gmail.com

1 Faculty of Engineering, School of Chemical and Process Engineering, University of Leeds, United Kingdom

2 Department of Basic and Medical Sciences, Neurosciences and Sense Organs, University of Bari, Italy

References

[1] Sofaer JA. Genetic approaches in the study of periodontal diseases. Journal of Clinical Periodontology [Internet]. 1990;**17**(7):401-408. Available from: http://doi.wiley.com/10.1111/j.1600-051X.1990.tb02337.x [Accessed: 19 March 2017]

[2] Johnson NW, Griffiths GS, Wilton JM, Maiden MF, Curtis MA, Gillett IR, et al. Detection of high-risk groups and individuals for periodontal diseases. Evidence for the existence of high-risk groups and individuals and approaches to their detection. Journal of Clinical Periodontology [Internet]. 1988;**15**(5):276-282. Available from: http://www.ncbi.nlm.nih.gov/pubmed/3292592 [Accessed: 19 March 2017]

[3] Lopez R, Hujoel P, Belibasakis GN. On putative periodontal pathogens: An epidemiological perspective. Virulence. 2015;**6**(3):249-257. [Internet]. Available from: http://www.ncbi.nlm.nih.gov/pubmed/25874553 [Accessed: 19 March 2017]

[4] Brunetti G, Oranger A, Mori G, Sardone F, Pignataro P, Coricciati M, et al. TRAIL effect on osteoclast formation in physiological and pathological conditions. Frontiers in Bioscience (Elite Ed). 2011;**3**:1154-1161. [Internet]. Available from: http://www.ncbi.nlm.nih.gov/pubmed/21622121 [Accessed: 17 September 2016]

[5] Chatzopoulos G-S, Doufexi A-E, Kalogirou F. Association of susceptible genotypes to periodontal disease with the clinical outcome and tooth survival after non-surgical periodontal therapy: A systematic review and meta-analysis. Medicina Oral, Patologia Oral Y Cirugia Bucal. 2016;**21**(1):e14–e29. [Internet]. Available from: http://www.ncbi.nlm.nih.gov/pubmed/26595831 [Accessed: 19 March 2017]

[6] Braun TM, Doucette-Stamm L, Duff GW, Kornman KS, Giannobile WV. Counterpoint: Risk factors, including genetic information, add value in stratifying patients for optimal preventive dental care. Journal of the American Dental Association. 2015;**146**(3):174-178. [Internet]. Available from: http://linkinghub.elsevier.com/retrieve/pii/S0002817715002378 [Accessed: 17 May 2017]

[7] Haber J, Wattles J, Crowley M, Mandell R, Joshipura K, Kent RL. Evidence for cigarette smoking as a major risk factor for periodontitis. Journal of Periodontology. 1993;**64**(1):16-23. [Internet]. Available from: http://www.ncbi.nlm.nih.gov/pubmed/8426285 [Accessed: 18 May 2017]

[8] Gupta N, Gupta ND, Goyal L, Moin S, Khan S, Gupta A, et al. The influence of smoking on the levels of matrix metalloproteinase-8 and periodontal parameters in smoker and nonsmoker patients with chronic periodontitis: A clinicobiochemical study. Journal of Oral Biology and Craniofacial Research. 2016;**6**(Suppl 1):S39–S43. [Internet]. Available from: http://www.ncbi.nlm.nih.gov/pubmed/27900249 [Accessed: 18 May 2017]

[9] Gupta N, Gupta ND, Garg S, Goyal L, Gupta A, Khan S, et al. The effect of type 2 diabetes mellitus and smoking on periodontal parameters and salivary matrix metalloproteinase-8 levels. Journal of Oral Science. 2016;**58**(1):1-6. [Internet]. Available from: http://www.ncbi.nlm.nih.gov/pubmed/27021533 [Accessed: 18 May 2017]

[10] Drisko CL. Periodontal debridement: Still the treatment of choice. Journal of Evidence-Based Dental Practice. 2014;**14**:33-41.e1. [Internet]. Available from: http://www.ncbi.nlm.nih.gov/pubmed/24929587 [Accessed: 17 May 2017]

[11] Socransky SS, Haffajee AD. The nature of periodontal diseases. Annals of Periodontology. 1997;**2**(1):3-10. [Internet]. Available from: http://www.ncbi.nlm.nih.gov/pubmed/9151538 [Accessed: 18 May 2017]

[12] Gkantidis N, Christou P, Topouzelis N. The orthodontic-periodontic interrelationship in integrated treatment challenges: A systematic review. Journal of Oral Rehabilitation. 2010;**37**(5):377-390. [Internet]. Available from: http://www.ncbi.nlm.nih.gov/pubmed/20202098 [Accessed: 19 March 2017]

[13] Needleman I, Worthington H V, Giedrys-Leeper E, Tucker R. Guided tissue regeneration for periodontal infra-bony defects. In: Needleman I, editor. Cochrane Database of Systematic Reviews. Chichester, UK: John Wiley & Sons, Ltd; 2006. p. CD001724 [Internet]. Available from: http://www.ncbi.nlm.nih.gov/pubmed/16625546 [Accessed: 18 May 2017]

[14] Ogihara S, Marks MH. Enhancing the regenerative potential of guided tissue regeneration to treat an intrabony defect and adjacent ridge deformity by orthodontic extrusive force. Journal of Periodontology. 2006;**77**(12):2093-2100 [Internet]. Available from: http://www.ncbi.nlm.nih.gov/pubmed/17209797 [Accessed: 18 May 2017]

[15] Scarano A, Crincoli V, Di Benedetto A, Cozzolino V, Lorusso F, Podaliri Vulpiani M, et al. Bone regeneration induced by bone porcine block with bone marrow stromal stem cells in a minipig model of mandibular "Critical Size" defect. Stem Cells International. 2017;**2017**:1-9 [Internet]. Available from: https://www.hindawi.com/journals/sci/2017/9082869/ [Accessed: 18 May 2017]

[16] Brunetti G, Oranger A, Mori G, Tamma R, Di Benedetto A, Pignataro P, et al. TRAIL is involved in human osteoclast apoptosis. Annals of the New York Academy of Sciences. 2007;**1116**(1):316-322 [Internet] Available from: http://doi.wiley.com/10.1196/annals.1402.011 [Accessed: 17 September 2016]

[17] Mori G, Brunetti G, Oranger A, Carbone C, Ballini A, Lo Muzio L, et al. Dental pulp stem cells: osteogenic differentiation and gene expression. Annals of the New York Academy of Sciences. 2011;**1237**:47-52 [Internet]. Available from: http://www.ncbi.nlm.nih.gov/pubmed/22082364 [Accessed: 18 September 2016]

[18] Mori G, Centonze M, Brunetti G, Ballini A, Oranger A, Mori C, et al. Osteogenic properties of human dental pulp stem cells. Journal of Biological Regulators and Homeostatic Agents. **24**(2):167-175 [Internet] Available from: http://www.ncbi.nlm.nih.gov/pubmed/20487630 [Accessed: 8 September 2016]

[19] Brunetti G, Colucci S, Pignataro P, Coricciati M, Mori G, Cirulli N, et al. T cells support osteoclastogenesis in an in vitro model derived from human periodontitis patients. Journal of Periodontology. 2005;**76**(10):1675-1680 [Internet]. Available from: http://www.ncbi.nlm.nih.gov/pubmed/16253089 [Accessed: 17 September 2016]

[20] Scarano A, Crincoli V, Di Benedetto A, Cozzolino V, Lorusso F, Podaliri Vulpiani M, et al. Stem Cells Int. 2017;**2017**:9082869

[21] Colucci S, Mori G, Brunetti G, Coricciati M, Pignataro P, Oranger A, et al. Interleukin-7 production by B lymphocytes affects the T cell-dependent osteoclast formation in an in vitro model derived from human periodontitis patients. International Journal of Immunopathology and Pharmacology. 18(3 Suppl):13-19. Available from: http://www.ncbi.nlm.nih.gov/pubmed/16848983 [Accessed: 17 September 2016]

[22] Di Benedetto A, Brunetti G, Posa F, Ballini A, Grassi FR, Colaianni G, et al. Osteogenic differentiation of mesenchymal stem cells from dental bud: Role of integrins and cadherins. Stem Cell Research. 2015;**15**(3):618-628 [Internet]. Available from: http://www.ncbi.nlm.nih.gov/pubmed/26513557 [Accessed: 20 May 2017]

[23] Martens LC. A decision tree for the management of exposed cervical dentin (ECD) and dentin hypersensitivity (DHS). Clinical Oral Investigations. 2013;**17**(S1):77-83 [Internet]. Available from: http://www.ncbi.nlm.nih.gov/pubmed/23262746 [Accessed: 19 May 2017]

[24] van Loveren C. Exposed cervical dentin and dentin hypersensitivity summary of the discussion and recommendations. Clinical Oral Investigations. 2013;**17**(S1):73-76 [Internet]. Available from: http://www.ncbi.nlm.nih.gov/pubmed/23224117 [Accessed: 2017 May 19]

[25] Zhu M, Li J, Chen B, Mei L, Yao L, Tian J, et al. The effect of calcium sodium phosphosilicate on dentin hypersensitivity: A systematic review and meta-analysis. Milgrom PM, editor. PLoS One [Internet]. 2015;**10**(11):e0140176. Available from: http://www.ncbi.nlm.nih.gov/pubmed/26544035 [Accessed: 19 May 2017]

[26] Anastasiou AD, Thomson CL, Hussain SA, Edwards TJ, Strafford S, Malinowski M, et al. Sintering of calcium phosphates with a femtosecond pulsed laser for hard tissue engineering. Materials & Design. 2016;**101**:346-354 [Internet]. Available from: http://www.sciencedirect.com/science/article/pii/S026412751630452X [Accessed: 18 May 2017]

[27] Anastasiou AD, Strafford S, Posada-Estefan O, Thomson CL, Hussain SA, Edwards TJ, et al. β-pyrophosphate: A potential biomaterial for dental applications. Materials Science and Engineering: C. 2017;**75**:885-894 [Internet]. Available from: http://www.sciencedirect.com/science/article/pii/S0928493116319129 [Accessed: 18 May 2017]

[28] Kalemaj Z, DebernardI CL, Buti J. Efficacy of surgical and non-surgical interventions on accelerating orthodontic tooth movement: A systematic review. European Journal of Oral Implantology. 2015;**8**(1):9-24 [Internet]. Available from: http://www.ncbi.nlm.nih.gov/pubmed/25738176 [Accessed: 29 November 2015]

[29] Kalemaj Z, Buti J, Deregibus A, Canuto RM, Maggiora M, Debernardi CL. Aligning effectiveness, secretion of interleukin 1β and pain control during fixed orthodontic treatment with Self-Ligating appliances and supplemental vibrational appliances. A randomized

controlled clinical trial. Journal of Biomedical. 2017;**2**(1):25-33 [Internet]. Available from: http://www.jbiomed.com/v02p0025.htm [Accessed: 20 May 2017]

[30] Melsen B. Tissue reaction to orthodontic tooth movement—A new paradigm. European Journal of Orthodontics. 2001;**23**(6):671-681 [Internet]. Available from: http://www.ncbi. nlm.nih.gov/pubmed/11890063 [Accessed: 18 May 2017]

[31] Paolantonio M, Festa F, di Placido G, D'Attilio M, Catamo G, Piccolomini R. Site-specific subgingival colonization by Actinobacillus actinomycetemcomitans in orthodontic patients. American Journal of Orthodontics and Dentofacial Orthopedics. 1999;**115**(4):423-428 [Internet]. Available from: http://www.ncbi.nlm.nih.gov/pubmed/ 10194288 [Accessed: 19 March 2017]

[32] Topaloglu-Ak A, Ertugrul F, Eden E, Ates M, Bulut H. Effect of orthodontic appliances on oral microbiota—6 month follow-up. Journal of Pediatric Dentistry. 2011;**35**(4):433-436 [Internet]. Available from: http://www.ncbi.nlm.nih.gov/pubmed/22046705 [Accessed: 19 March 2017]

[33] Diamanti-Kipioti A, Gusberti FA, Lang NP. Clinical and microbiological effects of fixed orthodontic appliances. Journal of Clinical Periodontology. 1987;**14**(6):326-333 [Internet]. Available from: http://www.ncbi.nlm.nih.gov/pubmed/3509967 [Accessed: 19 March 2017]

[34] Pan S, Liu Y, Zhang L, Li S, Zhang Y, Liu J, et al. Profiling of subgingival plaque biofilm microbiota in adolescents after completion of orthodontic therapy. Ojcius DM, editor. PLoS One [Internet]. 2017;**12**(2):e0171550. Available from: http://www.ncbi.nlm.nih.gov/ pubmed/28158292 [Accessed: 19 March 2017]

[35] Ren Y, Jongsma MA, Mei L, van der Mei HC, Busscher HJ. Orthodontic treatment with fixed appliances and biofilm formation—A potential public health threat? Clinical Oral Investigations. 2014;**18**(7):1711-1718 [Internet]. Available from: http://www.ncbi.nlm. nih.gov/pubmed/24728529 [Accessed: 19 March 2017]

[36] Azaripour A, Weusmann J, Mahmoodi B, Peppas D, Gerhold-Ay A, Van Noorden CJF, et al. Braces versus Invisalign®: Gingival parameters and patients' satisfaction during treatment: A cross-sectional study. BMC Oral Health. 2015;**15**(1):69 [Internet]. Available from: http://www.ncbi.nlm.nih.gov/pubmed/26104387 [Accessed: 19 March 2017]

[37] Tatakis DN, Chambrone L, Allen EP, Langer B, McGuire MK, Richardson CR, et al. Periodontal soft tissue root coverage procedures: A consensus report from the AAP regeneration workshop. Journal of Periodontology. 2015;**86**(2–s):S52–S55 [Internet]. Available from: http://www.ncbi.nlm.nih.gov/pubmed/25315018 [Accessed: 16 March 2017]

[38] Bueno Rossy LA, Chambrone L. Management of multiple recession-type defects after orthodontic therapy: A clinical report based on scientific evidence. American Academy of Periodontology. 2016;**6**(2):70-75 [Internet]. Available from: http://www.joponline.org/ doi/10.1902/cap.2015.150034 [Accessed: 16 March 2017]

[39] Melsen B, Allais D. Factors of importance for the development of dehiscences during labial movement of mandibular incisors: A retrospective study of adult orthodontic patients. American Journal of Orthodontics and Dentofacial Orthopedics. 2005;127(5):552-561; quiz 625 [Internet]. Available from: http://linkinghub.elsevier.com/retrieve/pii/S0889540604011126 [Accessed: 19 May 2017]

[40] Yared KFG, Zenobio EG, Pacheco W. Periodontal status of mandibular central incisors after orthodontic proclination in adults. American Journal of Orthodontics and Dentofacial Orthopedics. 2006;130(1):6.e1-8 [Internet]. Available from: http://linkinghub.elsevier.com/retrieve/pii/S0889540606002940 [Accessed: 19 May 2017]

[41] Pini Prato G, Baccetti T, Magnani C, Agudio G, Cortellini P. Mucogingival interceptive surgery of buccally-erupted premolars in patients scheduled for orthodontic treatment I. A 7-year longitudinal study. Journal of Periodontology. 2000;71(2):172-181 [Internet]. Available from: http://www.ncbi.nlm.nih.gov/pubmed/10711607 [Accessed: 19 May 2017]

[42] Redlich M, Shoshan S, Palmon A. Gingival response to orthodontic force. American Journal of Orthodontics and Dentofacial Orthopedics. 1999;116(2):152-158 [Internet]. Available from: http://www.ncbi.nlm.nih.gov/pubmed/10434088 [Accessed: 19 May 2017]

[43] Murakami T, Yokota S, Takahama Y. Periodontal changes after experimentally induced intrusion of the upper incisors in Macaca fuscata monkeys. American Journal of Orthodontics and Dentofacial Orthopedics. 1989;95(2):115-126 [Internet]. Available from: http://www.ncbi.nlm.nih.gov/pubmed/2916468 [Accessed: 19 May 2017]

[44] Corrente G, Abundo R, Re S, Cardaropoli D, Cardaropoli G. Orthodontic movement into infrabony defects in patients with advanced periodontal disease: A clinical and radiological study. Journal of Periodontology. 2003;74(8):1104-1109 [Internet]. Available from: http://www.ncbi.nlm.nih.gov/pubmed/14514223 [Accessed: 19 March 2017]

[45] Cardaropoli D, Re S, Corrente G, Abundo R. Intrusion of migrated incisors with infrabony defects in adult periodontal patients. American Journal of Orthodontics and Dentofacial Orthopedics. 2001;120(6):671-675 [Internet]. Available from: http://www.ncbi.nlm.nih.gov/pubmed/11742313 [Accessed: 19 March 2017]

[46] Neustadt E. The orthdontist's responsibility in the prevention of periodontal disease. Journal of the American Dental Association. 1930;17:1329

[47] Dummet CO. Orthodontics and periodontal disease. Journal of Periodontology. 1951;22:34-41

[48] Scopp IW, Bien SM. The principles of correciton of simple malocclusion in the treatment of periodontal disease. Journal of Periodontology. 1952;23:135-143

[49] Polson A, Caton J, Polson AP, Nyman S, Novak J, Reed B. Periodontal response after tooth movement into intrabony defects. Journal of Periodontology. 1984;55(4):197-202 [Internet]. Available from: http://www.ncbi.nlm.nih.gov/pubmed/6585537 [Accessed: 19 March 2017]

[50] Wennström JL, Stokland BL, Nyman S, Thilander B. Periodontal tissue response to orthodontic movement of teeth with infrabony pockets. American Journal of Orthodontics and Dentofacial Orthopedics. 1993;**103**(4):313-319 [Internet]. Available from: http://www.ncbi.nlm.nih.gov/pubmed/8480696 [Accessed: 19 March 2017]

[51] Harrel SK, Nunn ME, Hallmon WW. Is there an association between occlusion and periodontal destruction?: Yes—Occlusal forces can contribute to periodontal destruction. Journal of the American Dental Association. 2006;**137**(10):1380, 1382, 1384 passim [Internet]. Available from: http://www.ncbi.nlm.nih.gov/pubmed/17012716 [Accessed: 18 May 2017]

[52] Ingber JS. Forced eruption: Part I. A method of treating isolated one and two wall infrabony osseous defects—Rationale and case report. Journal of Periodontology. 1974; **45**(4):199-206 [Internet]. Available from: http://www.ncbi.nlm.nih.gov/pubmed/4522455 [Accessed: 18 May 2017]

[53] Joo J-Y, Kwon E-Y, Lee J-Y. Intentional passive eruption combined with scaling and root planing of teeth with moderate chronic periodontitis and traumatic occlusion. Journal of Periodontal & Implant Science. 2014;**44**(1):20 [Internet]. Available from: http://www.ncbi.nlm.nih.gov/pubmed/24616830 [Accessed: 18 May 2017]

[54] Rotundo R, Bassarelli T, Pace E, Iachetti G, Mervelt J, Pini Prato G. Orthodontic treatment of periodontal defects. Part II: A systematic review on human and animal studies. Progress in Orthodontics. 2011;**12**(1):45-52 [Internet]. Available from: http://linkinghub.elsevier.com/retrieve/pii/S1723778511000137 [Accessed: 19 March 2017]

[55] Mayer T, Basdra EK. A combined surgical and orthodontic treatment of Class III furcations. Report of a case. Journal of Clinical Periodontology. 1997;**24**(4):233-236 [Internet]. Available from: http://www.ncbi.nlm.nih.gov/pubmed/9144045 [Accessed: 18 May 2017]

[56] Re S, Cardaropoli D, Abundo R, Corrente G. Reduction of gingival recession following orthodontic intrusion in periodontally compromised patients. Orthodontics & Craniofacial Research. 2004;**7**(1):35-39 [Internet]. Available from: http://www.ncbi.nlm.nih.gov/pubmed/14989753 [Accessed: 18 May 2017]

[57] Martegani P, Silvestri M, Mascarello F, Scipioni T, Ghezzi C, Rota C, et al. Morphometric study of the interproximal unit in the Esthetic Region to correlate anatomic variables affecting the aspect of soft tissue embrasure space. Journal of Periodontology. 2007;**78**(12):2260-2265 [Internet]. Available from: http://www.ncbi.nlm.nih.gov/pubmed/18052697 [Accessed: 18 May 2017]

[58] Kurth JR, Kokich VG. Open gingival embrasures after orthodontic treatment in adults: Prevalence and etiology. American Journal of Orthodontics and Dentofacial Orthopedics. 2001;**120**(2):116-123 [Internet]. Available from: http://www.ncbi.nlm.nih.gov/pubmed/11500652 [Accessed: 18 May 2017]

[59] Reitan K. Principles of retention and avoidance of posttreatment relapse. American Journal of Orthodontics. 1969;**55**(6):776-790 [Internet]. Available from: http://www.ncbi.nlm.nih.gov/pubmed/4890739 [Accessed: 19 May 2017]

[60] Manni A, Pasini M, Mazzotta L, Mutinelli S, Nuzzo C, Grassi FR, et al. Comparison between an Acrylic Splint Herbst and an Acrylic Splint Miniscrew-Herbst for Mandibular Incisors Proclination Control. International Journal of Dentistry. 2014;**2014**:1-7 [Internet]. Available from: http://www.ncbi.nlm.nih.gov/pubmed/24963293 [Accessed: 20 May 2017]

[61] Will LA. Stability and retention. Frontiers of Oral Biology [Internet]. 2016:56-63. Available from: http://www.ncbi.nlm.nih.gov/pubmed/26599118 [Accessed: 19 May 2017]

[62] Al-Moghrabi D, Pandis N, Fleming PS. The effects of fixed and removable orthodontic retainers: a systematic review. Progress in Orthodontics. 2016;**17**(1):24 [Internet]. Available from: http://www.ncbi.nlm.nih.gov/pubmed/27459974 [Accessed: 19 May 2017]

[63] Bourzgui F, Aghoutan H, Diouny S. Craniomandibular disorders and mandibular reference position in orthodontic treatment. International Journal of Dentistry. 2013;**2013**:1-6 [Internet]. Available from: http://www.ncbi.nlm.nih.gov/pubmed/24101929 [Accessed: 19 May 2017]

Permissions

All chapters in this book were first published in PERIODONTITIS, by InTech Open; hereby published with permission under the Creative Commons Attribution License or equivalent. Every chapter published in this book has been scrutinized by our experts. Their significance has been extensively debated. The topics covered herein carry significant findings which will fuel the growth of the discipline. They may even be implemented as practical applications or may be referred to as a beginning point for another development.

The contributors of this book come from diverse backgrounds, making this book a truly international effort. This book will bring forth new frontiers with its revolutionizing research information and detailed analysis of the nascent developments around the world.

We would like to thank all the contributing authors for lending their expertise to make the book truly unique. They have played a crucial role in the development of this book. Without their invaluable contributions this book wouldn't have been possible. They have made vital efforts to compile up to date information on the varied aspects of this subject to make this book a valuable addition to the collection of many professionals and students.

This book was conceptualized with the vision of imparting up-to-date information and advanced data in this field. To ensure the same, a matchless editorial board was set up. Every individual on the board went through rigorous rounds of assessment to prove their worth. After which they invested a large part of their time researching and compiling the most relevant data for our readers.

The editorial board has been involved in producing this book since its inception. They have spent rigorous hours researching and exploring the diverse topics which have resulted in the successful publishing of this book. They have passed on their knowledge of decades through this book. To expedite this challenging task, the publisher supported the team at every step. A small team of assistant editors was also appointed to further simplify the editing procedure and attain best results for the readers.

Apart from the editorial board, the designing team has also invested a significant amount of their time in understanding the subject and creating the most relevant covers. They scrutinized every image to scout for the most suitable representation of the subject and create an appropriate cover for the book.

The publishing team has been an ardent support to the editorial, designing and production team. Their endless efforts to recruit the best for this project, has resulted in the accomplishment of this book. They are a veteran in the field of academics and their pool of knowledge is as vast as their experience in printing. Their expertise and guidance has proved useful at every step. Their uncompromising quality standards have made this book an exceptional effort. Their encouragement from time to time has been an inspiration for everyone.

The publisher and the editorial board hope that this book will prove to be a valuable piece of knowledge for researchers, students, practitioners and scholars across the globe.

List of Contributors

Vishakha Grover
Department of Periodontology and Oral Implantology, Dr. Harvansh Singh Judge Institute of Dental Sciences and Hospital, Panjab Univeristy, Chandigarh, India

Anoop Kapoor
Department of Periodontology and Oral Implantology, Shri Sukhmani Dental College and Hospital, Derabassi, Punjab, India

Zoe Rutter-Locher and Nidhi Sofat
Musculoskeletal Research Group, Institute of Infection and Immunity, St George's University of London, London, UK

Nicholas Fuggle
MRC Lifecourse Epidemiology Unit, University of Southampton, UK

Marco Orlandi and Francesco D'Aiuto
Unit of Periodontology, UCL Eastman Dental Institute, London, UK

Zvi G. Loewy
Touro College of Pharmacy, New York Medical College, New York, NY, USA

Shoshana Galbut
Lander College for Women, Touro College, New York, NY, USA

Ephraim Loewy
University of Maryland School of Dentistry, Baltimore, Maryland, USA

David A. Felton
University of Mississippi School of Dentistry, Jackson, MS, USA

Ana Maria Sell, Josiane Bazzo de Alencar and Jeane Eliete Laguila Visentainer
Department of Analysis Clinical and Biomedicine, Maringa State University, Parana, Brazil

Cleverson de Oliveira e Silva
Department of Dentistry, Ingá University Center (Uningá), Parana, Brazil

Veronica Lazar, Lia-Mara Ditu, Carmen Curutiu, Irina Gheorghe, Alina Holban and Carmen Chi iriuc
Department of Microbiology and Immunology, Faculty of Biology, University of Bucharest, Bucharest, Romania

Veronica Lazar, Lia-Mara Ditu, Carmen Curutiu, Irina Gheorghe, Alina Holban, Marcela Popa and Carmen Chi iriuc
Research Institute of the University of Bucharest, Bucharest, Romania

Fabrizia d'Apuzzo, Ludovica Nucci and Letizia Perillo
Multidisciplinary Department of Medical-Surgical and Dental Specialties, University of Campania "Luigi Vanvitelli", Naples, Italy

Abdolreza Jamilian
Orthodontic Department, Craniomaxillofacial Research Center, Tehran Dental Branch, Islamic Azad University, Tehran, Iran

Thanaphum Osathanon, Phunphimp Chanjavanakul, Pattanit Kongdecha and Panipuk Clayhan
STAR in Craniofacial Genetics and Stem Cells Research, Faculty of Dentistry, Chulalongkorn University, Bangkok, Thailand

Thanaphum Osathanon
Department of Anatomy, Faculty of Dentistry, Chulalongkorn University, Bangkok, Thailand

Nam Cong-Nhat Huynh
Department of Dental Basic Sciences, Faculty of Odonto-Stomatology, University of Medicine and Pharmacy, Ho Chi Minh City, Vietnam

Ahmed Zuhair Jasim Alwaeli
Department of Pathological Analysis Technique, University of Altoosi college, An-Najaf, Iraq

Hazem Khalaf, Eleonor Palm and Torbjörn Bengtsson
School of Medical Sciences, Örebro University, Örebro, Sweden

Zamira Kalemaj, Antonios D. Anastasiou and Animesh Jha
Faculty of Engineering, School of Chemical and Process Engineering, University of Leeds, United Kingdom

Felice R. Grassi
Department of Basic and Medical Sciences, Neurosciences and Sense Organs, University of Bari, Italy

Index

www.ingramcontent.com/pod-product-compliance
Lightning Source LLC
Chambersburg PA
CBHW061954190326
41458CB00009B/2872